Management of Nutritional and Metabolic Complications of Bariatric Surgery

Aparna Govil Bhasker • Nimisha Kantharia
Sarfaraz Baig • Pallawi Priya
Mariam Lakdawala • Miloni Shah Sancheti
Editors

Management of Nutritional and Metabolic Complications of Bariatric Surgery

Springer

Editors
Aparna Govil Bhasker
Bariatric and Laparoscopic Surgery
Global Hospital
Mumbai, India

Bariatric and Laparoscopic Surgery
Currae Hospital
Mumbai, India

Bariatric and Laparoscopic Surgery
Namaha Hospital
Mumbai, India

Bariatric and Laparoscopic Surgery
Apollo Hospital
Mumbai, India

Bariatric and Laparoscopic Surgery
Suchak Hospital
Mumbai, India

Bariatric and Laparoscopic Surgery
Saifee Hospital
Mumbai, India

Bariatric and Laparoscopic Surgery
Dr. Aparna's—Laparoscopy & Bariatric
Surgery Centre
Mumbai, India

Sarfaraz Baig
Belle Vue Clinic
Kolkata
India

Mariam Lakdawala
Dr. Aparna's - Laparoscopy & Bariatric
Surgery Centre
Currae Specialty Hospital
Mumbai
India

Nimisha Kantharia
Bhatia Hospital
Mumbai
India

Pallawi Priya
Belle Vue Clinic
Kolkata
India

Miloni Shah Sancheti
Dr. Aparna's - Laparoscopy & Bariatric
Surgery Centre
Sterling hospital
Mumbai
Maharashtra
India

ISBN 978-981-33-4701-4 ISBN 978-981-33-4702-1 (eBook)
https://doi.org/10.1007/978-981-33-4702-1

This Springer imprint is published by the registered company Springer Nature Singapore Pte Ltd.
The registered company address is: 152 Beach Road, #21-01/04 Gateway East, Singapore 189721, Singapore

Dedicated to all my patients who inspire me to become a better doctor every day and teach me more than I could ever learn from any book. Also, to my son Arvin and my husband Bhasker who make it all worth it.

—Aparna Govil Bhasker

Dedicated to Tara for permitting me sometimes to work on this book, and to Krunal for his timely facilitation of those rare moments.

—Nimisha Kantharia

Dedicated to my wife and all my patients who taught me that I should be a better listener. And to the Almighty who always listened.

—Sarfaraz Baig

Dedicated to Mom and Dad—Couldn't do anything without that genetic material you gave me- also because of my guilt since you only hear from me when I need something.

—Pallawi Priya

Dedicated to my four months old whose little fingers held my hands and taught me that even tiny steps can do wonders.

—Mariam Lakdawala

Dedicated to Mom- All that I am or hope to be, I owe to you and to my naughty little daughter who wants to be just like me when she grows up.

—Miloni Shah Sancheti

Foreword

It is always a challenge when one sets out to write about the topic as wide as bariatric surgery. This is because it is not just about the surgery that determines the success of the procedure. For a successful outcome, one must understand about the chronic multifactorial disease of obesity, the health burden to the individual and health stakeholders and how to manage the patient in the long term.

This book sets out to consolidate on the management of the nutritional and metabolic complications of bariatric surgery. It is appropriate timing as the numbers of bariatric surgery performed globally continue to increase to meet the demands of the obesity epidemic. Furthermore, since the turn of the century with the easy adoption of minimally invasive surgical techniques, bariatric surgery has been established to be safe and effective for the management of obesity. Bariatric surgery not only results in meaningful and sustained weight loss over the medium to long term but also effective in reversing or improving obesity-related risks and complications in patients, including type 2 diabetes and hypertension.

Whilst highly effective, bariatric surgery is not without risks and complications. Over the last 2 decades, bariatric surgery has been extensively studied in clinical trials and RCTs; its mechanism on gut physiology has been systematically studied and refined. Nutritional deficiencies and metabolic complications in the long term have emerged as significant concerns. The timing of this book to consolidate the existing literature about nutritional and metabolic complications of bariatric/metabolic surgery along with their management is perfect. It will serve as a good reference for all the bariatric and metabolic surgical teams around the world.

October 2020

Lilian Kow
President- International Federation for Surgery of Obesity
and Metabolic Surgery (IFSO)
Adelaide, Australia

Foreword

"The entirety of my career has been dedicated to the same purpose as the team of dedicated and gifted practitioners who have curated this book". The complexity and variation of how different people react to bariatric/metabolic surgery is indeed a pertinent topic and needs to be addressed with expertise. In my experience and ordeal in this field, so far I have not come across any other informative book on this subject. Anyone who is concerned with the rising issue of obesity knows how crucial it is to acquire and collect case studies and factual data about the hormonal shifts, metabolic complications and nutritional deficiencies involved post-surgery in order to understand issues in the context of every distinctive patient. Upon the recommendation of the editors of this book *Management of Nutritional and Metabolic Complications of Bariatric Surgery* came to me as a delight. It is by far one of the most comprehensive and meticulously curated books in the field of bariatric nutrition. This book comprises analyses and expert opinions from globally renowned practitioners. It starts off with the basics of what obesity is, to every aspect of the surgery, from the impact and drawbacks of the same. Upon reading it, I came across detailed chapters backed up with authentic researched data: from neurological, cardiovascular and gastrointestinal complications to psychological changes and recurring morbidities post-surgery. I highly recommend this book and it definitely deserves the spotlight. I am sure it will be extremely beneficial for studying diverse cases in the future to ensure the safety and proper care of every patient who comes to us with hope.

Best regards

Manish Khaitan
President- Obesity & Metabolic Surgery Society of India (OSSI)
Nobesity Bariatric & Metabolic Surgery Centre at KD Hospital
Ahmedabad, India

Preface

The idea of this book has been conceived over endless cups of mostly coffee, consumed in the breaks between lectures attended and courses conducted at various conferences over the last couple of years. Based as we all were in different cities, it was these conferences that provided a meeting point for many, many informal discussions about the common but less often described challenges our patients faced in the postoperative periods. All those stolen minutes built up to hours of wonder about the astonishing range and frequency of neurological complaints post-bariatric surgery. Technology was put to good use when we eagerly forwarded images of rashes seen, speculated on their variable aetiology and shared the intricacies of reaching a diagnosis. All of this eventually led us to develop the concept of this book, which was precisely what we were seeking in the give and take of our discussions.

As surgeons we spend so much time focusing on the technical aspects of surgery. We have lectures and books devoted to a single surgery type with a thousand variations in technique. We spend hours in the operating room mastering those nuances. We debate about limb lengths and number of ports and staplers. But beyond the operating table, we see our patients live with the permanently altered gastrointestinal systems that we have so meticulously sculpted, and we see the consequences of those alterations, mostly good, but sometimes bad and rarely grievous. This book is an attempt to take a close look at those lived consequences in their entirety. For instance, the hair loss that is such a common sequel of weight loss can be devastating for some patients undergoing it. Musculoskeletal and neurological issues that crop up can be debilitating for some. In other words, we wanted to create a reference book to cover all the metabolic and nutritional complications and sequelae (common or rare) that may occur post-bariatric surgery.

In our quest for this comprehensive knowledge, we were fortunate to have access to and be able to approach so many professionals in the international bariatric community, both surgeons and non-surgeons, dedicated to the care of patients suffering from obesity, especially post-bariatric surgery. Nearly every author is a teacher, mentor, colleague or a friend to one or all of us. It was a great pleasure as editors to reach out to each author to request their contribution. It was an even greater pleasure to read through the chapters, filled as they are with information that accrues from the authors' tremendous clinical experiences, backed by evidence-based research. We are extremely thankful to each and every author in this book for their contribution.

Each of the editors has his or her own special interest in metabolic and nutritional aspects of bariatric surgery. Dr. Sarfaraz Baig and Dr. Pallawi Priya are bariatric surgeons based in Kolkata, India. They have previously co-authored the book *Nutrition, Obesity and Bariatric Surgery* which covers the nutritional care in obesity and post-bariatric surgery. Dr. Aparna Govil Bhasker is a bariatric and laparoscopic surgeon based in Mumbai, India. She is also the course director of "Advanced Bariatric Nutrition Course". Dr Nimisha Kantharia is a bariatric and laparoscopic surgeon based in Mumbai, India, and has always had a keen interest in nutrition of surgical patients, and now specifically in relation to obesity. Ms. Mariam Lakdawala and Ms. Milioni Shah Sancheti are both Registered Dieticians and Bariatric Nutritionists, practising in Mumbai. They are also co-directors of the "Advanced Bariatric Nutrition Course", along with Dr. Bhasker. It is an immense interest in the postoperative care and well-being of the post-bariatric patients that binds all of us together.

We hope that with this book, we have created a reference manual for health professionals involved with patients with obesity and bariatric surgery, that would help in improving the follow-up of these patients.

With best regards,
Editors

Mumbai, India	Nimisha Kantharia
Mumbai, India	Aparna Govil Bhasker
Kolkata, India	Sarfaraz Baig
Kolkata, India	Pallawi Priya
Mumbai, India	Miloni Shah Sancheti
Mumbai, India	Mariam Lakdawala

Contents

The Disease That Is Obesity

1

James Senturk and Scott Shikora

Worldwide obesity has nearly tripled since 1975. Most of the world's population live in countries where overweight and obesity kills more people than underweight.

– World Health Organization

1.1 Introduction

Obesity may be best understood in the healthcare milieu as a chronic disease, with multiple contributing factors and multiple downstream consequences for individual health and longevity. More technically, however, obesity can be described as a phenotype that arises from a complex and dynamic interplay between an individual's inherited metabolic and neurohormonal predispositions and his or her environment [1]. For diagnostic and epidemiologic purposes, the disease is defined as an excess of body fat, which itself is characterized by a body mass index (BMI) of greater than or equal to 30 kg/m^2 for the western population and greater than or equal to 27 kg/m^2 for Asian population [2, 3].

The use of BMI for the measurement and tracking of obesity in the United States has been ongoing since the 1960s [4]. The usefulness of this metric rests on the relative ease of its calculation and its well-validated correlation with body fat [5]. As the field of obesity research has grown, other metrics including the distribution of body fat and the increasingly noted effects of gender, racial, and ethnic background on the morbidity associated with obesity have gained traction [6]. Indeed, BMI has been shown to discriminate against on the basis of muscle mass, gender, age, and certain

J. Senturk (✉) · S. Shikora
Department of Surgery, Brigham and Women's Hospital, Boston, MA, USA
e-mail: JSENTURK@PARTNERS.ORG; SSHIKORA@BWH.HARVARD.EDU

A. G. Bhasker et al. (eds.), *Management of Nutritional and Metabolic Complications of Bariatric Surgery*,
https://doi.org/10.1007/978-981-33-4702-1_1

ethnic groups including Asians and African Americans [7]. Anthropometric and epidemiologic tools continue to evolve, particularly with the rapid expansion of large-scale genetic analyses [8]. Nevertheless, at the present time, BMI alone remains well-correlated with obesity-associated morbidity and mortality and is an effective tool for both diagnosis and screening [9].

The classification of obesity as a disease is not trivial. While a BMI cutoff may offer a rapid diagnosis, the absence of a consistent and coincident set of signs, symptoms, or impairments stands at odds with more traditional definitions of disease [10]. Conversely, it has been argued that the broad burden of untoward metabolic and cardiovascular outcomes associated, at least longitudinally if not concomitantly, with obesity should substantiate its status as a disease [11, 12]. Indeed, the latter is the position taken by The Obesity Society. Formalized in 2012, a special committee from the group argued that labeling obesity a disease was both appropriate and necessary for the "benefit [of] the greater good by soliciting more resources into prevention, treatment, and research of obesity; encouraging more high-quality caring professionals to view treating the obese patient as a vocation worthy of effort and respect' and reducing the stigma and discrimination heaped on many obese persons [13]."

1.2 The Epidemiology of Obesity in 2019

Over the past two decades, there has been a wealth of academic writing on the epidemiology of obesity both in the United States and worldwide. Particularly in the developed world, the widespread dissemination and adoption of electronic medical and public health records, and information gathering has become both increasingly objective and facile. Whereas studies at the beginning of the millennium relied on in-person, mail, electronic, or telephone surveys, more recent work has drawn from population-based data sources [14–17].

Two large and authoritative studies that have laid the groundwork for the current prevalence and trends in obesity in the United States are the Behavioral Risk Factor Surveillance System (BRFSS) and the National Health and Nutrition Examination Survey (NHANES). The former suggested at the turn of the millennium that obesity prevalence in the Unites States had already reached 20% and is seen as a bellwether for the public health community at the time [18]. Investigators from the NHANES group have subsequently released regular reports on the subject. A recent study examining nearly 30,000 adults over a 10-year period reported the sobering finding that the age-standardized prevalence in obesity had climbed from 33.7 to 39.6%.

Globally, a study examining the records of 19 million adults 18 years of age or older across 186 countries that comprise 99% of the world's population concluded that the global prevalence of morbid obesity was 0.64% in men and 1.6% in women [14]. Of these, 18.4% (nearly 120 million people) lived in high-income English-speaking countries, which also harbored 27.1% (50 million people) of the world's severely obese (BMI $\geq$ 35 kg/m^2). Conversely, those populations with the largest proportions of underweight people were found in large countries in Asia and sub-Saharan Africa. When examining trends over a 40-year period, the authors observed that populations from middle-income countries including China, Russia, and India saw increases in the prevalence of obesity that rivaled the United States' in 2014. "[In 40 years,] we have transitioned," the authors conclude, "from a world in which underweight prevalence was more than double that of obesity to one in which more people are obese than underweight, both globally and in all regions except parts of sub-Saharan Africa and Asia" [14].

1.3 Causes of Obesity

The root causes of obesity on both an individual level as well as with an eye toward the progress of human societies are the subjects of substantial bodies of work that are impossible to encompass in a single text. Nevertheless, it is axiomatic in any discussion centered on disease to visit the prevailing contemporary theories regarding its causative factors. There is no question that the twentieth century bore witness to an unprecedented pace of technological advancement that transformed the production and distribution of food into an industry unlike that ever before seen in human history [19]. Naturally, as developed and developing societies churned out the machinery and logistical enterprises to all but squash famine, new realities came to light almost in concert. With increased mechanization, the extent of labor necessary to grow, harvest, and deliver foods declined while the availability of nourishment was all but guaranteed [20, 21]. The rise in the prevalence of obesity across societies has closely followed these enabling changes in logistics, technology, and agriculture [22]. Similarly, dietary patterns and food environments have not been immune to these radical shifts. Increased portion sizes, added fats, sweeteners, refined sugars, and low-cost, high-energy foods coupled with the rise of prepared foods and a decline of home-cooked meals have together crafted the obesogenic landscape of the modern period [23–27]. It would be remiss to omit the reality that the socioeconomically disadvantaged are disproportionately vulnerable to these trends [28, 29]

As the availability of low-cost, high-calorie food has grown exponentially, caloric expenditure has declined. Work has become increasingly sedentary and, in developed nations, labor-intense occupations have either been outsourced elsewhere or completely automated [12]. On the whole, there has been a trend toward decreased physical activity, both with regards to daily occupation as well as time spent away from employment [30–32]. With the increasing popularity of such conveniences as telecommuting and ready access to on-demand entertainment, these trends are expected to continue with increasing awareness and participation of an at-risk public.

Lastly, it is difficult to overlook the contribution of heritable factors to obesity. Genetics is likely to account for the documented heritability of obesity seen in twin studies, as well as the psychosocial factors that contribute to the individual relationship with food environments [8, 33, 34]. As is the emerging paradigm for the overwhelming majority of human diseases, there is not likely to be a single gene-single phenotype correlate, but rather a broad array of genetic, transcriptomic, noncoding, and epigenetic factors that predispose a given individual to excess adiposity and ultimately obesity [35–38]. While potential racial and ethnic determinants of obesity have been pursued as a corollary to these heritable predispositions, such demographic variables have been difficult to study outside of the United States and, when looked at within the U.S. population, are often challenging to dissociate from associated socioeconomic variables [39–42].

1.4 Consequences of Obesity

The consequences of obesity on physical well-being are well-studied and have been the foundation upon which public health campaigns have been built. There are obvious direct consequences, including a heightened risk of early diagnosis, early development of complications and death from pulmonary disease, chronic kidney disease, liver disease, and cardiovascular disease, including diabetes, hypertension, heart attack, stroke, and heart failure [43, 44]. By conservative estimates, population studies have suggested a 30% increase in mortality for every 5 kg/m^2 increase in BMI above 25 [45, 46]. The severity and even the presence of those cardiovascular morbidities associated with obesity and their attendant mortality risks are offset by weight loss, strengthening these long-observed associations [47, 48].

Practically speaking, obesity can have untoward consequences for the delivery of what might otherwise be standard medical care. Obesity in pregnancy confers added risk to both the fetus and mother [49]. Imaging studies carried out on patients with obesity may be limited on account of artifactual findings with increased adiposity and certain equipment may not be able to accommodate the habitus of severely obese patients [50]. The provision of anesthesia in the setting of morbid obesity, particularly in the critically ill, often requires additional expertise and awareness of technical challenges (e.g., mechanical ventilation, vascular access) [51]. In this population, morbid obesity has been shown to be an independent risk factor for death, particularly in surgical patients[52]. On a fundamental level, physical exams are both difficult and often inaccurate in the obese patient, challenging the delivery of both routine and emergency care [53–56]. Truly, all aspects of medical care are more complicated. A list of potential challenges in caring for obese patients is provided in Table 1.1.

Mental well-being is similarly taxed by those with excess body fat. There is a long-studied and documented reciprocal relationship between depression and obesity [57]. Obesity has been associated with a spectrum of psychiatric disorders, including bipolar disorder, social phobias, and panic attacks, independent of underlying physical illnesses [58]. The relationship between obesity and suicidal ideation continues to draw much attention [59].

It is not surprising that the costs borne by individuals with obesity are often enormous, not least because of their burden of comorbid illness but also due to the potential for superimposed depression, anxiety, and associated limitations in the ability to care for oneself [60]. Individuals with obesity are often targets of bias and stigma, which negatively influence employment prospects and professional

Table 1.1 Challenges associated with the delivery of medical care in the obese population

Bedside care	Diagnostic studies	Treatment
• Challenging or nondiagnostic physical exams • Inaccurate trauma surveys and burn assessments • Effacement of anatomic landmarks • Unreliable prostate, rectal, and female pelvic assessments • Inadequate turning and repositioning when bed-bound	• Size and weight limits of conventional scanners (CT, MRI) • Decreased accuracy of ultrasonography and cross-sectional imaging • Lower diagnostic yield of noninvasive cardiac testing	• Difficulty in airway and vascular access in critical care and perioperative settings • Compromised surgical ergonomics and exposure • Unpredictable pharmacokinetics and implications for drug dosing • Increased risk of death and major morbidity after surgery

progress [61, 62]. Obesity has been associated with higher sick leave and disability usage, which only adds to the stigma [63].

On a grander scale, the price of obesity to society can be staggering. Nearly a decade ago, investigators in the United States concluded that obesity-related costs amounted to nearly $150 billion (up from $75 billion from 5 years prior), with a combined total of 42% financed by government insurance programs (Medicare and Medicaid) [64]. Similar work from the European Union, though more dated, suggests costs at roughly 33 billion € from the previous decade. Buried in these figures are indirect costs, which include exercise programs, food provisions, equipment, and multispecialty clinics. These data alone highlight the importance of cost control in measuring the success of programs that aim to prevent or treat obesity.

1.5 Discussion

Obesity has rightfully been referred to as “the disease of the twenty-first century” [12]. As familiarity with obesity and its consequences has evolved from what may have historically been considered mere “corpulence,” the resources leveraged against obesity have increased dramatically. Obesity is now in the crosshairs of multiple medical specialties and societies. Physicians and surgeons alike have committed entire careers to serve patients afflicted by this disease. Importantly, research into the causative factors and the natural history of obesity have pushed the needle toward earlier and earlier screening and intervention. Childhood and adolescent obesity are now considered fundamental public health concerns worldwide [65].

Cultural and dietary habits have been historically difficult to change, all the more so when there is uncertainty or equipoise with regards to cause, effect, and urgency [66]. As researchers continue to dissect out cultural attitudes, practices, and food relationships that have and continue to contribute to obesity, so too is the public consciousness expected to grow aware of its dangers. Already in the United States and other high-income countries, the rate of increase in BMI since 2000 has been slower than in preceding decades, a finding that has been attributed to both a growing and increasingly visible public health enterprise [14]. It is not difficult to imagine far-reaching social programs that encourage healthy relationships with food and prioritization of physical fitness, for example. Unfortunately, the acceptance and adoption of such programs are less predictable. Therefore, the prevention of obesity remains a challenging goal.

Treating obesity, on the other hand, is clearly the focus of much healthcare attention and expenditure in 2019. There has been a wide and rapid expansion in the role of surgery in obesity in the past two decades, to which this volume calls attention. By affording individuals with obesity the opportunity to see decrements in their BMI and offset the deleterious metabolic and cardiovascular sequelae of obesity, surgery holds the promise of a "reset." Patients have the opportunity to engage in healthier dietary and lifestyle habits that may otherwise have been out of reach due to poor functional status [67]. Surgery alone, however, is neither sufficient for long-term weight control in the individual nor an appropriate approach to the population-wide treatment of obesity. Although outside the scope of this chapter, the costs, risks, adverse outcomes, and recidivism associated with obesity surgery together mandate that the field of bariatrics remains multidisciplinary. The old saying, "It takes a village" certainly applies to the care of the obese patient, which is best served by collaboration among multiple specialists including dietetics, endocrinology, surgery, and psychology.

1.6 Conclusion

Obesity is a disease of the twenty-first century that remains a problem with broad ramifications throughout the world. The causes of obesity are complex and continue to elude attempts at management at the level of populations. Individuals with obesity sustain numerous negative physical and psychological consequences and both, the costs and challenges associated with their care are significant. Managing obesity requires the involvement of multiple professionals from multiple disciplines. Additionally, the importance of social awareness and public health measures cannot be overstated.

Key Points

- *Obesity can be described as a phenotype that arises from a complex and dynamic interplay between an individual's inherited metabolic and neurohormonal predispositions and his or her environment.*
- *Although Body Mass Index has long been used to predict obesity, other parameters such as body composition, waist–hip ratio are being recognized as better measures of adiposity.*
- *The rise in the prevalence of obesity across societies has closely followed these enabling changes in logistics, technology, and agriculture. Socioeconomically disadvantaged are disproportionately vulnerable to these trends.*

- *Majority of the world's obese and morbidly obese population reside in high-income countries. However, current trends suggest alarmingly increasing obesity rates in middle-income countries as well.*
- *Trends over a 40-year period show that populations from middle-income countries including China, Russia, and India have seen increases in the prevalence of obesity that rivaled the United States' in 2014.*
- *By conservative estimates, population studies have suggested a 30% increase in mortality for every 5 kg/m^2, increase in BMI above 25.*
- *By affording individuals with obesity the opportunity to see decrements in their BMI and offset the deleterious metabolic and cardiovascular sequelae of obesity, bariatric surgery holds the promise of a "reset."*
- *Surgery alone, however, is neither sufficient for long-term weight control in the individual nor an appropriate approach to population-wide treatment of obesity.*
- *Last but not the least—"It takes a village" to take care of the patient with obesity.*

References

1. Smith GP. Critical introduction to obesity. In: Blass EM, editor. Obesity. 1st ed. Sunderland, MA: Sinauer; 2008. p. 1–17.
2. Centers for Disease Control and Prevention. Defining adult overweight and obesity, Centers for Disease Control and Prevention; 2016.
3. Seidell JC. Assessing obesity: Classification and epidemiology. Br Med Bull. 1997; https://doi.org/10.1093/oxfordjournals.bmb.a011611.
4. Ljungvall Å, Zimmerman FJ. Bigger bodies: Long-term trends and disparities in obesity and body-mass index among U.S. adults, 1960-2008. Soc Sci Med. 2012; https://doi.org/10.1016/j.socscimed.2012.03.003.
5. Mei Z, et al. Validity of body mass index compared with other body-composition screening indexes for the assessment of body fatness in children and adolescents. Am J Clin Nutr. 2002;75(6):978–85.
6. Nuttall FQ. Body mass index: Obesity, BMI, and health: A critical review. Nutr Today. 2015; https://doi.org/10.1097/NT.0000000000000092.
7. Moore EC, Pories WJ. The BMI: is it time to scratch for a more accurate assessment of metabolic dysfunction? Curr Obes Rep. 2014; https://doi.org/10.1007/s13679-014-0093-z.
8. Locke AE, et al. Genetic studies of body mass index yield new insights for obesity biology. Nature. 2015; https://doi.org/10.1038/nature14177.
9. Markowitz JS. Body mass index (BMI). Springer Briefs Public Health. 2018; https://doi.org/10.1007/978-3-319-77203-5_5.
10. Heshka S, Allison DB. Is obesity a disease? Int J Obes. 2001;25(10):1401–4.
11. Kopelman PG, Finer N. Reply: Is obesity a disease? Int J Obes. 2001; https://doi.org/10.1038/sj.ijo.0801791.
12. Rössner S. Obesity: The disease of the twenty-first century. Int J Obes. 2002; https://doi.org/10.1038/sj.ijo.0802209.
13. Allison DB, et al. Obesity as a disease: A white paper on evidence and arguments commissioned by the council of the obesity society. Obesity. 2008; https://doi.org/10.1038/oby.2008.231.
14. Di Cesare M, et al. Trends in adult body-mass index in 200 countries from 1975 to 2014: A pooled analysis of 1698 population-based measurement studies with 19.2 million participants. Lancet. 2016; https://doi.org/10.1016/S0140-6736(16)30054-X.

15. Flegal KM, et al. Overweight and obesity in the United States: Prevalence and trends, 1960-1994. Int J Obes. 1998; https://doi.org/10.1038/sj.ijo.0800541.
16. Flegal KM, et al. Prevalence and trends in obesity among US adults, 1999-2000. J Am Med Assoc. 2002; https://doi.org/10.1001/jama.2012.39.
17. Flegal KM, et al. Prevalence and trends in obesity among US adults, 1999-2008. JAMA. 2010; https://doi.org/10.1001/jama.2009.2014.
18. Mokdad AH, et al. Prevalence of obesity, diabetes, and obesity-related health risk factors, 2001. J Am Med Assoc. 2003; https://doi.org/10.1001/jama.289.1.76.
19. Eknoyan G. A history of obesity, or how what was good became ugly and then bad. Adv Chronic Kidney Dis. 2006; https://doi.org/10.1053/j.ackd.2006.07.002.
20. Caballero B. The global epidemic of obesity: An overview. Epidemiol Rev. 2007; https://doi.org/10.1093/epirev/mxm012.
21. Swinburn BA, et al. The global obesity pandemic: Shaped by global drivers and local environments. Lancet. 2011; https://doi.org/10.1016/S0140-6736(11)60813-1.
22. Popkin BM, Gordon-Larsen P. The nutrition transition: Worldwide obesity dynamics and their determinants. Int J Obes. 2004; https://doi.org/10.1038/sj.ijo.0802804.
23. Drewnowski A. The real contribution of added sugars and fats to obesity. Epidemiol Rev. 2007; https://doi.org/10.1093/epirev/mxm011.
24. Drewnowski A. Obesity, diets, and social inequalities. Nutr Rev. 2009; https://doi.org/10.1111/j.1753-4887.2009.00157.x.
25. Drewnowski A, Specter SE. Poverty and obesity: The role of energy density and energy costs. Am J Clin Nutr. 2004;79:6–16.
26. Nicklas TA, et al. Eating patterns, dietary quality and obesity. J Am Coll Nutr. 2001; https://doi.org/10.1080/07315724.2001.10719064.
27. Satija A, et al. Dietary patterns in India and their association with obesity and central obesity. Public Health Nutr. 2015; https://doi.org/10.1017/S1368980015000312.
28. Dinsa GD, et al. Obesity and socioeconomic status in developing countries: A systematic review. Obes Rev. 2012; https://doi.org/10.1111/j.1467-789X.2012.01017.x.
29. McLaren L. Socioeconomic status and obesity. Epidemiol Rev. 2007; https://doi.org/10.1093/epirev/mxm001.
30. Hu FB, et al. Television watching and other sedentary behaviors in relation to risk of obesity and type 2 diabetes mellitus in women. J Am Med Assoc. 2003; https://doi.org/10.1001/jama.289.14.1785.
31. Lopez-Zetina J, Lee H, Friis R. The link between obesity and the built environment. Evidence from an ecological analysis of obesity and vehicle miles of travel in California. Health Place. 2006; https://doi.org/10.1016/j.healthplace.2005.09.001.
32. Ng SW, Popkin BM. Time use and physical activity: A shift away from movement across the globe. Obes Rev. 2012; https://doi.org/10.1111/j.1467-789X.2011.00982.x.
33. Choquet H, Meyre D. Genetics of Obesity: What have we Learned? Curr Genomics. 2012; https://doi.org/10.2174/138920211795677895.
34. Lyon HN, Hirschhorn JN. Genetics of common forms of obesity: a brief overview. Am J Clin Nutr. 2005;82(1 Suppl):215S–17S.
35. Van Dijk SJ, et al. Epigenetics and human obesity. Int J Obes. 2015; https://doi.org/10.1038/ijo.2014.34.
36. Pigeyre M, et al. Recent progress in genetics, epigenetics and metagenomics unveils the pathophysiology of human obesity. Clin Sci. 2016; https://doi.org/10.1042/CS20160136.
37. Yang W, Kelly T, He J. Genetic epidemiology of obesity. Epidemiol Rev. 2007; https://doi.org/10.1093/epirev/mxm004.
38. Youngson NA, Morris MJ. What obesity research tells us about epigenetic mechanisms. Philos Trans R Soc B Biol Sci. 2013; https://doi.org/10.1098/rstb.2011.0337.
39. Carroll JF, et al. Visceral fat, waist circumference, and BMI: Impact of race/ethnicity. Obesity. 2008; https://doi.org/10.1038/oby.2007.92.

40. Cossrow N, Falkner B. Race/ethnic issues in obesity and obesity-related comorbidities. J Clin Endocrinol Metab. 2004; https://doi.org/10.1210/jc.2004-0339.
41. Krueger PM, Reither EN. Mind the gap: race/ethnic and socioeconomic disparities in obesity. Curr Diabetes Rep. 2015; https://doi.org/10.1007/s11892-015-0666-6.
42. Zhang Q, Wang Y. Trends in the association between obesity and socioeconomic status in U.S. adults: 1971 to 2000. Obes Res. 2004; https://doi.org/10.1038/oby.2004.202.
43. Afshin A, et al. Health effects of overweight and obesity in 195 countries over 25 years. N Engl J Med. 2017; https://doi.org/10.1056/NEJMoa1614362.
44. Khan SS, et al. Association of body mass index with lifetime risk of cardiovascular disease and compression of morbidity. JAMA Cardiol. 2018; https://doi.org/10.1001/jamacardio.2018.0022.
45. De Gonzalez AB, et al. Body-mass index and mortality among 1.46 million white adults. N Engl J Med. 2010; https://doi.org/10.1056/NEJMoa1000367.
46. MacMahon S, et al. Body-mass index and cause-specific mortality in 900 000 adults: Collaborative analyses of 57 prospective studies. Lancet. 2009; https://doi.org/10.1016/S0140-6736(09)60318-4.
47. Haslam D, James WP. Seminar—obesity. Lancet. 2005; https://doi.org/10.1016/S0140-6736(05)67483-1.
48. Rueda-Clausen CF, Ogunleye AA, Sharma AM. Health benefits of long-term weight-loss maintenance. Annu Rev Nutr. 2015; https://doi.org/10.1146/annurev-nutr-071714-034434.
49. Catalano PM. Management of obesity in pregnancy. Obstet Gynecol. 2007; https://doi.org/10.1097/01.AOG.0000253311.44696.85.
50. Uppot RN. Impact of obesity on radiology. Radiol Clin N Am. 2007; https://doi.org/10.1016/j.rcl.2007.03.001.
51. Huschak G, Busch T, Kaisers UX. Obesity in anesthesia and intensive care. Best Pract Res Clin Endocrinol Metab. 2013; https://doi.org/10.1016/j.beem.2013.02.001.
52. Nasraway SA, et al. Morbid obesity is an independent determinant of death among surgical critically ill patients. Crit Care Med. 2006; https://doi.org/10.1097/01.CCM.0000205758.18891.70.
53. Budiansky AS, Margarson MP, Eipe N. Acute pain management in morbid obesity—an evidence based clinical update. Surg Obes Relat Dis. 2017; https://doi.org/10.1016/j.soard.2016.09.013.
54. Pucher PH, et al. Demand for specialised training for the obese trauma patient: National ATLS expert group survey results. Injury. 2017; https://doi.org/10.1016/j.injury.2017.02.027.
55. Sheth SS. Super flexion position for difficult speculum examination. Int J Gynecol Obstet. 2013; https://doi.org/10.1016/j.ijgo.2012.11.005.
56. Shikora SA, et al. Relationship between obesity and uterine leiomyomata. Nutrition (Burbank, Los Angeles County, Calif.). 1991;7(4):251–5.
57. Luppino FS, et al. Overweight, Obesity, and Depression. Arch Gen Psychiatry. 2010; https://doi.org/10.1001/archgenpsychiatry.2010.2.
58. Mather AA, et al. Associations of obesity with psychiatric disorders and suicidal behaviors in a nationally representative sample. J Psychosom Res. 2009; https://doi.org/10.1016/j.jpsychores.2008.09.008.
59. Klinitzke G, et al. Obesity and suicide risk in adults—a systematic review. J Affect Disord. 2013; https://doi.org/10.1016/j.jad.2012.07.010.
60. Seidell JC. Societal and personal costs of obesity. Exp Clin Endocrinol Diabetes. 1998;106(Suppl. 2):7–9.
61. Morris S. The impact of obesity on employment. Labour Econ. 2007; https://doi.org/10.1016/j.labeco.2006.02.008.
62. The Obesity Society. Obesity, bias, and stigmatization. The Obesity Society; 2015.
63. Schmier JK, Jones ML, Halpern MT. Cost of obesity in the workplace. Scand Work Environ Health. 2006; https://doi.org/10.5271/sjweh.970.

64. Finkelstein EA, et al. Annual medical spending attributable to obesity: Payer-and service-specific estimates. Health Affairs. 2009; https://doi.org/10.1377/hlthaff.28.5.w822.
65. Lobstein T, et al. Child and adolescent obesity: Part of a bigger picture. Lancet. 2015; https://doi.org/10.1016/S0140-6736(14)61746-3.
66. Kumanyika SK. The obesity epidemic: Looking in the mirror. Am J Epidemiol. 2007; https://doi.org/10.1093/aje/kwm169.
67. Miras AD, et al. Obesity surgery makes patients healthier and more functional: real world results from the United Kingdom National Bariatric Surgery Registry. Surg Obes Relat Dis. 2018; https://doi.org/10.1016/j.soard.2018.02.012.

Associated Co-morbid Conditions of Clinically Severe Obesity

2

Maurizio De Luca, Nicola Clemente, Giacomo Piatto, Alberto Sartori, Cesare Lunardi, and Natale Pellicanò

A thorough knowledge of the associated co-morbid conditions of clinically severe obesity is warranted for every health care professional interested in bariatric therapy.

Maurizio De Luca

2.1 Introduction

Obesity has become an important public health problem. Its prevalence has progressively increased worldwide [1] to an extent that it is now a significant problem not only in affluent societies but also in developing countries [2–5].

Accurate assessment of total body fat requires sophisticated technology which is not readily available on a large scale [6, 7]. Consequently, the World Health Organisation (WHO) adopted body mass index (BMI), which is calculated by dividing the body weight in kilograms (kg) by the square of the height in metres (m), as a surrogate measure of total body fat [3]. BMI correlates fairly well with the percentage of body fat in the young and middle-aged people among whom obesity is most prevalent [6, 7]. According to this index, obesity is defined in the case of BMI value equal to or greater than 30 kg/m^2 in the western population and 27.5 kg m^2 in the Asian population.

Several large studies have demonstrated increased mortality above this threshold of BMI. In the Framingham study, a prospective cohort study, male and female

M. De Luca (✉) · N. Clemente · G. Piatto · A. Sartori · C. Lunardi · N. Pellicanò
Department of General and Metabolic Surgery, Montebelluna and Castelfranco Hospitals, Treviso, Italy
e-mail: nicola.clemente@ulss2.veneto.it; alberto.sartori@aulss2.veneto.it; cesare.lunardi@aulss2.veneto.it; natale.pellicano@aulss2.veneto.it

A. G. Bhasker et al. (eds.), *Management of Nutritional and Metabolic Complications of Bariatric Surgery*,
https://doi.org/10.1007/978-981-33-4702-1_2

non-smokers aged 40 years who suffered from obesity lived 5.8 and 7.1 years less than their non-obese counterparts [8]. Another study by Fontaine et al. which used data from the National Health and Nutrition Examination Survey (NHANES I and II) and the NHANES III Mortality Study found a marked reduction in life expectancy in young adults with obesity compared to non-obese adults.

However, apart from total body fat, the pattern of fat distribution has great relevance. Excess visceral fat, also referred to as central obesity, has a stronger association with cardiovascular disease than subcutaneous fat which is deposited mainly around the hips and buttocks [9]. Central obesity produces a characteristic body shape that resembles an apple and thus is also referred to as "apple-shaped" obesity as opposed to "pear-shaped" obesity in which fat is deposited on the hips and buttocks. This distribution is also reflected in the waist circumference and Waist: Hip Ratio (WHR) [10].

The INTERHEART study, similarly to other studies, showed that hip fat distribution assessed by hip circumference had a negative predictive effect on myocardial infarction (MI) whereas waist fat distribution assessed by waist circumference was associated with high rates of MI [9].

Body fat distribution, assessed using magnetic resonance imaging in leading research institutions, and its effects on mortality and morbidity is currently a topic of scientific research.

The reason for the increased mortality in obesity is related to the great burden of its associated co-morbidities [11]. It has been demonstrated that obesity treatment and especially bariatric surgery can heal or improve most of the associated diseases and, as a consequence, can increase life expectancy. As a consequence, co-morbidities in combination with BMI have been placed at the basis of the indication for bariatric surgery. In 1991 the Consensus Statement of the NIH Consensus Development Conference codified the first universally accepted guidelines for surgery for obesity and weight-related disease [12]. They asserted that a candidate for surgery for obesity and weight-related diseases is a patient suffering from obesity with:

1. BMI >40 kg/m^2
2. BMI >35 kg/m^2 in the presence of specific co-morbidities:
   - Hypertension
   - Ischemic heart diseases
   - Type 2 diabetes (T2DM)
   - Obstructive sleep apnea syndrome
   - Obesity syndrome/hypoventilation (Pickwickian syndrome)
   - Non-alcoholic fatty liver disease and steatohepatitis
   - Dyslipidemia
   - Gastroesophageal reflux diseases
   - Venous stasis diseases
   - Severe urinary incontinence

These inclusion criteria for bariatric surgery have been adopted by multiple other national guidelines as well [13].

This chapter aims to elucidate the main co-morbid conditions of clinically severe obesity.

2.2 Impaired Glucose Tolerance and Diabetes Mellitus

There is currently no controversy that obesity is associated with impaired glucose tolerance or type 2 diabetes mellitus. Insulin resistance is advocated as the underlying mechanism.

The association of obesity with diabetes has been demonstrated in several studies. In one of the biggest cohort studies, in which 84,941 female patients were followed up for 16 years, there were 3300 new cases of diabetes mellitus. Importantly, the study revealed that overweight or obesity were the main predictors of type 2 diabetes mellitus [14]. In men, there were similar findings from the Health Professional follow-up study. A 60.9% age-adjusted relative risk of developing diabetes was found in those with a BMI ≥ 35 kg/m^2 in comparison to those with BMI <23 kg/m^2 [15].

There is strong and consistent evidence that obesity management can delay the progression from pre-diabetes to type 2 diabetes [16, 17] and may be beneficial in the treatment of type 2 diabetes [18, 19]. In overweight and obese patients with type 2 diabetes, mild and sustained weight loss has been shown to improve glycaemic control and to reduce the need for glucose-lowering medications [18–20]. Small studies have demonstrated that in patients with obesity and type 2 diabetes more extreme dietary energy restriction with very-low-calorie diets can reduce HbA1c to <6.5% (48 mmol/mol) and fasting glucose to <126 mg/dL (7.0 mmol/L) in the absence of pharmacological therapy or ongoing procedures [21]. Weight loss-induced improvements in glycaemia are most likely to occur early in the natural history of type 2 diabetes when a still reversible β-cell dysfunction exists but insulin secretory capacity remains relatively preserved [22].

A substantial body of evidence has now accumulated, including data from several randomised controlled clinical trials, demonstrating that bariatric surgery achieves superior glycaemic control and reduction of cardiovascular risk factors in patients suffering from obesity with type 2 diabetes as compared with other lifestyle/medical interventions [23]. It is obvious that for surgery, to be effective, it should be coupled with optimal medical treatment and lifestyle adjustment [24].

The superiority of bariatric surgery in the treatment of diabetes holds from the economic point of view as well. Indeed, according to the analysis conducted by the International Federation of the Surgery of Obesity and Metabolic Disorders (IFSO), bariatric surgery is cost-effective and, in some instances, a cost-saving approach for the management of patients suffering from obesity and T2DM [24]. With a mild degree of evidence (level 2), a different efficacy of each bariatric procedure in improving glycaemic control has emerged. Diabetic obese patients undergoing biliopancreatic diversion/duodenal switch (BPD/DS) achieve the greatest rate of T2DM resolution when compared to other surgical procedures. Gastric Bypass (GBP) and Sleeve Gastrectomy (SG) have a similar short- to mid-term effectiveness on the improvement of glycaemic control, while the anti-diabetic effects of Laparoscopic Adjustable Gastric Banding (LAGB) are lower [24].

Based on this accrued evidence, several organisations and government agencies have expanded the indications for metabolic surgery to include patients with inadequately controlled type 2 diabetes and BMI as low as 30 kg/m^2 (27.5 kg/m^2 for Asians) [24, 25]. Even IFSO stated that there was a level 1 of evidence that surgery for obesity and weight-related diseases had an excellent short and mid-term risk/benefit ratio in patients with class I obesity (BMI 30–35 kg/m^2) suffering from T2DM and/or other co-morbidities.

The benefits of surgery can also be encountered in patients with T1DM and morbid obesity. Even if no recovery of the ß-cell function itself is expected, patients with obesity and T1DM are likely to experience a reduction in the daily insulin requirements as a result of the decrease in insulin resistance that is seen after weight loss. Positive effects on other weight-related diseases are a reasonable expectation as well [24].

2.3 Hypertension

The data available so far shows a strong association between obesity and hypertension. In one large cohort study of 82,473 participants, BMI was positively associated with hypertension at age 18 and midlife. There was also a marked increase in the risk of developing hypertension with weight gain [26]. In the Framingham study, the relative risk of hypertension in overweight men and women were 1.46 and 1.75, respectively, even after age adjustment [27]. In the same study, weight reduction in women with obesity aged 18 or older, reduced the risk of hypertension.

Recently, waist circumference (WC) has been considered as a reliable marker in assessing obesity and the risk of hypertension. When WC and BMI were compared as continuous variables in the same regression model, WC was found to be a better predictor of obesity-related hypertension, than BMI [28]. Moreover, WC is comparatively easier and faster to apply than BMI, which requires a weighing scale and subsequent calculation of the index.

Several pathophysiological mechanisms are believed to be at the basis of the association between obesity and hypertension. The most convincing one is the increase of the circulating plasmatic volume as a consequence of the reduced clearance of the Atrial Natriuretic Peptide (ANP); indeed, the physiologic inactivation of this hormone by fat tissue seems to be impaired by hyperinsulinemia and insulin resistance. Moreover, hyperinsulinemia is responsible for hyperplasia of the muscular layer of arterioles with a consequent increase of peripheral vascular resistance. Another possible explanation of hypertension is that hyperinsulinemia and insulin resistance impair endothelial function and the production of nitric oxide (NO). This, in turn, results in peripheral vasoconstriction.

2.4 Heart Disease

There is unequivocal evidence that there is an increased risk of coronary artery disease (CAD) in obesity. In the Asian Pacific Cohort Collaboration study in which more than 300,000 participants were followed up, there was a 9% increased incidence of ischaemic heart disease for every unit change in BMI. Increased risk of CAD was also found in the Framingham and Nurses Health Studies [27–29]. Indeed, obesity and in particular "central obesity" is associated with hypertriglyceridemia, decreased HDL and increased LDL levels; atherogenesis and consequent coronaropathy are also triggered by hypertension and impaired glucose tolerance.

Obesity can be associated with congestive heart failure (CHF). When the risk of heart failure (HF) was evaluated in the Framingham study, it was twofold higher in the group with obesity than in the non-obese group [30]. The increase of the body mass requires a bigger left ventricular ejection volume. This leads to an eccentric left ventricular hypertrophy which progressively becomes insufficient and decompensated, and CHF becomes clinically overt at this point.

Paradoxically, the analysis of the data retrieved from the Framingham study shows that a higher BMI is associated with longer survival in patients with congestive heart failure (CHF). In a retrospective analysis of 7767 patients with CHF who were categorised into 4 BMI ranges including obesity (BMI > 30 kg/m^2), there was reduced overall mortality within higher BMI groups in an almost linear trend. After further analysis, overweight and obese patients had a hazard ratio of 0.88 compared to healthy weight patients (taken as the reference group) whereas underweight patients with stable CHF had a 1.21 risk of death when they were compared to the same reference group [31]. The reason for this so-called "obesity paradox" is not clear. Probably other concomitant cardiovascular diseases linked to obesity may have led to the diagnosis of HF in its earlier stages, thus reducing the risk of death from CHF. On the other hand, the results of cardiopulmonary testing in overweight and healthy weight patients suffering from CHF were found to be similar [32, 33]. Therefore, the explanation of the paradox remains still unclear.

Considering the well-known noxious effects of obesity and the incomplete understanding of the mechanism of this "paradox", treatment of obesity is still recommended to reduce CHF associated mortality. Elucidating the mechanism of this paradox is still an area of scientific research.

On this aforementioned basis, it's simple to understand why weight loss induced by surgery is associated with a reduction in the incidence of major cardiovascular events, including myocardial infarction and stroke. As stated by the IFSO commission in 2016, cardiovascular event reductions after weight loss are more relevant in patients with a high cardiovascular risk [24]. There is also evidence that the resolution of obesity is associated with improvement of functional status and symptoms in patients with pre-existing ischemic heart disease or heart failure; however, the effects on long-term prognosis are not known [24].

Weight loss after bariatric surgery is associated with regression or improvement of early structural markers of atherosclerosis (carotid intima-media thickness, brachial flow-mediated dilation, and coronary artery calcium score) [24]. A lower degree of evidence exists about the issue of heart transplantation in the population with obesity. Preliminary results regarding this issue suggest that, in patients with severe obesity and end-stage heart failure, bariatric surgery may be useful as a bridge to successful heart transplantation [24].

2.5 Dyslipidemia

Dyslipidemia, consisting of reduced high-density lipoprotein (HDL) and increased triglycerides, is associated with obesity [34]. The underlying mechanism is largely due to insulin resistance. Very low-density lipoprotein (VLDL) clearance in plasma is dependent on the rate of hepatic synthesis and catabolism by the lipoprotein lipase, an enzyme that is also involved in the synthesis of HDL [34, 35]. In obesity, insulin resistance is associated with the increased hepatic synthesis of VLDL and impaired lipoprotein lipase function [36].

There is evidence that dyslipidemia, in obesity, can occur even in the absence of insulin resistance. In 1998, Gary et al. showed a significant association between obesity, particularly central obesity, and dyslipidemia after adjustment for insulin resistance.

2.6 Cerebrovascular Disease

Currently, available evidence shows that the risk of haemorrhagic and ischaemic stroke is increased in men with obesity. In women this association holds as far as ischaemic stroke is concerned; haemorrhagic stroke, on the other hand, lacks correlation with obesity. In the Korean prospective study involving 234,863 men who were followed up for 9 years, a significant positive association was found between BMI and the risk of ischemic stroke; in the case of haemorrhagic stroke, a "J-shaped" association was found, showing that its risk increased more than that of ischaemic stroke at the upper and lower extremes of BMI [37].

In a prospective study of 39,053 participants (all women) who were followed up for an average of 10 years, 432 strokes occurred. 307 were ischaemic, 81 haemorrhagic and 4 undefined. In obese subjects (BMI > 30 kg/m^2), the hazard ratios (95% CI) for total stroke, ischaemic stroke and haemorrhagic stroke were 1.5 (1.16–1.94), 1.72 (1.30–2.28) and 0.82 (0.43–1.58), respectively.

The reason for the different risk of haemorrhagic stroke between men and women with obesity is not fully understood and is under the scrutiny of the scientific community.

It is noteworthy that, central obesity (where fat is preferentially distributed around the trunk) is important in predicting mortality after stroke. In the Israel heart disease study, stroke mortality was predicted by central obesity alone, independently of BMI, hypertension, diabetes and socioeconomic status [38].

2.7 Metabolic Syndrome

According to the National Cholesterol Education Program's Adult Treatment Panel III (NCEP: ATP III), the metabolic syndrome is defined when at least 3 of the following 5 features are present: (1) waist circumference above 40 inches for men and above 35 inches for women, (2) triglycerides above 150 mg/dL, (3) HDL cholesterol below 40 mg/dL for men and 50 mg/dL for women, (4) blood pressure above 130/85 mmHg, (5) fasting glucose above 100 mg/dL.

Insulin resistance, which leads to an abnormal lipid and glucose metabolism, appears to be at the basis of metabolic syndrome [39]. This syndrome was initially believed to be an independent risk factor of cardiovascular disease; however, this has recently been challenged as the sum of the combined risk factors at the basis of the metabolic syndrome does not outnumber the sum of individual factors [40].

A moderate (level 2) level of evidence exists that bariatric surgery can achieve greater improvement in each component of the Metabolic Syndrome compared with non-surgical weight loss therapies [24].

2.8 Pulmonary Diseases

Several studies have linked obesity and obstructive sleep apnea (OSA). In the Wisconsin Sleep Cohort study, obesity showed a strong association with OSA [41]. In another study, increased neck circumference, which correlates with obesity, had a strong connection with obstructive sleep apnea [42]. The mechanism responsible for OSA in obesity is the external compression by the fat tissue on the airways with consequent narrowing of their lumen [43].

Asthma is another condition that is likely to occur in obesity. There is evidence that obesity increases the risk of asthma. In one prospective multicentre study, the prevalence of asthma was observed to increase in patients with obesity. Indeed, in recent clinical research, 75% of the patients who sought medical care for asthmatic respiratory distress were reported to be either obese or overweight [44]. The mechanism linking obesity and asthma is chronic systemic inflammation driven by increased inflammatory cytokines and chemokines, and other adipocytes-derived factors [45]. In turn, the chronic inflammation increases airway hyper-responsiveness which is typical of asthma.

The association of Obstructive Sleep Apnea Syndrome (OSAS) and asthma with obesity requires an accurate assessment of the respiratory function before surgery; instrumental investigations such as chest X-ray, pulmonary function tests, arterial blood gas are mandatory [24]. If the diagnosis of sleep apnea syndrome is suspected nocturnal oximetry or polysomnographic examination is suggested to assess whether a respiratory therapy device such as C-PAP (Continuous Positive Airways Pressure), should be used peri-operatively [24].

In 2016, IFSO implemented in its Position Statements the results of several studies demonstrating that bariatric surgery for obesity may result in resolution or improvement of (OSAS) and significant improvement of asthma management, defined as symptoms, level of lung function, and use of medication in asthmatic patients.

2.9 Gastrointestinal Diseases

A great part of the epidemiological studies to date have found an association between obesity and increased risk of Gastroesophageal Reflux Disease (GERD). In one large cross-sectional population study, which was part of a randomised trial, involving 10,537 subjects, the adjusted odds ratios for heartburn and acid regurgitation in obese patients were 2.91 (95% CI 2.07–4.08) and 2.23 (95% 1.44–1.99) respectively, compared with those with normal BMI. Recent evidence from a meta-analysis involving data from studies between 1966 and 2004 has demonstrated that obesity is significantly associated with GERD, oesophageal cancer and erosive esophagitis and that the severity of these disorders increases with increasing weight [46].

Another gastrointestinal disease that has been linked to obesity is cholelithiasis. Data from the literature shows that females with a BMI of more than 45 kg/m^2 had a sevenfold increase in the risk of gallstone disease compared to those with a BMI of less than 24 kg/m^2 [47].

Consequently IFSO, in 2016, issued the grade B recommendation to perform cholecystectomy during bariatric surgery for patients with biliary symptoms or patients with gallstones documented during pre-operative ultrasonography [24].

Liver disease is a common feature in the obese population, in the form of the so-called Non-Alcoholic Fatty Liver Disease (NAFLD). NAFLD consists of a spectrum of disease manifestations that have in common the absence of excessive alcohol consumption. On one end of the spectrum, there is simple steatosis, also referred to as non-alcoholic fatty liver (NAFL) disease. Patients with simple steatosis or NAFL just have steatosis without histologic evidence of hepatocellular injury. At the other end of the spectrum, there is Non-Alcoholic Fatty Liver Steato-Hepatitis (NASH) which combines steatosis and hepatocellular injury and which may be associated with hepatic fibrosis also. Prognosis changes dramatically whether patients have NASH or non-NASH disease. It is generally accepted that patients with simple steatosis progress very slowly, if at all. On the other hand, patients with NASH are more likely than the non-NASH group to have progressive liver disease and can experience complications such as cirrhosis and HCC. There is probably a wide range of factors that predispose patients to progress from simple steatosis to NASH; however, the exact rate of progression is unknown. Lebovics and Rubin, in their recent review of NAFLD, report a 20% rate of conversion from simple steatosis to NASH over a 15-year follow-up [48, 49]. Some genomics studies to date, have implicated genetic factors associated with the progression of NAFLD, although these factors lack clinical application at the moment. It is also interesting to note that while hepatic injury induced by NASH is similar to that seen in patients with alcoholic liver disease, NASH does appear to progress more slowly and is less severe on histology than steatohepatitis caused by alcohol [50, 51]. Indeed, over a relatively short period of follow-up, only 2% of NASH patients on average progressed to decompensated liver disease and cirrhosis [52, 53]. Once cirrhosis develops in NASH patients, their overall prognosis appears to be dismal. The clinical course of patients who had NASH-related cirrhosis was found by Ratziu et al. to be similar to those with cirrhosis from hepatitis C [54].

It is accepted by most experts that while patients with steatosis alone are not at risk for HCC, patients with cirrhosis from NASH are at risk for HCC. So far, the exact pathogenesis of NASH-related HCC remains unclear although experts do agree that age and advanced fibrosis are established risk factors for HCC in NASH. Even if there are variations from study to study on the overall incidence of NASH-related HCC, there is consistent evidence that the risk of HCC is lower than hepatitis C-related cirrhosis. For example, Yatsuji et al. calculated an incidence of HCC of 11.3% in 5 years for patients with cirrhosis secondary to NASH; which is lower than the incidence of HCC in patients with hepatitis C-related cirrhosis [55].

Recent reports indicate that weight loss induced by surgery could be beneficial for NASH although the lack of randomised clinical trials precludes a precise assessment of this benefit. As a consequence of this mild level of evidence (level 2), IFSO issued a grade B recommendation that weight loss after bariatric surgery could provide improvement or resolution of non-alcoholic fatty liver disease (NAFLD) and non-alcoholic steatohepatitis (NASH) [24].

2.10 Reproductive Disease

Obesity has a detrimental effect on female fertility [56]. In women over the age of 18 whose BMI is higher than 32 kg/m^2, the relative risk of anovulatory cycles and consequent infertility is 2.7 times higher [57]. For women having ovulatory cycles, the chance of conceiving a child is decreased by 5% for every BMI-unit increase [58].

The reasons for the decreased fertility are multiple and include higher leptin and lower adiponectin levels. Additionally, the production of steroids in the ovaries is compromised and in association with the elevated insulin levels, this leads to an inhibition of the sex hormone-binding globulin synthesis by the liver and hyperandrogenemia [59]. Reduced fertility is also due to the higher incidence of polycystic ovary syndrome (characterised by anovulation, hyperandrogenism and a polycystic ovary) in women with obesity [60]. Weight loss in women with polycystic ovary syndrome, obtained by lifestyle therapy, pharmacological therapy and surgery for obesity, improves spontaneous ovulation and pregnancy rates [61]. Since weight loss improves the chances of conception, it has to be considered the first-line therapy for women with this condition [62]. This grade B recommendation was issued by IFSO in the context of 2016 Position Statements with a level 2 of evidence; in particular, IFSO members pointed out that weight loss as a treatment for infertility should be considered in the first line regardless of the presence or absence of polycystic ovary syndrome and that weight loss could be achieved by lifestyle therapy, pharmacologic therapy or surgery.

There are other reproductive complications of obesity that can occur during pregnancy and labour. These include gestational diabetes, macrosomia, dystocia and increased rates of caesarean sections [63].

In addition to the effects on female reproductive physiology, obesity also has an impact on male reproduction [64]. MOSH or Male Obesity Secondary Hypogonadism is a well-known entity. The detailed effects of obesity on reproductive physiology are discussed in another chapter.

2.11 Psychosocial and Psychiatric Problems

Obesity in the affluent society has been associated with several untoward outcomes in terms of psychosocial or socioeconomic well-being. Women with obesity, for example, were found to be more likely to drop out from school, had a 20% lower chance of getting married, earned lower salaries in comparison to females who were not overweight [65]. However, the cause–effect relationship can be either way since socioeconomic status can be responsible for obesity and viceversa [66].

Overt psychiatric disorders have been linked to obesity. These disorders include schizophrenia and schizoaffective disorders, psychosis, bipolar disorder, substance abuse disorders, eating disorders (Bulimia, BED, and NES), neurocognitive disorders and personality disorders. Treatment with certain psychotropic medications, including antipsychotics and mood stabilisers, previous psychiatric hospitalisations, as well as a history of suicide attempts or other self-injurious behaviours also are widely considered risk factors for poor post-operative outcomes. Some of these conditions, in particular severe, uncontrolled psychosis, bipolar disorder, and substance abuse are widely considered contraindications to surgery [67–69].

Minor mental health problems such as mood and anxiety disorders are very common; they are considered negative predictors for the outcome of surgery for obesity, but not a contraindication for treatment, provided the patient is receiving appropriate mental health treatment [24].

2.12 Osteoarthritis

Osteoarthritis (OA) is strongly associated with obesity. In the Framingham cohort study, data from 1420 participants indicated that obesity was an important independent risk factor for OA after adjustment for age, physical activity and levels of uric acid [70].

The mechanism of OA has been attributed to direct chronic strain on the joints related to the overweight. However, some authors have raised the hypothesis that non-mechanical aetiologies may contribute to OA in obesity because the same changes of OA present in weight-bearing joints have also been demonstrated in non-weight bearing joints. There is growing evidence that dysregulation of adipokines (hormones from adipose tissue) such as adiponectin, visfatin and resistin may trigger OA, suggesting that osteoarthritis may be a systemic disease in obesity [71, 72].

2.13 Cancer

There is considerable evidence of an association between obesity and some cancers [73]. These include cancer of the gallbladder, oesophagus (adenocarcinoma), thyroid, kidney, uterus, colon and breast [74, 75]. In the USA, 14% of cancer deaths are attributed to obesity; this percentage reaches 20% in female individuals.

This link has further been strengthened by the observation that a reduced incidence of cancer and reduced mortality from cancer is registered after weight loss [76, 77]. It was estimated that the hypothetical correction of the excess weight in the US population [78] would have been able to prevent about 900,000 cancer deaths.

So far, the underlying mechanism linking these cancers to obesity is not clear. In the case of uterus and breast cancers, it is thought to be the higher oestrogen levels synthesised from adipose tissue [79, 80].

Considering that there are no randomised clinical trials on this topic, IFSO attributed a grade C level to the statement that surgery for obesity can reduce the incidence of some malignancies and the mortality related to them [24].

2.14 Conclusions

Obesity is an epidemic disease not only affecting industrialised societies but also developing countries. It is associated with a reduced life expectancy because of the great burden of associated diseases. These can affect virtually every organ from cardiovascular to the respiratory, reproductive and gastrointestinal system. Metabolism is also negatively affected by obesity as demonstrated by the high prevalence of diabetes, dyslipidemia and endocrine pathologies. Even several psychosocial and psychiatric diseases have been pathogenetically linked to obesity. Moreover, there is growing evidence that obesity increases the likelihood of some cancers; this is far from being a sheer statistical connection because several scientific studies have demonstrated a clear pathogenetic mechanism connecting obesity and cancer.

Most of these pathologies can regress or at least improve with weight loss interventions and especially with bariatric surgery. Thus, these co-morbidities and their resolution represent, along with BMI, a keystone in the indication for bariatric surgery. Moreover, the presence of these diseases can modify the operative risk and, as a consequence, careful pre-operative evaluation is required and, when possible, optimisation of the patient. Last, but not least, post-operative results, weight loss included, can be affected by the pre-existing pathologies; patients operated on for obesity should be followed up on a patient-tailored rather than a standardised schedule.

For all these above-mentioned reasons, it is important for every healthcare professional involved in the therapy for obesity to have a thorough knowledge of these diseases.

Key Points

- *The resolution or improvement of co-morbidities has to be considered as another goal of bariatric surgery and must be given the same importance as weight loss in its outcomes.*
- *Excess visceral fat, also referred to as central obesity, has a stronger association with cardiovascular disease than subcutaneous fat.*
- *Weight loss-induced improvements in glycaemia are most likely to occur early in the natural history of type 2 diabetes when a still reversible β-cell dysfunction exists and insulin secretory capacity remains relatively preserved.*
- *In the Asian Pacific Cohort Collaboration study in which more than 300,000 participants were followed up, there was a 9% increased incidence of ischaemic heart disease for every unit change in BMI*
- *Available evidence shows that the risk of haemorrhagic and ischaemic stroke is increased in men with obesity.*
- *For women having ovulatory cycles, the chance of conceiving a child is decreased by 5% for every BMI-unit increase*
- *A moderate (level 2) level of evidence exists that bariatric surgery can achieve greater improvement in each component of the Metabolic Syndrome compared with non-surgical weight loss therapies.*
- *Obesity treatment and especially bariatric surgery can heal or improve most of the diseases associated with obesity and as a consequence can increase life expectancy.*
- *According to the analysis conducted by the International Federation of the Surgery of Obesity and Metabolic Disorders (IFSO), bariatric surgery is cost-effective and, in some instances, a cost-saving approach for the management of patients suffering from obesity and T2DM.*

References

1. Flegal KM, Carroll MD, Ogden CL, Johnson CL. Prevalence and trends in obesity among US adults, 1999–2000. JAMA. 2002;288(14):1723–7.
2. The Malawi STEPS survey for chronic non-communicable diseases and their risk factors. 2010 [Google Scholar].
3. Lopez AD, Mathers CD, Ezzati M, Jamison DT, Murray CJL. Global burden of disease and risk factors. The World Bank and Oxford University Press; 2006. Available http://www.dcp2.org/pubs/GBD [Google Scholar].
4. Murray C, Lopez A. The global burden of disease: a comprehensive assessment of mortality and disability from diseases, injuries, and risk factors in 1990 and projected to 2020, vol. 1. Geneva: World Health Organization; 1996.
5. Baingana FK, Bos ER. Changing patterns of disease and mortality in sub-Saharan Africa: An overview. In: Jamison DT, Feachem RG, Makgoba MW, Bos ER, Baingana FK, et al., editors.

Disease and mortality in sub-Saharan Africa. 2nd edn. World Bank; 2008. pp. 1–9 [Google Scholar].
6. World Health Organization. Report of a WHO Consultation on Obesity. Geneva, Switzerland: World Health Organization; 1998. Obesity: preventing and managing the global epidemic [Google Scholar].
7. NHLBI Expert Panel. Clinical guidelines on the identification, evaluation, and treatment of overweight and obesity in adults: evidence report. Bethesda, MD: NIH; 2002 (NIH publication no. 02-4084) [Google Scholar].
8. Peeters A, Barendregt JJ, Willekens F, Mackenbach JP, Al Mamun A, Bonneux L. Obesity in adulthood and its consequences for life expectancy: a life-table analysis. Ann Intern Med. 2003;138:24–32.
9. Dhana K, Kavousi M, Ikram MA, Tiemeier HW, Hofman A, Franco OH. Body shape index in comparison with other anthropometric measures in prediction of total and cause-specific mortality. J Epidemiol Community Health. 2016;70(1):90–6. https://doi.org/10.1136/jech-2014-205257. Epub 2015 Jul 9
10. Krakauer JC. Untangling waist circumference and hip circumference from body mass index with a body shape index, hip index, and anthropometric risk indicator. Metab syndr Related Disord. 2018;16(4):160–5. https://doi.org/10.1089/met.2017.0166. Epub 2018 Mar 13
11. Dietz WH, Robinson TN. Clinical practice. Overweight children and adolescents. N Engl J Med. 2005;352:2100.
12. NIH conference. Gastrointestinal surgery for severe obesity. Consensus development conference panel. Ann Intern Med. 1991;115(12):956–61.
13. Forestieri P, et al. Linee guida e stat dell'arte della chirurgia bariatrica e metabolica in Italia. EDISES s.r.l. – Napoli; 2008. ISBN: 978 88 7959 455 4.
14. Frank B, Hu FB, Manson JE, Stumpfer MJ, Colditz G, Liu S, Solomon CG, Willett WC. Diet, Lifestyle, and the risks of type 2 diabetes in women. N Engl J Med. 2001;345(11):790–7.
15. Koh-Banerjee P, Wang Y, Hu FB, Spiegelman D, Willett WC, Rimm EB. Changes in body weight and body fat distribution as risk factors for clinical diabetes in US men. Am J Epidemiol. 2004;159(12):1150–9.
16. Tuomilehto J. The emerging global epidemic of type 1 diabetes. Curr Diab Rep. 2013;13:795–804.
17. Knowler WC, Barrett-Connor E, Fowler SE, et al. Diabetes Prevention Program Research Group. Reduction in the incidence of type 2 diabetes with lifestyle intervention or metformin. N Engl J Med. 2002;346:393–403.
18. UK Prospective. Diabetes Study 7. UK Prospective Diabetes Study 7: response of fasting plasma glucose to diet therapy in newly presenting type II diabetic patients, UKPDS Group. Metabolism. 1990;39:905–12.
19. Rothberg AE, McEwen LN, Kraftson AT, Fowler CE, Herman WH. Very-low-energy diet for type 2 diabetes: an underutilized therapy? J Diabetes Complication. 2014;28:506–10.
20. Pastors JG, Warshaw H, Daly A, Franz M, Kulkarni K. The evidence for the effectiveness of medical nutrition therapy in diabetes management. Diabetes Care. 2002;25:608–13.
21. Day JW, Ottaway N, Patterson JT, et al. A new glucagon and GLP-1 co-agonist eliminates obesity in rodents. Nat Chem Biol. 2009;5:749–57.
22. Steven S, Hollingsworth KG, Al-Mrabeh A, et al. Very low-calorie diet and 6 months of weight stability in type 2 diabetes: pathophysiological changes in responders and nonresponders. Diabetes Care. 2016;39:808–15.
23. Rubino F, Nathan DM, Eckel RH, et al. Delegates of the 2nd Diabetes Surgery Summit. Metabolic surgery in the treatment algorithm for type 2 diabetes: a joint statement by international diabetes organizations. Diabetes Care. 2016;39:861–77.
24. De Luca M, Angrisani L, et al. Indications for surgery for obesity and weight-related diseases: position statements from the International Federation for the Surgery of Obesity and Metabolic Disorders (IFSO). Obes Surg. 2016;26:1659–96. https://doi.org/10.1007/s11695-016-2271-4.

25. Rubino F, Kaplan LM, Schauer PR, Cummings DE, Delegates DSS. The Diabetes Surgery Summit consensus conference: recommendations for the evaluation and use of gastrointestinal surgery to treat type 2 diabetes mellitus. Ann Surg. 2010;251:399–405.
26. Cohen JB. Hypertension in obesity and the impact of weight loss. Curr Cardiol Rep. 2017;19(10):98. https://doi.org/10.1007/s11886-017-0912-4.
27. Wilson PW, D'Agostino RB, Sullivan L, Parise H, WB K. Overweight and obesity as determinants of cardiovascular risk; the Framingham experience. Arch Intern Med. 2002;162:1867–72.
28. Janssen I, Katzmarzyk PT, Ross R. Waist circumference and not body mass index explains obesity-related health risk. Am J Clin Nutr. 2004;79:379–84.
29. Luo J, Rossouw J, Margolis KL. Smoking cessation, weight change and coronary heart disease among postmenopausal women with and without diabetes. JAMA. 2013;310(1):94–6. https://doi.org/10.1001/jama.2013.6871.
30. Kenchaiah S, Evans JC, Levy D, Wilson PW, Benjamin EJ, Larson MG, et al. Obesity and the risk of heart failure. N Engl J Med. 2002;347:305–13.
31. Curtis JP, Selter JG, Wang Y, Rathore SS, Jovin IS, Jadbabaie F, et al. The obesity paradox. Body mass index and outcomes in patients with heart failure. Arch Intern Med. 2005;165:55–61.
32. Davos CH, Doehner W, Rauchhaus M, et al. Body mass and survival in patients with chronic heart failure without cachexia: the importance of obesity. J Card Fail. 2003;929–35.
33. Lavie CJ, Osman AF, Mlani RV, Mehra MR. Body composition and prognosis in chronic systolic heart failure: the obesity paradox. Am J Cardiol. 2003:91891–4.
34. Piché ME, Vasan SK, Hodson L, Karpe F. Relevance of human fat distribution on lipid and lipoprotein metabolism and cardiovascular disease risk. Curr Opin Lipidol. 2018;29(4):285–92. https://doi.org/10.1097/MOL.0000000000000522.
35. Sun L, Ishida T, Miyashita K, Kinoshita N, Mori K, Yasuda T, Toh R, Nakajima K, Imamura S, Hirata K. Plasma activity of endothelial lipase impacts high-density lipoprotein metabolism and coronary risk factors in humans. J Atheroscler Thromb. 2014;21(4):313–21. Epub 2013 Dec 26
36. Despres JP, Moorjani S, Pouliot MC, Tremblay A, Nadeau A, Lupien PJ, Bouchard C. Correlates of plasma very-low-density lipoprotein concentration and composition in premenopausal women. Metabolism. 1990;39:577–83.
37. Song YM, Sung J, Davey Smith G, Ebrahim S. Body mass index and ischemic and hemorrhagic stroke; a prospective study in Koreanmen. Stroke. 2004;35:831–6.
38. Tanne D, Medalie JH, Goldbourt U. Body fat distribution and long-term risk of stroke mortality. Stroke. 2005;36:1021–5.
39. Executive summary of the third report of the National Cholesterol Education Program (NCEP), author Expert Panel on Detection, Evaluation, and Treatment of High Blood Cholesterol In Adults (Adult Treatment Panel III). JAMA. 2001;285:2486–2497
40. Eckel RH, Albert KG, Grund SM. The metabolic syndrome. Lancet. 2010;375:181–3.
41. Young T, Palta M, Dempsey J, Skatrud J, Weber S, Badr S. The occurrence of sleep-disordered breathing among middle-aged adults. N Engl J Med. 1993;328:1230–5.
42. Genta PR, Schorr F, Eckert DJ, Gebrim E, Kayamori F, Moriya HT, Malhotra A, Lorenzi-Filho G. Upper airway collapsibility is associated with obesity and hyoid position. Sleep. 2014;37(10):1673–8. https://doi.org/10.5665/sleep.4078.
43. Isono S. Obesity and obstructive sleep apnoea: mechanisms for increased collapsibility of the passive pharyngeal airway. Respirology. 2012;17(1):32–42. https://doi.org/10.1111/j.1440-1843.2011.02093.x.
44. Weiss ST, Shore S. Obesity and asthma: directions for research. Am J Respir Care Med. 2004;169:963–8.
45. Shore SA, Fredberg JJ. Obesity, smooth muscle and airway hyper responsiveness. J Allergy Clin Immunol. 2005;115:925–7.
46. Hampel H, Abraham NS, El-Serag HB. Meta-analysis: obesity and the risk for gastroesophageal relux disease and its complications. Ann Intern Med. 2005;143:199–211.

47. Bonfrate L, Wang DQ, Garruti G, Portincasa P. Obesity and the risk and prognosis of gallstone disease and pancreatitis. Best Pract Res Clin Gastroenterol. 2014;28(4):623–35. https://doi.org/10.1016/j.bpg.2014.07.013.
48. Lebovics E, Rubin J. Non-alcoholic fatty liver disease (NAFLD): why you should care, when you should worry, what you should do. Diabetes Metab Res Rev. 2011;27:419–24.
49. Pais R, Pascale A, Fedchuck L, Charlotte F, Poynard T, Ratziu V. Progression from isolated steatosis to steatohepatitis and fibrosis in nonalcoholic fatty liver disease. Clin Res Hepatol Gastroenterol. 2011;35:23–8.
50. Kim MY. The progression of liver fibrosis in non-alcoholic fatty liver disease. Korean J Gastroenterol. 2017;69(6):341–7. https://doi.org/10.4166/kjg.2017.69.6.341.
51. Singh S, Allen AM, Wang Z, Prokop LJ, Murad MH, Loomba R. Fibrosis progression in non-alcoholic fatty liver vs nonalcoholic steatohepatitis: a systematic review and meta-analysis of paired-biopsy studies. Clin Gastroenterol Hepatol. 2015;13(4):643–54.e1–9; quiz e39–40. https://doi.org/10.1016/j.cgh.2014.04.014
52. Lee RG. Nonalcoholic steatohepatitis: a study of 49 patients. Hum Pathol. 1989;20:594–8.
53. Wree A, Broderick L, Canbay A, Hoffman HM, Feldstein AE. From NAFLD to NASH to cirrhosis-new insights into disease mechanisms. Nat Rev Gastroenterol Hepatol. 2013;10(11):627–36. https://doi.org/10.1038/nrgastro.2013.149.
54. Ratziu V, Bonyhay L, Di Martino V, et al. Survival, liver failure, and hepatocellular carcinoma is obesity-related cryptogenic cirrhosis. Hepatology. 2002;35:1485–93.
55. Yatsuji S, Hashimoto E, Tobari M, et al. Clinical features and outcomes of cirrhosis due to non-alcoholic steatohepatitis compared with cirrhosis caused by chronic hepatitis C. J Gastoenterol Hepatol. 2009;24:248–54.
56. Pandey S, Pandey S, Maheshwari A, Bhattacharya S. The impact of female obesity on the outcome of fertility treatment. J Hum Reprod Sci. 2010;3(2):62–7.
57. Delitala AP, Capobianco G, Delitala G, Cherchi PL, Dessole S. Polycystic ovary syndrome, adipose tissue and metabolic syndrome. Arch Gynecol Obstet. 2017;296(3):405–19. https://doi.org/10.1007/s00404-017-4429-2.
58. van der Steeg JW, Steures P, Eijkemans MJ, Habbema JD, Hompes PG, Burggraaff JM, et al. Obesity affects spontaneous pregnancy chances in subfertile, ovulatory women. Hum Reprod. 2008;23(2):324–8.
59. Gil-Campos M, Cañete RR, Gil A. Adiponectin, the missing link in insulin resistance and obesity. Clin Nutr. 2004;23(5):963–74.
60. Motta AB. The role of obesity in the development of polycystic ovary syndrome. Curr Pharm Des. 2012;18(17):2482–91.
61. Baeten JM, Bukusi EA, Lambe M. Pregnancy complications and outcomes among overweight and obese nulliparous women. Am J Public Health. 2001;91(3):436–40.
62. Cedergren MI. Maternal morbid obesity and the risk of adverse pregnancy outcome. Obstet Gynecol. 2004;103(2):219–24.
63. Dietl J. Maternal obesity and complications during pregnancy. J Perinat Med. 2005;33:100–5.
64. Esposito K, Giugliano F, Di Palo C, Giugliano G, Marfella R, D'Andrea F, et al. Effect of lifestyle changes on erectile dysfunction in obese men: a randomized controlled trial. JAMA. 2004;291:2978–84.
65. Gortmaker SL, Must A, Perrin JM, Sobol AM, Dietz WH. Social and economic consequences of overweight in adolescence and young adulthood. N Engl J Med. 1993;329:1008–12.
66. Juonala M, Harcourt BE, Saner C, Sethi M, Saffery R, Magnussen CG, Burgner DP, Sabin MA. Neighbourhood socioeconomic circumstances, adiposity and cardiometabolic risk measures in children with severe obesity. Obes Res Clin Pract. 2019;pii:S1871-403X(19)30068-7. https://doi.org/10.1016/j.orcp.2019.05.004.
67. Rosik CH. Psychiatric symptoms among prospective bariatric surgery patients: rates of prevalence and their relation to social desirability, pursuit of surgery, and follow-up attendance. Obes Surg. 2005;15:677–83.

68. Mitchell JE, Selzer F, Kalarchian MA, Devlin MJ, Strain GW, Elder KA, et al. Psychopathology before surgery in the longitudinal assessment of bariatric surgery-3 (LABS-3) psychosocial study. Surg Obes Relat Dis. 2012;8(5):533–41.
69. Livhits M, Mercado C, Yermilov I, Parikh JA, Dutson E, Mehran A, et al. Preoperative predictors of weight loss following bariatric surgery: systematic review. Obes Surg. 2012;22(1):70–89.
70. Georgiev T, Angelov AK. Modifiable risk factors in knee osteoarthritis: treatment implications. Rheumatol Int. 2019;39(7):1145–57. https://doi.org/10.1007/s00296-019-04290-z. Epub 2019 Mar 25. Review. PMID: 30911813
71. Herrero-Beaumont G, Pérez-Baos S, Sánchez-Pernaute O, Roman-Blas JA, Lamuedra A. Targeting chronic innate inflammatory pathways, the main road to prevention of osteoarthritis progression. Biochem Pharmacol. 2019;165:24–32. https://doi.org/10.1016/j.bcp.2019.02.030. Epub 2019 Feb 27
72. Aspeden RM, Scheven BA, Hutchison JD. Osteoarthritis as a systemic disorder including stromal cell differentiation and lipid metabolism. Lancet. 2001;357(9262):1118–20.
73. Baren-Engquist K, Chang M. obesity and cancer risk: recent review and evidence. Curr Oncol Resp. 2011;13(1):71–6.
74. Renehan AG, Tyson M, Egger M, Heller RF, Zwahlen M. Body mass index and the incidence of cancer: a systematic review and meta analysis of prospective observational studies. Lancet. 2008;371–578.
75. Kabat GC, Xue X, Kamensky V, Lane D, Bea JW. Risk of breast, endometrial, colorectal, and renal cancers in postmenopausal women in association with a body shape index and other anthropometric measures. Cancer Causes Control. 2015;26(2):219–29. https://doi.org/10.1007/s10552-014-0501-4. Epub 2014 Nov 28
76. Sjöström L, Gummesson A, Sjöström CD, et al. Effects of bariatric surgery on cancer incidence in obese patients in Sweden (Swedish Obese Subjects Study): a prospective, controlled intervention trial. Lancet Oncol. 2009;10:653–62.
77. Adams TD, Stroup AM, Gress RE, et al. Cancer incidence and mortality after gastric bypass surgery. Obesity (Silver Spring). 2009;17:796–802.
78. Calle EE, Rodriguez C, Walker-Thurmond K, Thun MJ. Overweight, obesity, and mortality from cancer in a prospectively studied cohort of U.S. adults. N Engl J Med. 2003;348(17):1625–38.
79. Tumminia A, Vinciguerra F, Parisi M, Graziano M, Sciacca L, Baratta R, Frittitta L. Adipose tissue, obesity and adiponectin: role in endocrine cancer risk. Int J Mol Sci. 2019;20(12). pii:E2863. https://doi.org/10.3390/ijms20122863
80. Schmandt RE, Iglesians DA, Co NN, Lu KH. Understanding Obesity and Endometrial Cancer Risk: Opportunities for prevention. Am J Obstet Gynecol. 2011;205:518–25.

Pre-existing Nutritional Deficiencies Associated with Obesity

3

Mariam Lakdawala, Miloni Shah Sancheti,
Nimisha Kantharia, and Aparna Govil Bhasker

We need a new definition of malnutrition. Malnutrition means-under and over nutrition. Malnutrition means emaciated and obese.

– Catherine Bertini

M. Lakdawala (✉)
Bariatric and Laparoscopic Surgery, Global Hospital, Mumbai, Maharashtra, India

Bariatric and Laparoscopic Surgery, Currae Hospital, Mumbai, Maharashtra, India

M. Shah Sancheti
Bariatric and Laparoscopic Surgery, Namaha Hospital, Mumbai, Maharashtra, India

Sterling Hospital, Mumbai, Maharashtra, India

N. Kantharia
Wockhardt Hospital, Mumbai, Maharashtra, India

Bhatia Hospital, Mumbai, Maharashtra, India

Jaslok Hospital, Mumbai, Maharashtra, India

A. G. Bhasker
Bariatric and Laparoscopic Surgery, Global Hospital, Mumbai, Maharashtra, India

Bariatric and Laparoscopic Surgery, Currae Hospital, Mumbai, Maharashtra, India

Bariatric and Laparoscopic Surgery, Namaha Hospital, Mumbai, Maharashtra, India

Bariatric and Laparoscopic Surgery, Apollo Hospital, Mumbai, Maharashtra, India

Bariatric and Laparoscopic Surgery, Suchak Hospital, Mumbai, Maharashtra, India

Bariatric and Laparoscopic Surgery, Saifee Hospital, Mumbai, Maharashtra, India

Bariatric and Laparoscopic Surgery, Dr. Aparna's—Laparoscopy & Bariatric Surgery Centre, Mumbai, Maharashtra, India

A. G. Bhasker et al. (eds.), *Management of Nutritional and Metabolic Complications of Bariatric Surgery*,
https://doi.org/10.1007/978-981-33-4702-1_3

3.1 Introduction

Obesity is defined as a condition with abnormal or excessive fat accumulation that poses a risk to health [1]. In the last 30 years, globalization has lifted millions out of poverty, hunger and infectious disease. While this has led to significant improvement in the quality of lives of common people, the same social and economic shifts have also led to an increase in waistlines. The prevalence of obesity has doubled between 1980 and 2014 worldwide [2]. Developing countries like India and China are at the brink of an obesity epidemic today [3].

A person is classified as being affected by clinically severe obesity when their body mass index (BMI) is greater than 40 kg/m^2 (37.5 for Asians), or they are more than 100 pounds over their ideal body weight. Additionally, individuals who have a BMI of 35 kg/m^2 (32.5 for Asians) or greater with an existing co-morbidity (i.e. diabetes, hypertension, etc.) are also classified as being severely obese [3]. Even moderate obesity is hazardous for health as it is associated with a number of health issues like type II diabetes mellitus, high blood pressure, dyslipidaemia, lung disease, liver disease, varicose veins, arthritis, cancers, cardiovascular diseases, gallbladder stones, hernias, etc. Paradoxically, although obesity is viewed as a state of overnutrition, patients suffering from obesity suffer from a number of nutritional deficiencies and obesity represents yet another spectrum of malnutrition.

The aim of this chapter is to provide an overview of the:

- Prevalence of pre-existing nutritional deficiencies associated with obesity
- Causes of nutritional deficiencies in individuals suffering from obesity
- An overview of the physiology of various nutrients in the body
- Signs and symptoms of nutrient deficiencies
  (a) Management of pre-operative nutritional deficiencies

3.2 Obesity: A State of Malnutrition

Malnutrition is defined as a condition that develops when the human body does not receive adequate quantities of energy-providing nutrients (protein, carbohydrates and fats), vitamins, minerals and water required for normal tissue and organ growth [4]. Though obesity is considered to be a state of "overnutrition", paradoxically in the past few years, malnutrition has become the new synonym of obesity due to its association with various nutritional deficiencies. There are multiple reasons for this paradox such as easy availability of processed and packaged foods at a low price, increased consumption of empty calorie and energy-dense foods, sedentary lifestyle, altered metabolism leading to poor bioavailability of nutrients [5], prolonged use of certain medications, food preferences [6] and obesity-associated inflammation [7].

3.3 Causes of Nutritional Deficiencies in Individuals Suffering from Obesity

An energy imbalance created as a result of excessive energy intake in relation to energy expenditure forms the pathophysiological basis of obesity in the majority of cases. At the same time, the quality of food consumed is equally important and must not be overlooked [8]. Nowadays, there is an increase in the consumption of processed foods which are generally low in vitamins and minerals. Increased intake of less nutritious food has been shown to proportionately decrease the intake of unprocessed nutritious food like fruits, vegetables, whole grains and legumes and protein-rich foods [9]. In developing countries like India, the dependence on less nutritious processed foods is more, as these foods are comparatively less expensive than the unprocessed nutritious foods. This holds true for many other parts of the world as well.

Obesity leads to a state of inflammation in the human body. Excess adipose tissue leads to the release of pro-inflammatory cytokine - interleukin 6 (IL-6) which may in turn lead to low-grade systemic inflammation [10]. Chronic inflammation causes increased hepcidin release in liver and fat tissue which inhibits iron absorption.

Obesity also leads to defective storage and bioavailability of certain nutrients. For example, it causes a deficiency of Vitamin D due to its sequestration in adipose tissue. This could also apply to other lipophilic vitamins. In a study that was done to assess micronutrient deficiencies in obese subjects undergoing a Low-Calorie Diet (LCD), a negative correlation was observed between lipophilic vitamins and body fat at baseline and a significant increase in serum Vitamin D concentrations following an LCD suggesting the release of the stored vitamin D during weight loss [11].

The risk of small intestinal bacterial overgrowth (SIBO) characterized by an excessive/abnormal growth of Gram-negative aerobic and anaerobic bacteria in the proximal small bowel [12] has shown to increase by 11 times in patients with obesity as compared to non-obese patients and is independent of small bowel transit time, gastric pH and small bowel pH [13]. An increase in the count of Firmicutes and a decrease in the Bacteroidetes bacterial group have been observed in the gut of individuals with obesity [14]. These may lead to better and more efficient energy extraction from food and also cause low grade inflammation [15].

In individuals with obesity, who are already at risk of developing Non-Alcoholic Fatty Liver Disease (NAFLD), SIBO further adds up to its risk and severity. This was supported by a recent study, in which bacterial overgrowth was more frequent in patients with clinically severe obesity as compared to normal-weight subjects and was associated with severe steatosis [16].

In addition to liver disease, hypothyroidism and the use of diuretics in this population also add to nutritional deficiencies.

Vegetarianism is another reason that could lead to inadequate intake of certain nutrients due to their reduced bioavailability in plant sources. This is a concern especially in the Indian population wherein 35% of the population is vegetarian [17]. A vegetarian diet, being rich in fibre and antioxidants, has shown to be beneficial in reducing the risk of non-communicable diseases [18]. However, it has been observed that vegetarians as compared to omnivores are deficient in certain nutrients and thus their requirement of supplementation is higher pre-operatively [19].

Patients suffering from obesity are also frequently on some or the other form of self-supervised low-calorie diet, thus increasing their susceptibility to micronutrient deficiencies. In a recent study, obese subjects ($n = 32$) underwent a low-calorie formula diet covering their dietary reference intake (DRI) for a period of 3 months. At baseline and after 3 months their micronutrient levels were assessed, it was found that even more subjects were deficient in certain micronutrients after 3 months of diet intervention, suggesting that their demands are higher than the normal weight population. The possible reasons for this could be metabolic alterations during the period of weight loss, unequal distribution of lipophilic compounds, enhanced oxidative stress induced by the excess adipose tissues and electrolyte imbalance due to fluid changes in the body [11].

Low micronutrient levels can also be attributed to the volumetric dilution factor as obesity causes expansion of the total body water in the extracellular compartment [20].

Lastly, micronutrient deficiencies and excessive caloric intake disturb the normal biochemical pathway which leads to the accumulation of toxic by-products resulting in further weight gain or development of associated metabolic diseases [11].

3.4 An Overview on Physiology of Various Nutrients in the Body

3.4.1 Iron

Iron is an active part of haemoglobin in red blood cells and is also a constituent of the muscle protein myoglobin and a variety of proteins that speed up chemical reactions within the body. Once iron is absorbed from the food it is carried in the blood via the transport protein transferrin. Much of this is transported to the bone marrow where it is used for haemoglobin formation. Extra iron is then stored in the liver in the form of ferritin and hemosiderin.

The cause of iron deficiency in individuals with obesity could be attributed to multiple factors such as a state of chronic inflammation in response to the excessive amounts of fat tissues, dilution effect due to increased plasma volume [21], poor food choices and vegetarianism.

Hepcidin—is a protein and a key regulator for the entry of iron in blood circulation. Its levels are higher in individuals with obesity and are linked to subclinical inflammation; which may reduce iron absorption and blunt the effects of iron fortification. Increased pro-inflammatory cytokines, such as leptin, interleukin-6 (IL-6),

C-Reactive Protein (CRP) stimulate hepcidin production by the liver and adipose tissues. Hepcidin excess has been suggested to decrease dietary iron absorption and increase iron sequestration from reticulo-endothelial macrophages [22].

Thus, low iron status in overweight individuals may result from a combination of nutritional (reduced absorption) and functional (increased sequestration) iron deficiency [23]. In addition to poor absorption, nutritional deficiency could also be due to poor dietary choices, vegetarianism and poor access to foods rich in iron.

The absorption of iron is influenced by many other factors. Absorption of ingested iron increases in proportion to an increase in the body's need. For example: blood loss during an injury, accident or during pregnancy.

There are two sources of iron: Heme iron and non-heme iron. The absorption of heme form is much better than the non-heme form of iron.

The following factors would enhance the absorption of non-heme iron:

- Gastric acid is required to increase the solubility of iron and favours the ferrous form of iron.
- Vitamin C, when consumed with the source of iron, increases the solubility of iron in the duodenum.
- Citric acid or citrus juices and fruits, at acidic pH absorption of iron is better. Commonly seen at the proximal small intestine.

The following factors reduce the absorption of iron:

- Tannic acid, as from tea
- Antacids of any type
- Calcium and phosphate salts taken as medicine

Dietary sources of iron: All types of meat contains heme iron, bajra, poha, green leafy vegetables.

Signs and symptoms of iron deficiency: General fatigue, breathlessness, giddiness, dimness of vision, anorexia, koilonychia, glossitis, stomatitis, palpitation and decreased physical activity

Prevention of these symptoms is dietary changes and proper supplementation

3.5 Calcium and Vitamin D

Calcium and phosphorus are best known for their contribution to the strength of the skeleton, body metabolism, muscle activity and functioning of nerves. Factors that influence the amount of calcium in the blood are likely to influence the phosphorus levels as well. Parathyroid hormone (PTH) and vitamin D play a very important role in calcium regulation. Vitamin D promotes calcium absorption from the small intestine:

- It works with PTH to increase the mobilization of calcium from the bones to the blood.

- PTH and vitamin D together help renal reabsorption of calcium.
- PTH increases urinary excretion of phosphorus. In turn, a drop in serum phosphorus levels results in an increase in serum calcium levels.

Normally the amount of PTH released is affected by calcium levels. A low calcium serves as a stimulus for the release of PTH. As soon as the calcium level rises, the secretion of PTH ceases temporarily.

Obesity is associated with vitamin D deficiency, hyperparathyroidism and secondary hypercalcemia [24]. Vitamin D deficiency is seen in approximately 57–94% of individuals suffering from obesity [25].

Exposure to sunlight is the only known source of vitamin D. Cultural and social taboos on clothing in some regions may limit the exposure to sun.

A vegetarian diet also limits dietary intake of vitamin D. Poor nutrition and a sedentary lifestyle have led this deficiency to be an epidemic. The availability of Vitamin D fortified foods has increased, but lack of awareness and less affordability makes it difficult to access these foods. Fortification of staple foods with vitamin D may prove to be a more viable solution towards attaining vitamin D sufficiency.

Individuals suffering from obesity have low plasma concentrations of 25-hydroxyvitamin D [25(OH) D], which is associated with increased plasma concentrations of parathyroid hormone. It has been proposed that production of the active vitamin D metabolite 1, 25-dihydroxy vitamin D increases in high BMI individuals and this, in turn, exerts negative feedback control on the hepatic synthesis of 1, 25-dihydroxy vitamin D. It has also been suggested that the metabolic clearance of vitamin D may increase in obesity, possibly with enhanced uptake by adipose tissue. Although the explanation for the increased risk of vitamin D deficiency in obesity is unknown, it has been postulated that individuals suffering from obesity may avoid exposure to solar ultraviolet (UV) radiation, which is indispensable for the cutaneous synthesis of vitamin D3. If the increased risk of vitamin D deficiency in obesity were the result of a primary alteration or a direct consequence of obesity itself then a rational intervention could be instituted [24]. As vitamin D is fat-soluble and is readily stored in adipose tissue, it could be sequestered in the larger body pool of fat of individuals suffering from obesity. It is observed that blood vitamin D3 concentrations increased in both the obese and non-obese subjects after exposure to an identical amount of UV-B irradiation. Further, the alteration of the vitamin D endocrine system in obese subjects is characterized by secondary hyperparathyroidism which is associated with enhanced renal tubular reabsorption of calcium and increased circulating 1,25(OH)2D.

Dietary sources of Vitamin D: Milk and milk products, fatty fish, like tuna, mackerel, salmon, fortified food with vitamin D, beef liver, egg yolk, few grains, beans and lentils.

Signs and symptoms of vitamin D deficiency: Fatigue, bone and back or joint pain, impaired wound healing, bone loss, hair loss, muscle pain, rickets, tetany, osteomalacia, osteoporosis.

3.6 Water Soluble: B-Vitamins

All the B-Vitamins play a very crucial role in various haematological and neurological functions in the body. Elevated levels of homocysteine as a result of low levels of folic acid and Vitamin B12 is said to be an independent risk factor for oxidative stress and cardiovascular diseases [26].

There is a lot of variation in vitamin B status across different countries and this is mainly due to the differences in the level of food fortification. It could also be due to food choices and supplementation [27]. Chronic alcoholism is another factor that can lead to Vitamin B1 and folate deficiency by interfering with its active transport across the intestinal wall and causing its excretion in urine [28–30].

Folic acid has a low storage capacity and is found in leafy vegetables, whole meat products and legumes. Similarly, thiamine (Vitamin B1), a coenzyme involved in many biochemical pathways, is stored in small amounts in skeletal muscles, liver, kidney, heart and brain and can get depleted within a week. Whereas vitamin B12 found in meat, eggs and milk products has comparatively more storage capacity, hence a deficiency would suggest a low intake over a long period of time [31].

The availability of thiamine is limited to yeast, whole grains, beef, lean pork and legumes. It gets destroyed easily in an alkaline environment ($pH > 8$), at high temperature and when consumed with ethanol- or thiaminase-containing foods like caffeinated or decaffeinated tea/coffee, raw fish and shellfish [4]. Pre-operative thiamine deficiency was seen in 29% of 379 patients, in which the deficiency was higher in African American (31%) and Hispanics (47%) compared to the Caucasian population (7%) [32]. Another study observed low levels of thiamine in 47 (15.5%) out of 303 patients undergoing bariatric surgery. Another observation made in this study was that none of the patients with pre-operative thiamine deficiency developed neurological manifestation post bariatric surgery. This was attributed to their pre-operative protocol for thiamine supplementation. Since the incidence of thiamine deficiency is higher post bariatric surgery due to recurrent episodes of vomiting and is associated with irreversible neurological sequelae, it is very important to correct it pre-operatively [4].

A recent study revealed that B12 deficiency is observed in one-fifth of the population suffering from obesity and is positively correlated with BMI [21]. While the prevalence of Vitamin B12 deficiency has been reported to be 18% pre-operatively in patients suffering from obesity [9, 33], in India it is found to be as high as 56.7% [6]. Vitamin B12 deficiency if not corrected can lead to pernicious anaemia [21].

3.7 Fat-Soluble Vitamins: Vitamin A, E and K

Fat-soluble vitamin deficiency is more commonly observed post malabsorptive surgeries. The antioxidant vitamins - A (beta-carotene and retinol) and E (alpha-tocopherol) have shown to be deficient in both children and adults suffering from obesity. Pre-existing Vitamin A deficiency of 14% has been reported in adults undergoing bariatric surgery [34]. Screening for Vitamin E and K is discounted in the bariatric population owing to the lack of data on pre-operative deficiencies. A study reported 2.2% ($n = 89$) Vitamin E deficiency in patients undergoing bariatric surgery [35].

3.8 Zinc

Zinc is the second most prevalent trace element found in the human body and is crucial for normal cell function and metabolism. It also functions as an antioxidant and regulates immune function, taste and appetite [36]. Studies have suggested that zinc deficiency was present in 28% of the patients pre-operatively.

Dietary sources of zinc: Beef, chicken, fish, liver, wheat germ, and whole grains.

3.9 Management of Pre-operative Nutritional Deficiencies

Micronutrient deficiencies can contribute to the risk of developing many obesity-associated diseases if not assessed and corrected in a timely manner. Vitamin D deficiency has been shown to increase the risk for diabetes, cardiovascular diseases and several types of cancers [32, 37]. Zinc deficiency can lead to the development of certain types of cancers [38, 39] and could promote both acute and chronic liver diseases [40].

Nutritional deficiencies, if not detected and corrected pre-operatively, have also been shown to have a great impact on the post-operative morbidity and mortality [41]. As per the ASMBS guidelines, pre-operative investigations including nutritional assessment are mandatory for a bariatric surgery candidate [42]. Unfortunately, these tests are being carried out in less than 25% of the population undergoing bariatric surgery [43].

Given below is the list of tests that may be advised to patients undergoing bariatric surgery.

Blood tests	Radiological	Others
Complete blood count	Chest X-ray PA View	Upper GI endoscopy with *H. pylori* testing
Kidney function tests	ECG	Pulmonary function test
Sr. uric acid	2-D Echocardiography	Polysomnography (Sleep study)
Liver function test	USG abdomen and pelvis	
Fasting and post prandial blood sugars	Bilateral venous colour doppler of lower limbs	
Fasting and post prandial insulin levels	Liver elastography	
Fasting and post prandial C-peptide levels		
Glycosylated haemoglobin (HbA1c)		

Blood tests	Radiological	Others
Lipid profile		
Blood group		
Coagulation profile		
HIV, HCV, HBsAg (Elisa)		
Thyroid profile		
Serum PTH		
Serum ionized calcium		
Serum homocysteine		
Serum folic acid		
Serum vitamin B 12		
Serum vitamin D 3		
Serum iron studies		
Urine routine and microscopy/ microalbuminuria, urinary calcium		

Nutritional parameters in the above list help us to identify the nutritional status of the patient and in case of deficiencies supplement them in the pre-surgery period.

Given below is the supplementation protocol in case of nutritional deficiencies before undergoing bariatric surgery:

Nutrient	Cut-offs at which supplementation is initiated	Supplement dosage
Vitamin D	< 30 ng/mL < 10 ng/mL	Vitamin D3 injection 3 lakh units intramuscular - Stat Vitamin D3 injection 6 lakh units intramuscular - Stat
Vitamin B12	< 300 pg/mL	Injection Cyanocobalamin 1000 mcg + 100 mg thiamine intramuscular - Stat [44]
Calcium	Sr. Calcium <8.8 mg/dL Or Ionized calcium < 1.12 mmol/L	Calcium citrate 1000 mg per oral once daily
Iron profile	Sr. Iron <65 µg/dL (For men) Sr. Iron <50 µg/dL (For women) Or Hb < 10.0 g/dL	Injection Ferric carboxymaltose 500 mg in 250 mL NS over 3 h IV - Stat
Folic acid	< 3 ng/mL	Folic acid 5 mg per oral daily
Total protein, serum albumin	Total protein < 6.5 g/dL Sr. Albumin < 3.5 g/dL	Patients are advised to be on a high protein diet for 7–14 days pre-operatively as per their clinical profile

The pre-operative investigations include only vitamin B12 and vitamin B9 (folic acid). Other B vitamin tests are expensive and their dietary reference intake is comparatively lower. B vitamins being water-soluble do not cause toxicity when taken in excess. Thus, in addition to vitamin B12, we suggest that patients must be supplemented empirically with vitamin B6 (pyridoxine—50–100 mg), vitamin B1 (thiamine—100 mg), d-panthenol (50 mg), vitamin B3 (nicotinamide—100 mg), etc. to ensure good nutritional status pre-operatively.

Assessment of fat-soluble vitamins—Vitamin A, E and K is not done pre-operatively as the deficiency of these nutrients is not commonly observed in the population suffering from obesity. Also, post-operatively the deficiency of these vitamins is seen more often after mal-absorptive procedures like bilio-pancreatic diversion due to fat malabsorption.

3.10 Conclusion

The rise in the incidence of obesity has led to a proportionate increase in the number of bariatric surgeries. Nutritional deficiencies are not only a common concern post bariatric surgery but are seen commonly in the pre-operative phase. It has been observed that a nutritionally sufficient patient recovers faster as compared to a patient with a poor nutritional status. Thus, pre-operative nutritional screening is crucial for identifying the nutritional deficiencies. These deficiencies must be corrected in the pre-surgery phase with adequate supplementation to ensure a smooth post-operative recovery, better weight loss outcomes and decreased morbidity and mortality.

Key Points

- *Although obesity is viewed as a state of overnutrition, patients suffering from obesity paradoxically suffer from a number of nutritional deficiencies. Obesity represents another spectrum of malnutrition.*
- *Increased intake of less nutritious food has been shown to proportionately decrease the intake of unprocessed nutritious food like fruits, vegetables, whole grains and legumes and protein-rich foods.*
- *Chronic inflammation causes increased hepcidin release in liver and fat tissue which inhibits iron absorption in patients suffering from obesity.*
- *Obesity leads to defective storage and bioavailability of certain nutrients like Vitamin D and other lipophilic vitamins.*
- *The risk of small intestinal bacterial overgrowth (SIBO) characterized by an excessive/abnormal growth of Gram-negative aerobic and anaerobic bacteria in the proximal small bowel is said to be 11 times higher in patients suffering from obesity.*
- *Nutritional deficiencies if not detected and corrected pre-operatively, have shown to have a great impact on the post-operative morbidity and mortality*
- *Nutritionally sufficient patients recover faster after bariatric surgery as compared to patients with a poor nutritional status*
- *Nutritional deficiencies must be corrected in the pre-surgery phase with adequate supplementation to ensure a smooth post-operative recovery, better weight loss outcomes and a decreased morbidity and mortality* (Table 3.1).

Table 3.1 Pre-operative nutritional deficiencies observed in patients suffering from obesity

Reference	Remedios et al. [6]	Flancbaum et al. [44]	Moizé et al. [45]	Sánchez et al. [46]	Schweiger et al. [47]	Krzizek et al. [31]	Ernst et al. [35]	Lee et al. [48]
Sample size	2740	379 (320 Women & 59 Men)	231	103	114 (83 Women & 31 men)	1732 (1339 Women & 393 Men)	232	577
Study population	Indians	Whites, Hispanics, African Americans	Spanish	Morbidly obese Chilean women	Israel	Austria	Switzerland	Singapore (Asia)
Study year	2016	2006	2011	2016	2006–2008	2018	Nov 2005–Dec 2007	Sept 2008–Nov 2017
BMI range (kg/m^2)		51.8 ± 10.6	48.2 ± 7.8	43.1 ± 5.3	44.3	44 ± 9	>35	42.4 ± 8.4
% Def of Iron (μg/dL)	43	43.9		12.6	35	9.6		32.7
% Def of Vit B12 (pg/mL)	56.7			10.6	3.6	5.1	18.1	9.5
% Def of Vit D (ng/mL)	35	68.1	94	71.7		97.5	89.7	57.5
% Def of Calcium (mg/dL)	11			13.3	0.9			1.8
% Def of Proteins (g/dL)	10							
% Def of albumin (g/dL)	9.38			0	0		12.5	47.1
Secondary hyperparathyroidism PTH (pg/mL)	42.45		41	66.6	39	30.2	36.6	34.7
% Def of Ferritin		8.4		8.7	24		6.9	29.3
% Def of Hb		22		7.7	19		6.9	23.3 (Male), 15.8 (Female)
% Def of Thiamine		29						
% Def of zinc				2.9			24.6	
% Def of Folic acid					24	63.2	3.4	31

References

1. Tortora GJ, Derrickson BH. Principles of anatomy and physiology. Hoboken, NJ: Wiley; 2008.
2. www.who.int/mediacentre/factsheets/fs311/en/
3. Dixit S, Zirpe K, Khatib K. Principles in critical care nutrition. New Delhi: Jaypee; 2019.
4. Carrodeguas L, Kaidar-Person O, Szomstein S, Antozzi P, Rosenthal R. Preoperative thiamine deficiency in obese population undergoing laparoscopic bariatric surgery. Surg Obes Relat Dis. 2005;1(6):517–22.
5. Kaidar-Person O, Person B, Szomstein S, Rosenthal RJ. Nutritional deficiencies in morbidly obese patients: a new form of malnutrition? Obes Surg. 2008;18(7):870–6.
6. Remedios C, Bhasker AG, Dhulla N, Dhar S, Lakdawala M. Bariatric nutrition guidelines for the Indian population. Obes Surg. 2016;26(5):1057–68.
7. McClung JP, Karl JP. Iron deficiency and obesity: the contribution of inflammation and diminished iron absorption. Nutr Rev. 2009;67(2):100–4.
8. Westerterp-Plantenga MS, Wijckmans-Duijsens NE, Verboeketvan de Venne WP, de GK, van het Hof KH, Weststrate JA. Energy intake and body weight effects of six months reduced or full fat diets, as a function of dietary restraint. Int J Obes Relat Metab Disord. 1998;22:14–22.
9. Xanthakos SA. Nutritional deficiencies in obesity and after bariatric surgery. Pediatr Clin. 2009;56(5):1105–21.
10. Visser M, Bouter LM, McQuillan GM, Wener MH, Harris TB. Elevated C-reactive protein levels in overweight and obese adults. JAMA. 1999;282:2131–5.
11. Damms-Machado A, Weser G, Bischoff SC. Micronutrient deficiency in obese subjects undergoing low calorie diet. Nutr J. 2012;11(1):34.
12. Stein J, Stier C, Raab H, Weiner R. Review article: the nutritional and pharmacological consequences of obesity surgery. Aliment Pharmacol Ther. 2014;40(6):582–609.
13. Roland BC, Lee D, Miller LS, Vegesna A, Yolken R, Severance E, et al. Obesity increases the risk of small intestinal bacterial overgrowth (SIBO). Neurogastroenterol Motil. 2018;30(3):e13199.
14. Ley RE, Turnbaugh PJ, Klein S, ecology GJIM. human gut microbes associated with obesity. Nature. 2006;444:1022–3. https://doi.org/10.1038/4441022a.
15. Turnbaugh PJ, Ley RE, Mahowald MA, Magrini V, Mardis ER, Gordon JI. An obesity-associated gut microbiome with increased capacity for energy harvest. Nature. 2006;444:1027–31. https://doi.org/10.1038/nature05414.
16. Sabaté JM, Jouët P, Harnois F, Mechler C, Msika S, Grossin M, Coffin B. High prevalence of small intestinal bacterial overgrowth in patients with morbid obesity: a contributor to severe hepatic steatosis. Obes Surg. 2008;18(4):371–7.
17. Key TJ, Appleby PN, Rosell MS. Health effects of vegetarian and vegan diets. Proc Nutr Soc. 2006;65(1):35–41. https://doi.org/10.1079/PNS2005481.
18. Shridhar K, Dhillon PK, Bowen L, Kinra S, Bharathi AV, Prabhakaran D, et al. Nutritional profile of Indian vegetarian diets—the Indian Migration Study (IMS). Nutr J. 2014;13(1):55.
19. Sherf-Dagan S, Hod K, Buch A, Mardy-Tilbor L, Regev Z, Ben-Porat T, et al. Health and nutritional status of vegetarian candidates for bariatric surgery and practical recommendations. Obes Surg. 2018;28(1):152–60.
20. Waki M, Kral JG, Mazariegos M, Wang J, Pierson RN Jr, Heymsfield SB. Relative expansion of extracellular fluid in obese vs. nonobese women. Am J Physiol Endocrinol Metab. 1991;261(2):E199–203.
21. Arshad M, Jaberian S, Pazouki A, Riazi S, Rangraz MA, Mokhber S. Iron deficiency anemia and megaloblastic anemia in obese patients. Rom J Intern Med. 2017;55(1):3–7.
22. Cepeda-Lopez AC, Osendarp SJ, Melse-Boonstra A, Aeberli I, Gonzalez-Salazar F, Feskens E, et al. Sharply higher rates of iron deficiency in obese Mexican women and children are predicted by obesity-related inflammation rather than by differences in dietary iron intake. Am J Clin Nutr. 2011;93(5):975–83.

23. Cepeda-Lopez AC, Aeberli I, Zimmermann MB. Does obesity increase risk for iron deficiency? A review of the literature and the potential mechanisms. Int J Vitam Nutr Res. 2010;80(4):263.
24. Shah P, Chauhan AP. Impact of obesity on vitamin D and calcium status. Int J Med Res Rev. 2016;4(02).
25. Gebler L, Charuvastra M, Silver D. Nutritional deficiencies associated with obesity. J Obes Weight Loss Ther. 2015;5(252):2.
26. Wald DS, Law M, Morris JK. Homocysteine and cardiovascular disease: evidence on causality from a meta-analysis. BMJ. 2002;325:1202.
27. Al-Mutawa A, Anderson A, Alsabah S, Al-Mutawa M. Nutritional status of bariatric surgery candidates. Nutrients. 2018;10(1):67.
28. Mahan L, Escott-Stump S. Krause's food nutrition therapy. 12th edn. St. Louis, MO: Saunders/Elsevier; 2008. p. 84–5, 414, 1229.
29. Gastaldi G, Casirola D, Ferrari G, Rindi G. Effect of chronic ethanol administration on thiamine transport in microvillous vesicles of rat small intestine. Alcohol Alcohol. 1989;24(2):83–9.
30. Food and Nutrition Board. Dietary reference intakes for thiamin, riboflavin, niacin, vitamin B b6 s, folate, vitamin Bb12 s, pantothenic acid, biotin, and choline; Washington, DC: National Academy Press; 1998. p. 81, 182, 203–4, 211, 273.
31. Krzizek EC, Brix JM, Herz CT, Kopp HP, Schernthaner GH, Schernthaner G, Ludvik B. Prevalence of micronutrient deficiency in patients with morbid obesity before bariatric surgery. Obes Surg. 2018;28(3):643–8.
32. Bischoff-Ferrari HA, Giovannucci E, Willett WC, Dietrich T, wson-Hughes B. Estimation of optimal serum concentrations of 25-hydroxyvitamin D for multiple health outcomes. Am J Clin Nutr. 2006;84:18–28.
33. Bhatti O, Bielefeldt KK, Nusrat S. Nutritional deficiencies in obesity and after weight reduction. Ann Nutr Disord Ther. 2015;2:1024–9.
34. Pereira S, Saboya C, Chaves G, Ramalho A. Class III obesity and its relationship with the nutritional status of vitamin A in pre-and postoperative gastric bypass. Obes Surg. 2009;19(6):738–44.
35. Ernst B, Thurnheer M, Schmid SM, Schultes B. Evidence for the necessity to systematically assess micronutrient status prior to bariatric surgery. Obes Surg. 2009;19(1):66–73.
36. Yuyama LKO, Yonekura L, Aguiar JPL, Rodrigues MLCF, Cozzolino SMF. Zinco. In: Cozzolino SMF, editor. Biodisponibilidade de Nutrientes, 3th edn. Barueri: Manole. p. 616–43.
37. Holick MF. Vitamin D deficiency. N Engl J Med. 2007;357:266–81, 24.
38. Chakravarty PK, Ghosh A, Chowdhury JR. Zinc in human malignancies. Neoplasma. 1986;85–90(27):33.
39. Guy NC, Garewal H, Holubec H, et al. A novel dietary-related model of esophagitis and Barrett's esophagus, a premalignant lesion. Nutr Cancer. 2007;59:217–27.
40. Stamoulis I, Kouraklis G, Theocharis S. Zinc and the liver: an active interaction. Dig Dis Sci. 2007;52:1595–612.
41. Shankar P, Boylan M, Sriram K. Micronutrient deficiencies after bariatric surgery. Nutrition (Burbank, Los Angeles County, Calif). 2010;26(11–12):1031–7.
42. Parrott J, Frank L, Rabena R, et al. American Society for Metabolic and Bariatric Surgery integrated health nutritional guidelines for the surgical weight loss patient, 2016 update: micronutrients. Surg Obes Relat Dis. 2017;13(5):727–41.
43. Gudzune KA, Huizinga MM, Chang H-Y, et al. Screening and diagnosis of micronutrient deficiencies before and after bariatric surgery. Obes Surg. 2013;23(10):1581–9.
44. Flancbaum L, Belsley S, Drake V, Colarusso T, Tayler E. Preoperative nutritional status of patients undergoing Roux-en-Y gastric bypass for morbid obesity. J Gastrointest Surg. 2006;10(7):1033–7.
45. Moizé V, Deulofeu R, Torres F, de Osaba JM, Vidal J. Nutritional intake and prevalence of nutritional deficiencies prior to surgery in a Spanish morbidly obese population. Obes Surg. 2011;21(9):1382–8.

46. Sánchez A, Rojas P, Basfi-fer K, Carrasco F, Inostroza J, Codoceo J, et al. Micronutrient deficiencies in morbidly obese women prior to bariatric surgery. Obes Surg. 2016;26(2):361–8.
47. Schweiger C, Weiss R, Berry E, Keidar A. Nutritional deficiencies in bariatric surgery candidates. Obes Surg. 2010;20(2):193–7.
48. Lee PC, Ganguly S, Dixon JB, Tan HC, Lim CH, Tham KW. Nutritional deficiencies in severe obesity: a multiethnic Asian Cohort. Obes Surg. 2019;29(1):166–71.

Bariatric Procedures: Anatomical and Physiological Changes

4

Almino Cardoso Ramos, Hugo V. Coca Jimenez Carraso, and Eduardo Lemos De Souza Bastos

In understanding the basics of digestion, you'll discover who's in charge. Here's a hint. It's not you.

– Nancy Mure

4.1 Introduction

Obesity is a chronic, multifactorial, disease with increasing incidence and prevalence, especially in countries with western lifestyles [1, 2]. Although dietary control, regular physical activity and/or drug therapy have been considered as the first line of therapeutic approach, bariatric surgery seems to be the most effective

A. C. Ramos (✉)
International Federation for the Surgery of Obesity and Metabolic Disorders (IFSO), Naples, Italy

Gastro-Obeso-Center, Advanced Institute for Metabolic Optimization, Sao Paulo, Brazil

Hugo V. Coca Jimenez Carraso
Intensive Care Unit, Santa Casa de Misericordia de Marilia Hospital, Marilia, Brazil

Nutrition Department, Santa Casa de Misericordia de Marilia Hospital, Marilia, Brazil

Federal University of Sao Paulo, Sao Paulo, Brazil

Eduardo Lemos De Souza Bastos
International Federation for the Surgery of Obesity and Metabolic Disorders (IFSO), Naples, Italy

Gastro-Obeso-Center, Advanced Institute for Metabolic Optimization, Sao Paulo, Brazil

Division of Gastrointestinal Surgery, Marilia Medical School (FAMEMA), Marilia, Brazil

Brazilian Society of Bariatric and Metabolic Surgery (SBCBM), Sao Paulo, Brazil

A. G. Bhasker et al. (eds.), *Management of Nutritional and Metabolic Complications of Bariatric Surgery*,
https://doi.org/10.1007/978-981-33-4702-1_4

approach for patients with higher body mass index (BMI) and/or with associated comorbidities. Studies comparing medical and surgical treatment in individuals with clinically severe obesity have shown better results in short, medium, and long term in favor of the surgical approach in terms of sustained weight loss, control of comorbidities, reduction in major macrovascular events and mortality [3–7].

Since the 1950s, several surgical procedures have been proposed to achieve the desired weight loss and control of comorbidities [8]. Roughly, they are categorized as predominantly restrictive, predominantly malabsorptive, and mixed procedures (combination of both). However, this classification is merely didactic, since only gastric restriction and/or nutrient malabsorption appear to be inaccurate to provide a full explanation of all successful outcomes attributed to most bariatric procedures currently in use. It has now been recognized that anatomical alterations directed at restricting the amount of food or reducing the absorptive intestinal surface are less relevant than substantial changes in neural and endocrine signaling pathways commonly seen after bariatric surgery [9–16].

Therefore, it is more appropriate to anatomically classify the bariatric procedures into two groups, according to the absence or presence of small bowel diversion. In the first group (without intestinal bypass), Laparoscopic Adjustable Gastric Band (LAGB), Vertical Banded Gastroplasty (VBG), and Laparoscopic Sleeve Gastrectomy (LSG) are well-fitted. Examples of the second (with intestinal bypass) are Roux-en-Y Gastric Bypass (RYGB), One-Anastomosis Gastric Bypass (OAGB), Biliopancreatic Diversion (BPD—Scopinaro's Surgery), Biliopancreatic Diversion with Duodenal Switch (BPD-DS), Single-Anastomosis Duodenoileal Bypass with Sleeve Gastrectomy (SADI-S), Ileal Interposition, Transit Bipartition and Jejunoileal Bypass (JIB). Currently, some of these techniques are no longer being used, for example, VBG and JIB. Still, there is a wide range of operative techniques, each procedure with its peculiarity in relation to the technical design and mechanism of action. Some procedures are time-honored, such as RYGB, while some new procedures are emerging and gaining acceptance among patients and surgeons, such as LSG and OAGB.

With or without small bowel diversion, surgical bariatric procedures modify the anatomy of the digestive system and have an impact on entire gastrointestinal (GI) physiology, by restricting the food intake, altering the digestive and absorptive process, changing the GI hormones, motility, microbiota balance, neural signaling among other lesser-known mechanism. In addition, bariatric surgeries can strongly alter the regulation of hunger/satiety in the central nervous system, change food preferences and taste, and modify energy expenditure [9, 17–19]. All these postoperative changes can be summarized in the so-called BRAVE effect, i.e., Bile flow alteration, Reduction of gastric size, Anatomical gut rearrangement and Altered flow of nutrients, Vagal manipulation, and Enteric and adipose hormones modulation [20].

Although most of these physiological changes are part of the therapeutic purpose and therefore expected, they can also cause adverse effects such as food intolerance, nutritional deficiencies, chronic abdominal pain, diarrhea, flatulence, dumping syndrome, gastroesophageal reflux disease, small intestinal bacterial overgrowth, among others [21–32]. Occasionally, adverse events can be clinically severe and impair the quality of life. In these situations, the attempt to restore normal anatomy may sometimes be the only viable therapeutic option. The changes caused by the adjustable gastric band (AGB) are completely reversible by simply withdrawing the device. LSG and BPD-DS are not subject to reversal, as both include partial gastrectomy. While it is technically feasible to restore the original food transit after RYGB and OAGB, since nothing is removed, the restoration includes new GI anastomoses. The anatomical configuration of the gastrointestinal tract is not completely normal and therefore, neither is the physiology.

Therefore, it is essential to know the anatomical and physiological changes caused in the digestive system by the different bariatric procedures. For understanding the expected outcomes and for the immediate recognition of their possible adverse events. In this chapter, only the anatomical changes associated with the most common bariatric procedures performed around the world will be addressed-LSG (45.9%), RYGB (39.6%), LAGB (7.4%), OAGB (OAGB) (1.8%), and BPD-DS (1.1%) [33], here sorted according to absence or presence of small bowel diversion.

4.2 Anatomical Changes of Procedures Without Small Bowel Diversion

4.2.1 Laparoscopic Adjustable Gastric Band

The LAGB is a restrictive procedure that consists of placing a silicone band around the upper stomach, very close to the cardia (Fig. 4.1). When left in place, the device provides a significant reduction in gastric capacity by creating a superior pouch of reduced size (10–20 mL) and a luminal narrowing that slows the emptying of ingested food to the lower portions of the stomach. Through a connection tube and a subcutaneous access port, it is possible to perform adjustments to the internal diameter of the device in order to manage the level of restriction and the emptying speed of the upper gastric pouch. LAGB is a completely reversible procedure, and the simple removal of the device totally restores the original anatomy and physiology of the GI tract.

4.2.2 Laparoscopic Sleeve Gastrectomy

The LSG is the fastest growing bariatric procedure in recent years, preferred by both surgeons and patients mainly due to excellent results in terms of weight loss, control of obesity-related comorbidities, and quality of life, which is achieved through a faster, technically less demanding surgical procedure [33, 34]. In addition, the absence of intestinal bypass preserves the original absorptive surface, significantly reducing adverse events related to nutrient malabsorption, which is a common concern associated with bypass procedures.

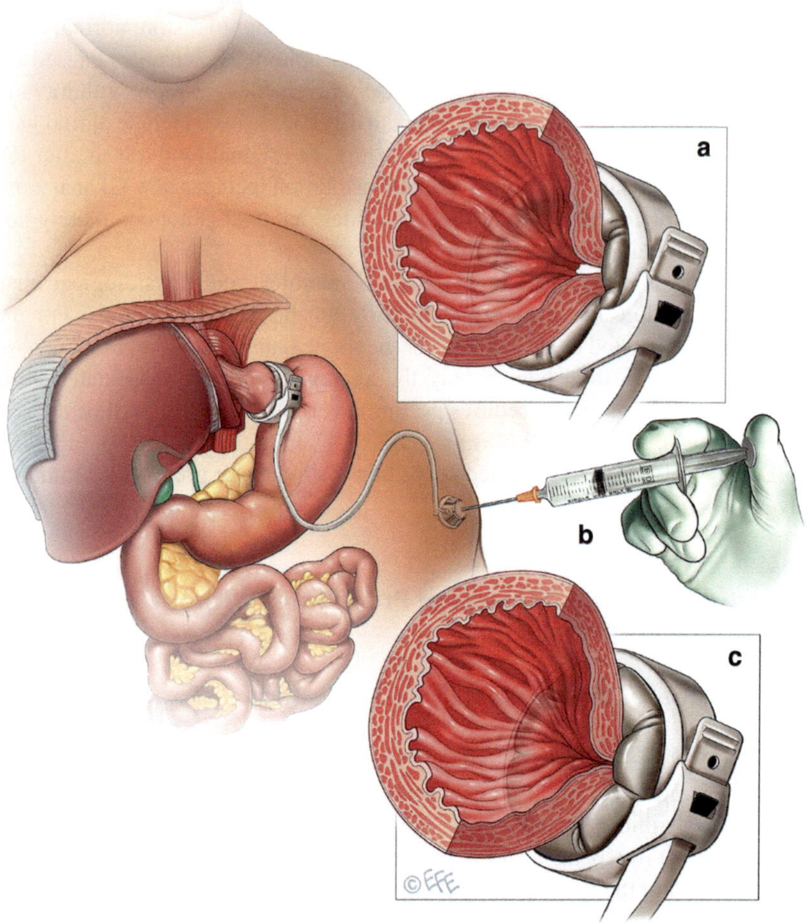

Fig. 4.1 Schematic drawing showing AGB in place. (**a**) Deflated band ("open"); (**b**) subcutaneous access port; (**c**) inflated band ("closed")

The operative technique can be summarized in the removal of about 70–80% of the stomach by means of stapled vertical gastrectomy, which includes a small part of the antrum, a large part of the body, and the entire gastric fundus (Fig. 4.2). The pylorus is preserved, and therefore, the gastric emptying mechanism is kept intact. The only anatomical change is a reduction in the size of the gastric reservoir, which is approximately 100–150 mL capacity. This single, "simple" anatomical alteration (partial gastrectomy), however, can cause deep modifications in the functioning of the entire digestive system. Because of a partial gastrectomy, LSG is an irreversible bariatric procedure.

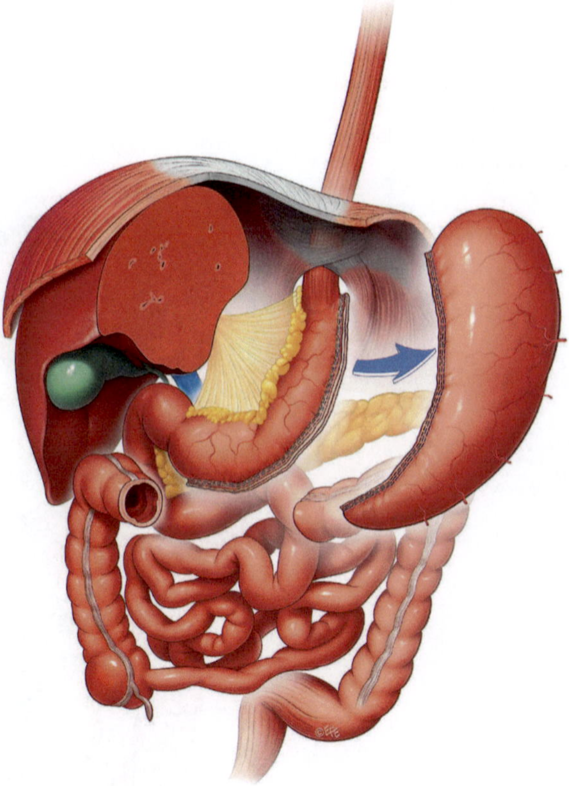

Fig. 4.2 Schematic drawing representative of the final surgical aspect of LSG highlighting the removed stomach, remaining only a long gastric tube (the Sleeve itself). The entire gut is kept untouched

4.3 Anatomical Changes in Procedures with Small Bowel Diversion

4.3.1 Roux-en-Y Gastric Bypass

A small pouch based on lesser gastric curvature is constructed in the upper stomach through linear staplers, excluding about 95% of the stomach. The alimentary pathway is reconstructed in Roux-en-Y fashion, using alimentary and biliopancreatic limbs, connected to each other by distal enteroenterostomy (Fig. 4.3). The alimentary limb usually is about 100–120 cm long, through which only food mixed with saliva and minimal gastric juices flow down. On the other hand, within the biliopancreatic limb (50–150 cm in length) only gastric and biliopancreatic secretions flow without food. Thus, the ingested food only meets gastric and biliopancreatic secretions after enteroenterostomy, in the common channel. The length of the common channel varies according to the total length of the small bowel since the surgeons usually work with fixed lengths of only the alimentary and biliopancreatic limbs.

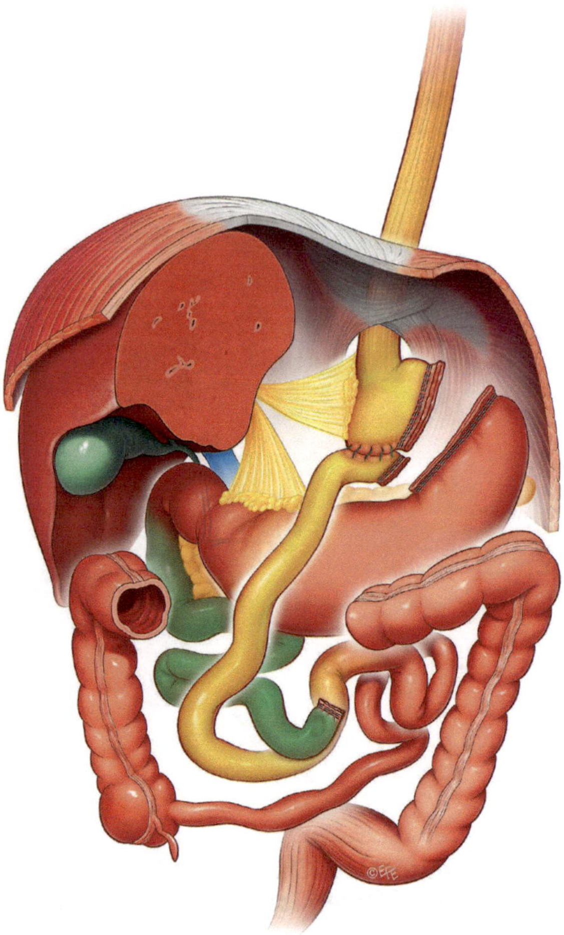

Fig. 4.3 Schematic drawing representative of the final surgical aspect of RYGB with small, vertical gastric pouch, Roux-en-Y reconstruction, and longer common channel

Therefore, the anatomic configuration of RYGB provides a reduced gastric capacity (20–30 mL), along with an exclusion of the stomach (95%), duodenum and a variable length of the jejunum (usually 50–150 cm). This causes a restriction, in addition to substantially altering the neurohormonal signaling of the GI tract and modifying the well-tuned processes of digestion and absorption. Although RYGB is prone to induce some nutrient deficiencies (mainly due to duodenal bypass), the malabsorptive component itself is generally mild.

4.3.2 One-Anastomosis Gastric Bypass

The OAGB was originally described in the early 2000s and is a procedure with principles similar to RYGB, but technically simpler and faster. The procedure involves the creation of a long and narrow pouch ("Sleeve-like") based on the lesser curvature of the stomach, followed by end-to-side anastomosis between the gastric pouch and the small bowel approximately 150–200 cm distal to the duodenojejunal flexure (angle of Treitz). Unlike the RYGB, there is not an alimentary limb, but rather afferent and efferent loops, since the reconstruction of the food transit occurs following the Billroth II design (Fig. 4.4). The capacity of the gastric reservoir is diminished (more than LSG, but less than RYGB), and the entire duodenum and the first 150 to 200 cm of the small bowel (jejunum) are bypassed.

The OAGB has been usually reported as a hypo absorptive procedure with a higher incidence of diarrhea, steatorrhea, deteriorated liver parameters, and nutritional adverse events [35, 36], although the amount of small bowel diversion is very similar to RYGB with long limbs. Thus, the pivotal anatomical and perhaps also physiological difference with RYGB is the absence of an alimentary limb (Roux-limb).

Fig. 4.4 Schematic drawing representative of the final surgical aspect of OAGB with long gastric pouch and Billroth II type reconstruction

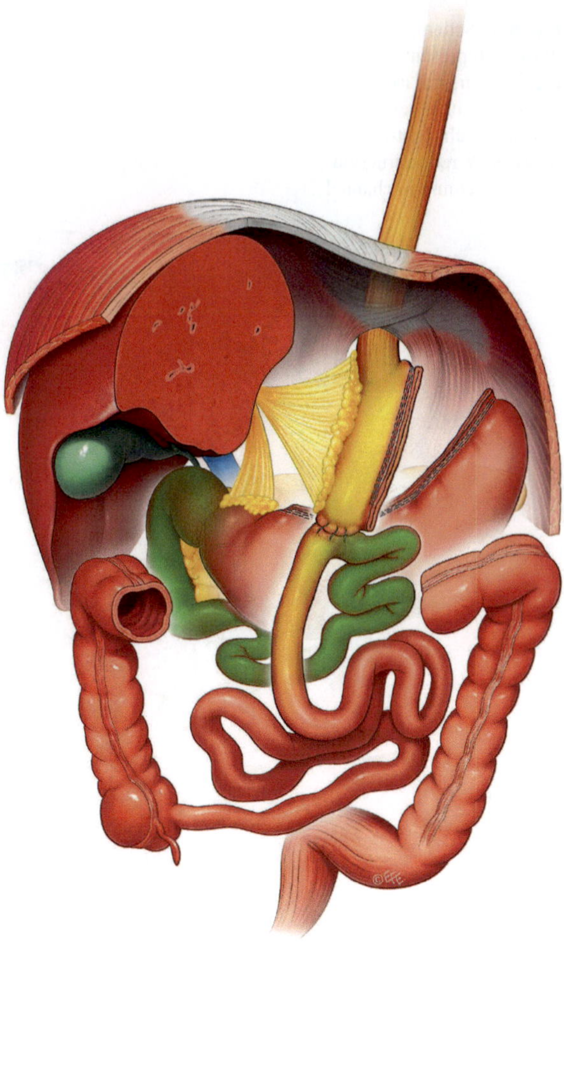

4.3.3 Biliopancreatic Diversion with Duodenal Switch

Rarely performed today, BPD-DS is a chiefly malabsorptive procedure. Recently, a new single-anastomosis-based BPD-DS design (Single-Anastomosis Duodenoileal bypass with Sleeve Gastrectomy—SADI-S) represents a current attempt to reduce side effects and provide a technical simplification [37, 38].

Usually described as a "malabsorptive" procedure, BPD-DS includes both restrictive and malabsorptive components. The restriction is due to a Sleeve gastrectomy. A linear stapled transection of the duodenum immediately after the pylorus is performed and the food transit is reconstructed by means of an end-to-side, hand-sewn Roux-en-Y duodenoileostomy. Enteroenterostomy is then performed at a distance of 50–120 cm from the ileocecal valve. The final configuration of the small bowel diversion in the BPD-DS (as well as the classic BPD and SADI-S) is longer alimentary and biliopancreatic limbs and shorter common channels (Figs. 4.5, 4.6

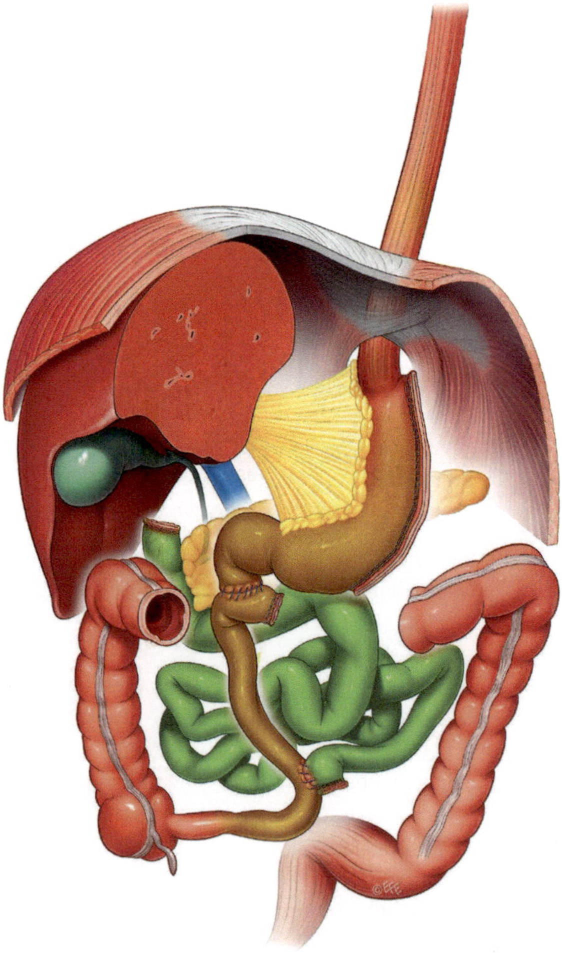

Fig. 4.5 Schematic drawing representative of the final surgical aspect of BPD-DS with sleeve gastric pouch, post-pyloric Roux-en-Y reconstruction, and short common channel

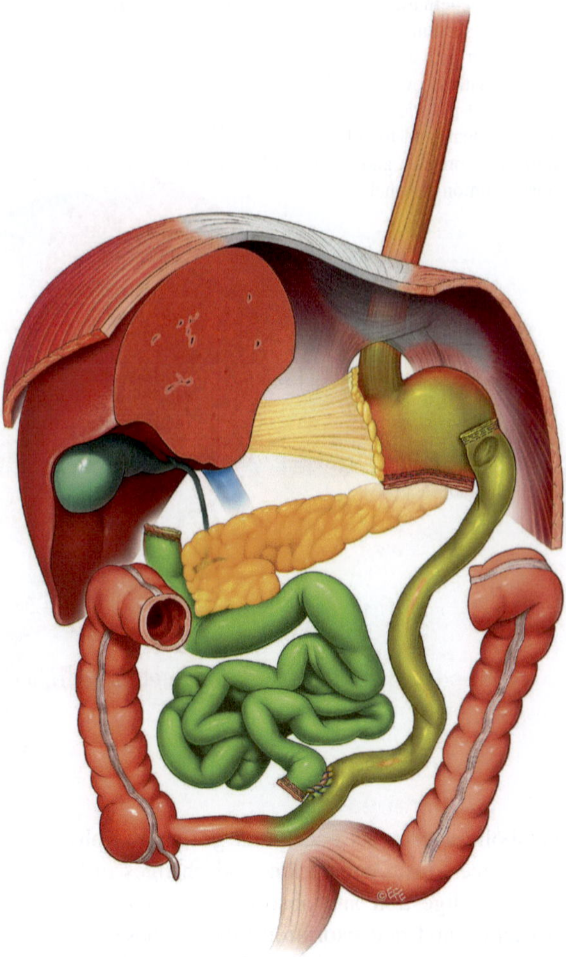

Fig. 4.6 Schematic drawing representative of the final surgical aspect of classic BPD (Scopinaro's Surgery) with partial gastrectomy, large horizontal gastric pouch, and short common channel

and 4.7). The length of the common channel (how short it is left) predominantly defines the degree of malabsorption and can be a factor for the severe and sometimes uncontrollable adverse effects.

4.4 Physiological Changes on GI Tract After Bariatric Procedures

The anatomical changes brought about by the various procedures also induce changes in the physiology of the digestive system in different ways and to different degrees. Bariatric surgery targets various organs and systems beyond the GIT, including the central nervous system, liver, pancreas, adipose tissue, and muscle, among others, impacting the whole metabolism of the human body. Profound

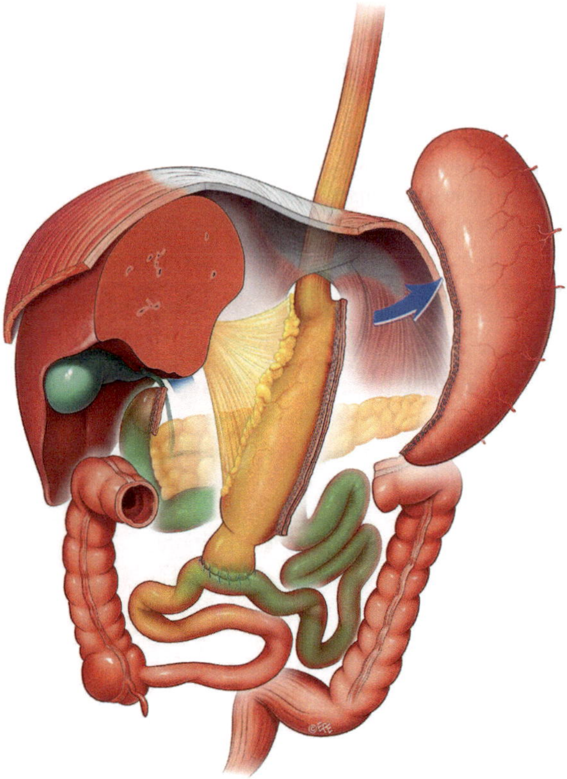

Fig. 4.7 Schematic drawing representative of the final surgical aspect of SADI-S with sleeve gastric pouch, post-pyloric (duodenoileal) end-to-side single anastomosis, and short common channel

metabolic alterations occur that go beyond physical restriction and involve food preferences, taste perception, and changes in hunger/satiety control signaling. In addition, digestion and absorption of nutrients is also affected. Apart from the restriction and malabsorption factors, these changes are mediated through neural pathways and substances like leptin, ghrelin, insulin, cytokines, and several gut-derived hormones, among others. Even in procedures considered purely restrictive, such as LAGB, the efficacy of weight loss may be associated with neurohormonal mechanisms [18, 19, 39–41].

In spite of the available literature, the actual impact of bariatric procedures on the physiology of the digestive system is far from completely understood and needs to be studied further.

4.5 Food Intake

In general, food intake is reduced following bariatric surgery. The impact on food intake starts from the cephalic phase itself. Hormones like ghrelin, insulin, and gastrin are released in response to the thought, sight and/or smell of food [19, 42]. Soon after bariatric procedure, patients usually show a significant reduction in fasting and postprandial ghrelin levels. However, these low levels appear not to be sustained in the long term. Therefore, although the significant drop in serum ghrelin may be contributory in the weight loss immediately after bariatric surgery, this may not have the same relevance in weight loss maintenance.

Return to baseline levels may also be implicated in recidivism in the long term. In this sense, the surgical impact of LSG on ghrelin levels seems to be more consistent and durable than RYGB, since most ghrelin secreting cells are irreversibly removed by the operation (gastric fundus) [12, 43–45]. However, it remains open to debate as the incidence of weight regain after LSG has been shown to be significant.

Changes in appetite, food preferences, and taste perception may also diminish food intake postoperatively, impacting on weight loss. An increased preference for low-sugar and low-fat diets have been frequently observed after bariatric procedures [46]. The exact underlying mechanism of this remarkable modification in food preferences and palatability is poorly understood since self-reporting is the most common method used to record food preferences after bariatric surgery, which gives inconsistent and less than reliable findings [47–50]. Interestingly these changes do not appear to be strongly related to the type of bariatric procedure. In addition, modification in chewing time should be also considered as a contributing factor in reducing food intake. Although dependent on the dental state and the type of food ingested, bariatric patients tend to increase chewing, especially for solid foods [51].

Given the reduced gastric capacity resulting from bariatric procedures, meal sizes are proportionally reduced after bariatric procedures [52]. However, in addition to the restriction, postoperative food intake reduction is also known to be related to an expressive shift in the signaling of the hunger/satiety neuronal center due to increased levels of GI satiety hormones, such as pancreatic polypeptide (PP), peptide YY (PYY), glucagon-like peptide 1 (GLP-1) and 2 (GLP-2), gastrin, secretin, obestatin, vasoactive intestinal polypeptide (VIP), gustducin, oxyntomodulin (OXM) and glucose-dependent insulinotropic polypeptide (GIP) [53]. Although it is a common effect of almost all procedures, changes on hunger/satiety center mediated by digestive substances seem to be more profound after diversionary procedures.

4.6 Gastric Emptying: Digestive Motility

Upper GI motility may also play a role in the pathophysiology of obesity, since accelerated gastric emptying may decrease the satiety time and consequently promote greater food intake. Therefore, it is interesting to evaluate the behavior of gastric emptying and upper GI motility after bariatric procedures. Esophageal motor dysfunction and dilation by emptying scintigraphy, esophageal dysmotility by manometry, and signals of esophagitis by upper endoscopy are the most common methods employed to clinically evaluate gastric emptying. Although GI motility can also be investigated by methods such as the migrating motor complex and postprandial motor pattern, the relationship between abnormalities usually found and clinical symptoms remains uncertain [54, 55].

Gastric emptying seems to be normal or accelerated after LSG (and probably also after BPD-DS). Although this acceleration in emptying of gastric sleeve may compromise the perception of postprandial satiety to some extent, a rapid delivery of the ingested food may also promote greater release of satiety gut hormones, such as GLP-1, contributing to the efficacy of the procedure [56]. Notwithstanding, it remains controversial whether the amount of antrectomy and Sleeve calibration influence weight loss. Another source of concern regarding the emptying of gastric sleeve is the occurrence of the dumping syndrome. Although believed to be less prevalent, mainly due to preservation of the pyloric sphincter, symptoms perceived as dumping may occur after LSG, depending on the type of food ingested [57]. The pathophysiology of this late dumping is probably linked to increased release of several enteric hormones such as neurotensin, VIP, GIP, and GLP-1, inducing disordered GI motility and hypoglycemia.

As for RYGB (and probably also OAGB), the major concern about gastric pouch emptying is indisputably the dumping syndrome. The pathophysiology of the early dumping observed after RYGB appears to be related to the absence of pylorus as a valve regulating gastric pouch emptying rather than increased motility [58]. At the same time, the rapid delivery of food ingested in the small bowel (alimentary limb and common channel) can co-produce symptoms of late dumping [32]. In this sense, calibrated gastroenteroanastomosis can mimic the barrier normally caused by the pylorus, providing greater stasis of the food ingested within the gastric pouch, increasing the feeling of satiety, possibly decreasing the occurrence of early dumping, and ultimately contributing to the postoperative weight loss after RYGB [59].

In AGB, as expected, several esophageal abnormalities associated with impaired gastric emptying are observed, depending on the amount of insufflation/deflation of the device. This dysmotility may be related to the mechanical barrier caused by the narrow lumen that separates the upper and lower gastric chambers when the device is in place. In some situations, the severity of disorders and symptoms of the upper digestive system may need withdrawal of the band, and some sequelae can persist in the long term [54].

4.7 Digestion and Absorption

The major alterations in the digestive and absorptive processes are related to the gastric volume reduction and length of bypass. The digestion begins in the mouth during chewing by mixing the food with the saliva. The salivary flow behavior following bariatric surgery is somewhat controversial, but there is some evidence to suggest that it remains unchanged after RYGB [60]. Gastrin and cholecystokinin (CCK) are homologous hormone systems that act synergistically in gastric acid secretion and in gastric and gallbladder emptying. Gastrin is released by G-cells located primarily in the gastric antrum and duodenum to stimulate the secretion of gastric acid by the parietal cells of the stomach and enhance gastric motility. Gastrin may impact on insulin secretion via gastrin receptors in the islet of the pancreas [61]. As one would expect, serum levels of gastrin are generally suppressed after techniques that provide wide gastric and duodenal exclusion, such as RYGB. The impact of LSG with preserved antrum on gastrin secretion appears to be lower, or even absent [62]. In turn, CCK behaves controversially. It is synthesized and secreted by I-cells localized in the duodenal mucosa, helps in satiety, and inhibits gastric motility and emptying. After LSG, given the non-exclusion of the food bolus from the lumen of the duodenum, CCK levels appear to be normally increased [63]. Paradoxically, similar observations have been noted after RYGB. Other factors for CCK release like parasympathetic signaling may be implicated in the increased levels of CCK following bariatric procedures with duodenal exclusion, like RYGB, OAGB, and BPD-DS [53, 61]. Pancreatic juice containing several enzymes is released into the duodenum in response to chime along with bile and helps in the digestion of proteins, carbohydrates, and lipids. The major enzymes are lipase (lipid decompositions in fatty acids and glycerol), trypsin (break proteins in minor fragments), and pancreatic amylase (starch decomposition). The secretion of these enzymes and their actions are usually impaired in procedures with small bowel (duodenum) diversion, such as RYGB, OAGB, and BPD-DS, impairing the absorption of these macronutrients.

The overall absorptive capacity of the digestive system is mainly due to the integrity of the small bowel, including the duodenum. In procedures without small bowel diversion, such as AGB and LSG, the absorptive surface remains intact, and therefore, limited change in the absorption is expected postoperatively. Nutritional deficiencies observed after exclusive gastric procedures such as LSG can be due to reduced food intake (mechanical restriction and/or early satiety), food intolerance (vomiting), and/or changes in the regulation and release of digestive enzymes. Surgical procedures with intestinal diversion can additionally lead to impaired absorption of macro and micronutrients, depending on the extent of the intestinal bypass. The larger the bypassed area, the greater is the impairment in the absorptive process. In this regard, malabsorptive procedures, such as BPD-DS and distal RYGB (longer alimentary and/or biliopancreatic limbs and shorter common channels) are more commonly associated with postoperative nutritional disorders. Severe, and sometimes clinically uncontrollable, nutritional disorders represent the high biological cost associated with this group of procedures for a greater efficacy in weight loss and control of comorbidities [64–67]. According to the recent literature, OAGB has also been associated with a higher rate of hypoalbuminemia and anemia [36, 68, 69]. However, regardless of small bowel diversion, all types of bariatric procedures can virtually cause nutritional deficiencies, each due to specific reasons [70].

Although specific deficiencies are expected according to the gut segments bypassed, due to disruption of the digestive sequence, additional deficiencies of macro- and micronutrients can manifest.

Micronutrients are essential dietary factors that are needed in minimal amounts to support various biochemical pathways and metabolic processes in the human body and include trace elements (chromium, copper, manganese, selenium, and zinc), essential minerals (calcium, iodine, iron, and magnesium), fat-soluble vitamins (vitamins A, D, E, and K) and water-soluble vitamins such as thiamine (vitamin B1), riboflavin (vitamin B2), niacin (vitamin B3), pantothenic acid (vitamin B5), pyridoxine (vitamin B6), biotin (vitamin B7), folic acid (vitamin B9), cobalamin (vitamin B12), and ascorbic acid (vitamin C). In turn, macronutrients are nutrients that provide daily energy and make up the structure of the human body and are therefore required in large quantities. Major components are proteins, fats, carbohydrates, and also water. The most common micronutrients deficiencies with clinical significance after bariatric procedures, especially after small bowel diversion, are related to iron (iron-deficiency anemia), vitamin B12 (pernicious anemia), folates (macrocytic anemia), thiamine (neurological commitment), and calcium and vitamin D (osteoporosis/fractures). In turn, protein malnutrition is the most common macronutrient deficiency associated with patients undergoing bariatric surgery [28, 71–74].

4.8 Micronutrient Deficiencies

Bariatric techniques that include either gastric resection or gastric exclusion, such as LSG and RYGB, respectively, may lead to hypochlorhydria and reduction in the intrinsic factor. Reduction of gastric acid decreases the bioavailability of vitamin B12 from food, while the quantitative reduction of gastric intrinsic factor may significantly compromise the absorption of B12 in the distal ileum. The result of these two mechanisms can be a low rate of serum vitamin B12. In addition, impairment in the pancreatic proteases action caused by duodenal exclusion may contribute to poor vitamin B12 absorption. Other secondary causes of B12 deficiency may include food intolerance (and therefore even more drastic reduction of food intake) and small intestinal bacterial overgrowth. Fortunately, body storage of vitamin B12 is substantial and clinical deficiencies usually only emerge in the late postoperative period (after 1 year) [28, 71, 72, 75].

A low-iron diet and chronic disease features associated with obesity predispose for iron deficiency and anemia in morbidly obese patients in the preoperative period. Post bariatric surgery, this situation may be worsened by hypochlorhydria, reduction in iron intake, and duodenojejunal bypass. The hypochlorhydria resulting from almost all bariatric procedures hinders the reduction of ferric iron into the absorbable ferrous form, reducing iron uptake. In addition, food intolerances, especially for red meat, maybe a relevant factor for low oral iron intakc. Finally, poor adherence to dietary guidelines and recommended supplementation may also reduce the luminal amount of iron available to be absorbed. Thus, even in procedures without small bowel diversion, such as LSG, there may be deficiencies in serum iron availability, albeit to a lesser extent [76]. However, techniques that bypass the primary site of iron absorption (duodenum), such as RYGB, OAGB, and BPD-DS, significantly increase the incidence of clinical or laboratory deficiency of iron, especially in menstruating women [77].

Folic acid is a micronutrient primarily absorbed in the duodenum and proximal jejunum. Although widely present in several types of foods, folate storage in the liver is generally not sufficient for more than 2–3 months of consumption. Folate deficiency has been associated with macrocytic anemia in patients following bariatric surgery, mainly after procedures with small bowel diversion (RYGB, OAGB, and BPD-DS). Poor intake can also be blamed as a source of deficiency after AGB and LSG. On the other hand, high serum levels of folic acid in the postoperative period may also occur and have been considered as a marker of small intestinal bacterial overgrowth following bariatric surgery [71, 74].

Thiamine deficiency is a worrisome nutritional complication after bariatric surgery, since this co-enzyme is essential for the metabolism of carbohydrates and amino acids, and in the reactions that produce energy (Krebs cycle). In addition, cerebral metabolism is highly dependent on thiamine. The major consequence of thiamine deficiency is beriberi, a clinical syndrome featured by psychiatric, neurologic, cardiac and/or gastrointestinal manifestations. The hallmark of neurological commitment associated with low levels of thiamine is the paresthesia of the hands or feet, motor impairment, or loss of balance soon after 1–3 months after bariatric surgery ("bariatric beriberi"). The presence of small intestinal bacterial overgrowth should always be considered when oral thiamine supplementation is not resolutive [78]. In addition, symptoms of Wernicke's encephalopathy or acute psychosis should be considered medical emergencies. Although thiamine can be absorbed throughout the small bowel (jejunum and ileum), an efficient absorptive process is also dependent on the duodenal mucosal enzymes [28, 71]. Thus, techniques with duodenal bypass may be more prone to the development of thiamine deficiency, such as RYGB [79]. However, reduced food intake, supplementation non-adherence, and especially recurrent vomiting also appear to be important factors, since thiamine deficiency has been reported after LSG as well [80].

Vitamin D is a prohormone steroid that has two main sources: skin (in response to ultraviolet radiation) and dietary. Intestinal absorption occurs primarily in the small bowel with an efficiency of approximately 50% in the normal digestive system and is facilitated by bile salts. After its synthesis or absorption, vitamin D is metabolically activated in the liver to form 25-hydroxyvitamin D (25OHD), and then into the kidney to generate the active circulating metabolite, 1,25-dihydroxy vitamin D (1,25(OH)2D), or calcitriol. Vitamin D is an essential modulator of calcium metabolism, maintaining adequate calcium and phosphate levels required for bone formation by promoting absorption in the intestines [81]. Based on this, low sunlight exposure, reduced food intake, and decrease in the gut absorptive surface are considered pivotal causes of post-bariatric vitamin D deficiency. The major impact of vitamin D deficiency is the decrease in calcium absorption, secondary hyperparathyroidism, hypophosphatemia, and increased bone turnover. Altogether, these alterations usually result in lower bone mineral density and can lead to the development of skeletal disorders, notably osteopenia, osteomalacia, and osteoporosis. Therefore, bariatric patients undergoing techniques that combine restriction in food intake with a significant decrease in the small bowel absorptive area (distal RYGB, OAGB, and BPD-DS) are more likely to exhibit impairment in the metabolic availability of vitamin D and, hence, the development of clinical features. In turn, calcium plays a crucial role in numerous biological processes, ranging from muscle contraction and blood clotting. Adequate intestinal absorption is essential for calcium acquisition and bone is the major calcium reservoir. Resorption is a physiological pathway in maintaining calcium homeostasis, closely regulated by the parathyroid hormone. When calcium absorption is declined and serum levels drop (due to low intestinal absorption related to hypochlorhydria, poor consumption of calcium-containing foods, and/or vitamin D deficiency), excessive resorption is triggered, generally at the expense of decreasing bone density mineralization and acceleration of bone remodeling, probably increasing the risk of osteoporosis and bone fractures mainly in unsupplemented situations [28, 71, 72, 74, 82, 83]. After LSG, where anatomical small bowel absorption area is not compromised, preoperative suboptimal levels (both calcium and vitamin D) plus postoperative restricted dietary intake may probably be the reasons for clinical deficiencies.

4.9 Macronutrient Deficiencies

Protein malnutrition is the principal macronutrient deficiency after bariatric surgery and is a major source of concern in the postoperative period since, unlike carbohydrates and fat, protein is not stored in the human body. Protein deficiencies may have a very broad clinical presentation ranging from mild laboratory hypoalbuminemia to generalized edema and death. Thus, protein malnutrition following bariatric surgery should be inspected periodically by serum albumin levels, which can accuse difficulties in protein uptake long before the arising of more serious clinical features. The incidence of postoperative hypoproteinemia depends on the type of bariatric surgery, being relatively smaller after restrictive procedures without intestinal bypass (AGB and LSG) and greater after procedures with a malabsorptive component. Notoriously, the greater the small bowel bypass the greater the risk of protein malnutrition [72, 84–86]. Pathogenesis is most commonly related to malabsorption due to bypassing segments of the small bowel where the protein is absorbed primarily (duodenum and proximal jejunum). To a lesser extent, limitation in food intake, substantial decrease in pepsinogen levels, and reduction of pancreatic secretion of proteolytic enzymes may also be unfavorable factors for digestion and protein absorption [18]. Dietetic counseling with increased protein intake in the daily diet and oral supplementation are the most effective management to prevent post-bariatric hypoproteinemia. If this fails consistently, reversion of the malabsorptive component of the surgery may be lifesaving in selected cases.

Fat uptake mainly depends on biliary and lipolytic enzymes released by the gallbladder and pancreas, which are primarily regulated by CCK. In bariatric procedures with small bowel diversion (RYGB, OAGB, and BPD-DS), dietary fats (triglycerides, phospholipids, cholesterol) remain almost intact until reaching the common channel (or distal segments of efferent limb, in case of OAGB). Later lipids breakdown with delayed formation of micelles strongly limiting the amount of fat available for absorption in the small bowel. Hence, undigested fat goes to the large intestine and produces fat malabsorption and steatorrhea. Although uncommon, this pathophysiology can be present even after procedures that comprise a weaker malabsorptive component, such as RYGB [87].

Although bariatric procedures can alter carbohydrate digestion and absorption, mainly due to the limited action of the pancreatic amylase to convert polysaccharides into oligosaccharides present in small bowel diversion techniques, deficiencies are virtually nonexistent, as this essential macronutrient is absorbed in the entire gut. Absorbed carbohydrates are stored in the liver and skeletal muscle as quickly available glycogen to serve as a major source of energy for body metabolism and, most importantly, for the brain and red blood cells. In addition, in the face of inadequate carbohydrate substrate (low food intake and/or some degree of malabsorption), fat and protein are broken down through gluconeogenesis to provide nutritional substrate for the brain and red blood cells. Thus, carbohydrate deficiency is always preceded by a marked loss of fat mass and severe protein deficiency [18].

Based on these expected adverse effects common to almost all types of bariatric procedures, periodic clinical and laboratory screening for nutritional deficiencies and, if needed, targeted and standardized supplementation both for macro and micronutrients, are recommended. A more intensive surveillance is recommended after malabsorptive procedures. In the long term, it is even admissible that small bowel adaptive mechanisms would attenuate mainly macronutrients deficiencies in post-bariatric patients.

4.10 Enterohormones

Undoubtedly, the growing understanding of the postoperative behavior of enterohormones may be considered as one of the major advances in bariatric surgery in recent years. These sets of knowledge gave rise to the principles of so-called metabolic surgery and anchored new pharmacological drugs for the clinical treatment of obesity and T2DM. Liraglutide, a glucagon-like peptide 1 agonist (GLP-1), is a prime example.

Fasting and postprandial levels of several enterohormones are significantly altered after bariatric surgery, with a well-documented impact on the hunger/satiety regulation and metabolic control in bariatric patients. Although all obesity-associated metabolic diseases may be positively affected, the incretin-mediated T2DM outcomes have been the most addressed to date.

The incretin effect is a very old concept in which the oral glucose administration promotes greater insulin secretion compared to a similar parenteral infusion [88, 89]. The insulinotropic gut-derived factors that could be responsible for this enhancement in insulin secretion after oral/enteral glucose intake were then denominated as incretins. Thus, the incretin effect is an amplification of insulin secretion driven by incretins and is recognized as the major mechanism for normal glucose tolerance. As expected, this effect is greatly reduced or totally missing in obese diabetic patients and the restoration of this physiological effect is one of the goals sought by bariatric procedures. To date, only glucose-dependent insulinotropic polypeptide (GIP) and GLP-1 fulfill the definition of an incretin hormone in humans. GIP and GLP-1 are produced by specialized enteroendocrine K- and L-cells, respectively. K- and L-cells are sensitive to mainly macronutrients (carbohydrates, fats, and proteins). By responding more to the nutrient uptake than to the presence in the gut lumen, increased enterohormones levels may accurately indicate the arrival of such nutrients into the bloodstream [90].

GIP was the first incretin identified and was initially nominated as a gastric inhibitory polypeptide, given its ability to delay gastric emptying (satiety hormone). Later, GIP was renamed to glucose-dependent insulinotropic polypeptide after recognition of its action as an enhancer of insulin secretion by the pancreas. GIP is secreted mainly by enteroendocrine K-cells, found at higher density in the duodenum. It was recognized that GIP alone could not fully explain the incretin effect commonly observed after bariatric surgery, since impairment of endogenous GIP activity attenuates but does not abolish the incretin effect. Given its controversial profile after bariatric procedures, with scarce data after procedures like LSG, the relevance of GIP in mediating weight loss and incretin effect remains to be better determined and therefore has currently been undervalued [53, 91, 92].

GLP-1 is undoubtedly the most powerful incretin associated with bariatric surgery [93]. This gut hormone is primarily secreted by enteroendocrine L-cells, which increase in number toward the distal small bowel, being also numerous in the large intestine [91, 92]. GLP-1 is a satiety hormone that delays gastric emptying, increases insulin release, and decreases glucagon production. Although fasting GLP-1 levels do not markedly change after bariatric surgery, postprandial levels of GLP-1 increase significantly after most bariatric procedures [93]. RYGB (and other procedures with small bowel bypass and hence, functional gut shortening such as OAGB and BPD-DS) have exhibited high postprandial levels of GLP-1, coinciding with high rates of glycemic control in diabetic patients. Indeed, bariatric surgery provides an expressive increase in GLP-1 release, normalizing the attenuated incretin effect generally presented in diabetic patients. The higher and earlier the stimulation of ileal L-cells by luminal content (secretions, bile salts, and foods), the greater the release of GLP-1. Thus, dramatically elevated postprandial levels of GLP-1 were measured after RYGB (10–20 times higher than normally observed in healthy people with original digestive tube) [11, 58], a phenomenon also observed after BPD-DS [94] but not after LAGB [95]. These high levels substantially contribute to both weight loss (suppression of appetite) and glucose homeostasis (incretin effect) [11]. After LSG, GLP-1 also rises, but at slightly lower levels [45, 58, 96]. Faster gastric emptying and lower small bowel transit time have been indicated as the key mechanism for sustained post-Sleeve stimulation of ileal L-cells, rising the GLP-1 levels and subsequently activating the ileal brake [56, 97, 98].

In addition to the well-documented effects of incretins (GIP and GLP-1), a plethora of enterohormones have also their fasting and postprandial profile significantly changed after bariatric surgery. Glucagon-like peptide 2 (GLP-2) is produced by enteroendocrine cells and also by neurons in the central nervous system. Intestinal GLP-2 is derived from proglucagon and co-secreted by L-cells along with GLP-1 upon nutrient uptake [11]. The main recognized action of GLP-2 in the digestive system is to promote intestinal villi hypertrophy and to downregulate apoptosis. In general, the post-bariatric GLP-2 profile has sparked little interest to date and therefore has been rarely addressed. After RYGB, high postprandial levels of GLP-2 have already been observed and interestingly correlated with aspects of satiety regulation [53, 99]. Oxyntomodulin (OXM) is an anorexigenic peptide also derived from proglucagon and co-secreted with GLP-1 by enteroendocrine L-cells. OXM appears to reduce hunger, food intake, and ghrelin levels, as well as decrease gastric acid secretion and GI motility (satiety hormone). Although high levels of OXM have been observed shortly after RYGB [100] no OXM-specific receptor has yet been well identified, and its relevance in bariatric outcomes remains to be better determined [19, 53]. Peptide YY (PYY) is also released by enteroendocrine L-cells in the distal small bowel and colon in response to feeding. In the bloodstream, PYY is converted to PYY(3-36), its active form. PYY(3-36) appears to be a satiety hormone, since circulating levels usually increase in the postprandial period, leading to a delayed gastric emptying, reduced insulin production, and altered GI motility. However, the major target of PYY(3-36) is the central regulation of appetite, reducing food intake. Serum levels of PYY(3–36) appear to be enhanced postprandially following bariatric surgery, regardless of procedure (RYGB, LSG, and BPD-DS). However, a better understanding of the PYY(3-36) physiology is still needed to establish the real impact of this enterohormone on weight loss and metabolic control after bariatric surgery [19, 53, 94, 101, 102].

In summary, the release of enterohormones and the interaction between them is profoundly altered after bariatric surgery, assuming a pivotal place in weight loss and improvement/remission of obesity-related comorbidities, and even surpassing in relevance the role of classic restrictive and malabsorptive mechanisms.

4.11 Gut Microbiota

As gut microbiota disarray has often been associated with obesity and its metabolic comorbidities [103, 104], there also has been a rising interest in gut microbiota behavior following bariatric surgery since some studies have suggested that gut microbial communities play a key role in mediating beneficial effects attributed to bariatric procedures, whether in relation to weight loss or to metabolic control [105–107]. The list of the gut microbiota modifications after bariatric surgery is already very long, but it is still far from complete or fully understood, since few studies have specifically addressed this relevant topic in humans at present. The increased relative abundance of the phylum Proteobacteria (class Gammaproteobacteria; genera Escherichia, Klebsiella, and Enterobacter), as well as an increase in members of the phylum Bacteroidetes and a general decrease in members of the phylum Firmicutes, are the major changes commonly observed [105, 108], regardless of the procedure.

The relevance in assessing the species Escherichia coli in studies involving gut microbial changes after bariatric surgery comes from the fact that it constitutes part of the "core microbiome," that is, bacterial species that can be found in most gut microbiota profiles of healthy individuals. Also, Escherichia coli is recognized by its high translocation ability which may impact chronic systemic inflammatory response. In turn, the assessment of the Bacteroidetes/Firmicutes ratio takes a leading role in the studies of gut microbiota after bariatric surgeries because these phyla correspond to about 90% of the gut microbial community [104, 109–111]. Although the profile of higher levels of several species in the Gammaproteobacteria class and lower levels in species belonging to Firmicutes phylum seem to be sustainable in the long term [112], the investigations that address the stability of microbial profile after bariatric surgery are still sturdy.

Interestingly, some studies involving morbidly obese individuals submitted to bariatric surgery have shown changes in gut microbiota profile soon after 3 months of surgery, therefore, long before the final weight loss [113, 114]. This finding is in agreement with prompt metabolic improvement usually observed after bariatric surgery, since gut microbial balance has been recognized as a hallmark of the host's health status [115–117]. In general, technical designs of bariatric surgeries appear to be a favoring factor to commonly observed changes in the gut microbial communities. These functional changes may be influenced by drastic changes in food intake, either in quantity or in quality/preferences [118, 119]. Thus, the intestinal microbiota would be forced to conform to this new pattern of food consumption. In addition, changes in luminal pH, nutrient supply, motility, and increased oxygen concentration in the small bowel can be implicated in the arising of a new microbiota profile, which would ultimately represent no more than an adaptation to the new anatomic and physiological configuration of GI tract.

Not surprisingly, most studies on changes in gut microbiota following bariatric surgery involve RYGB, the most traditional bariatric procedure worldwide and also the most commonly performed until very recently. This procedure may increase the richness of gut microbiota, especially the bacteria belonging to Proteobacteria [113]. Although the exact mechanism is still unclear, factors such as the luminal pH and modifications in the nutrient supply can be pivotal. On the other hand, few studies have addressed the postoperative gut microbial behavior after LSG to date. Notwithstanding, some data available have shown that LSG also affects both the microbiota profile and gut permeability [106, 120, 121]. The exact underlying mechanism also remains poorly understood, but, as expected, the LSG appears to provide a different and less pronounced impact on microbiota balance than procedures with small bowel diversion, such as RYGB and duodenojejunal bypass [106, 121, 122]. Even so, the alterations in gut microbiota after LSG appear to go beyond dietary restriction and consequent fat mass loss [123, 124]. Food preferences, decrease in energy intake, and alterations in GI motility may be underlying factors.

4.12 Conclusion

The anatomy and physiology of the digestive system are markedly altered after bariatric surgery. Most of these changes are expected and are the therapeutic target of surgical interventions, having a positive impact on obesity and related comorbidities. The same anatomical and physiological changes may also be the source of severe adverse effects following bariatric surgery. Therefore, all professionals involved in the surgical treatment of morbid obesity should be thoroughly familiar with the anatomical and physiological changes caused by a variety of procedures, to help them recognize the therapeutic targets as well as deal with the possible adverse outcomes.

Key Points

- *Bariatric surgery brings about changes in the GI system by means of Bile flow alteration, Reduction of gastric size, Anatomical gut rearrangement and Altered flow of nutrients, Vagal manipulation, and Enteric and adipose hormones modulation.*
- *Changes in appetite, food preferences, taste perception and chewing time may diminish food intake postoperatively, impacting weight loss. An increased preference for low-sugar and low-fat diet have been frequently observed after bariatric procedures.*
- *Gastric emptying time is reduced after sleeve gastrectomy and BPD-DS.*
- *Late dumping, commonly seen after the diversionary procedures, is also reported after Sleeve gastrectomy, probably secondary to accelerated gastric emptying. It is related to the increased release of several enterohormones such as neurotensin, VIP, GIP, and GLP-1, inducing disordered GI motility and hypoglycemia.*
- *A decrease in absorption is due to hypochlorhydria, decreased Intrinsic Factor, reduction in absorptive surface due to division, billow alteration, and reduced intestinal transit time.*
- *Increased delivery of nutrients to the distal intestine leads to increased levels of enterohormones like GLP1, GIP, PYY, and oxyntomodulin leading to an incretin effect.*
- *An increase in members of the phylum Bacteroidetes and a general decrease in members of the phylum Firmicutes are the commonly observed major changes in the gut microbiome. The changes precede the weight loss and are seen as soon as 3 months after the surgery. These changes have been observed in some studies after LSG as well.*

References

1. NCD Risk Factor Collaboration. Trends in adult body-mass index in 200 countries from 1975 to 2014: a pooled analysis of 1698 population-based measurement studies with 19.2 million participants. Lancet. 2016;387(10026):1377–96.
2. Ng M, Fleming T, Robinson M, Thomson B, Graetz N, Margono C, et al. Global, regional, and national prevalence of overweight and obesity in children and adults during 1980-2013: A systematic analysis for the Global Burden of Disease Study 2013. Lancet. 2014;384(9945):766–81.
3. Courcoulas AP, Yanovski SZ, Bonds D, Eggerman TL, Horlick M, Staten MA, et al. Long-term outcomes of bariatric surgery: a National Institutes of Health symposium. JAMA Surg. 2014;149(12):1323–9.

4. Fisher DP, Johnson E, Haneuse S, Arterburn D, Coleman KJ, O'Connor PJ, et al. Association between bariatric surgery and macrovascular disease outcomes in patients with type-2 diabetes and severe obesity. JAMA. 2018;320(15):1570–82.
5. Maciejewski ML, Arterburn DE, Van Scoyoc L, Smith VA, Yancy WS Jr, Weidenbacher HJ, et al. Bariatric surgery and long-term durability of weight loss. JAMA Surg. 2016;151(11):1046–55.
6. Schauer PR, Bhatt DL, Kirwan JP, Wolski K, Aminian A, Brethauer SA, et al. Bariatric surgery versus intensive medical therapy for diabetes - 5-year outcomes. N Engl J Med. 2017;376(7):641–51.
7. Sjöström L, Peltonen M, Jacobson P, Sjöström CD, Karason K, Wedel H, et al. Bariatric surgery and long-term cardiovascular events. JAMA. 2012;307(1):56–65.
8. Phillips BT, Shikora SA. The history of metabolic and bariatric surgery: development of standards for patient safety and efficacy. Metabolism. 2018;79:97–107.
9. Abdeen G, le Roux CW. Mechanism underlying the weight loss and complications of Roux-en-Y gastric bypass. Obes Surg. 2016;26(2):410–21.
10. Chakravartty S, Tassinari D, Salerno A, Giorgakis E, Rubino F. What is the mechanism behind weight loss maintenance with gastric bypass? Curr Obes Rep. 2015;4(2):262–8.
11. Holst JJ, Madsbad S, Bojsen-Møller KN, Svane MS, Jørgensen NB, Dirksen C, et al. Mechanisms in bariatric surgery: gut hormones, diabetes resolution, and weight loss. Surg Obes Relat Dis. 2018;14(5):708–14.
12. Kim KS, Sandoval DA. Endocrine function after bariatric surgery. Compr Physiol. 2017;7(3):783–98.
13. Miras AD, le Roux CW. Mechanisms underlying weight loss after bariatric surgery. Nat Rev Gastroenterol Hepatol. 2013;10(10):575–84.
14. Mulla CM, Middelbeek RJW, Patti ME. Mechanisms of weight loss and improved metabolism following bariatric surgery. Ann N Y Acad Sci. 2018;1411(1):53–64.
15. Pucci A, Batterham RL. Mechanisms underlying the weight loss effects of RYGB and SG: similar, yet different. J Endocrinol Invest. 2019;42(2):117–28.
16. Schlottmann F, Galvarini MM, Dreifuss NH, Laxague F, Buxhoeveden R, Gorodner V. Metabolic effects of bariatric surgery. J Laparoendosc Adv Surg Tech A. 2018;28(8):944–8.
17. Herron DM, Roohipour R. Bariatric surgical anatomy and mechanisms of action. Gastrointest Endosc Clin N Am. 2011;21(2):213–28.
18. Ponsky TA, Brody F, Pucci E. Alterations in gastrointestinal physiology after Roux-en-Y gastric bypass. J Am Coll Surg. 2005;201(1):125–31.
19. Quercia I, Dutia R, Kotler DP, Belsley S, Laferrère B. Gastrointestinal changes after bariatric surgery. Diabetes Metab. 2014;40(2):87–94.
20. Wabitsch M. Gastrointestinal endocrinology in bariatric surgery. Endocr Dev. 2017;32:124–38.
21. Boerlage TC, van de Laar AW, Westerlaken S, Gerdes VE, Brandjes DP. Gastrointestinal symptoms and food intolerance 2 years after laparoscopic Roux-en-Y gastric bypass for morbid obesity. Br J Surg. 2017;104(4):393–400.
22. Borbély YM, Osterwalder A, Kröll D, Nett PC, Inglin RA. Diarrhea after bariatric procedures: diagnosis and therapy. World J Gastroenterol. 2017;23(26):4689–700.
23. Borbély Y, Schaffner E, Zimmermann L, Huguenin M, Plitzko G, Nett P, et al. De novo gastroesophageal reflux disease after sleeve gastrectomy: role of preoperative silent reflux. Surg Endosc. 2019;33(3):789–93.
24. Bordalo LA, Mourão DM, Bressan J. Nutritional deficiencies after bariatric surgery: why they happen? Acta Med Port. 2011;4 (Suppl):1021–8.
25. Høgestøl IK, Chahal-Kummen M, Eribe I, Brunborg C, Stubhaug A, Hewitt S, et al. Chronic abdominal pain and symptoms 5-years after gastric bypass for morbid obesity. Obes Surg. 2017;27(6):1438–45.
26. Liakopoulos V, Franzén S, Svensson AM, Miftaraj M, Ottosson J, Näslund I, et al. Pros and cons of gastric bypass surgery in individuals with obesity and type 2 diabetes: nationwide, matched, observational cohort study. BMJ Open. 2019;9(1):e023882.

27. Mason ME, Jalagani H, Vinik AI. Metabolic complications of bariatric surgery: diagnosis and management issues. Gastroenterol Clin North Am. 2005;34(1):25–33.
28. Patel JJ, Mundi MS, Hurt RT, Wolfe B, Martindale RG. Micronutrient deficiencies after bariatric surgery: an emphasis on vitamins and trace minerals. Nutr Clin Pract. 2017;32(4):471–80.
29. Potoczna N, Harfmann S, Steffen R, Briggs R, Bieri N, Horber FF. Bowel habits after bariatric surgery. Obes Surg. 2008;18(10):1287–96.
30. Sabate JM, Coupaye M, Ledoux S, Castel B, Msika S, Coffin B, et al. Consequences of small intestinal bacterial overgrowth in obese patients before and after bariatric surgery. Obes Surg. 2017;27(3):599–605.
31. Souche R, de Jong A, Nomine-Criqui C, Nedelcu M, Brunaud L, Nocca D. Complications after bariatric surgery. Press Med. 2018;47(5):464–70.
32. van Beek AP, Emous M, Laville M, Tack J. Dumping syndrome after esophageal, gastric or bariatric surgery: pathophysiology, diagnosis, and management. Obes Rev. 2017;18(1):68–85.
33. Angrisani L, Santonicola A, Iovino P, Vitiello A, Higa K, Himpens J, et al. IFSO worldwide survey 2016: primary, endoluminal, and revisional procedures. Obes Surg. 2018;28(12):3783–94.
34. Bastos ELS. Why has laparoscopic sleeve gastrectomy become the most accomplished bariatric procedure? Interv Obes Diabetes. 2019;2(5). https://doi.org/10.31031/IOD.2019.02.000548.
35. Kruschitz R, Luger M, Kienbacher C, Trauner M, Klammer C, Schindler K, et al. The effect of Roux-en-Y vs. omega-loop gastric bypass on liver, metabolic parameters, and weight loss. Obes Surg. 2016;26(9):2204–12.
36. Robert M, Espalieu P, Pelascini E, Caiazzo R, Sterkers A, Khamphommala L, et al. Efficacy and safety of one anastomosis gastric bypass versus Roux-en-Y gastric bypass for obesity (YOMEGA): a multicentre, randomized, open-label, non-inferiority trial. Lancet. 2019;393(10178):1299–309.
37. Gebelli JP, Gordejuela AG, Ramos AC, Nora M, Pereira AM, Campos JM, et al. SADI-S with right gastric artery ligation: technical systematization and early results. Arq Bras Cir Dig. 2016;29(Suppl 1):85–90.
38. Topart P, Becouarn G. The single anastomosis duodenal switch modifications: a review of the current literature on outcomes. Surg Obes Relat Dis. 2017;13(8):1306–12.
39. Ellacott KL, Halatchev IG, Cone RD. Interactions between gut peptides ant the central melanocortin system in the regulation of energy homeostasis. Peptides. 2006;27:340–9.
40. Stefanidis A, Forrest N, Brown WA, Dixon JB, O'Brien PB, Kampe J, et al. An investigation of the neural mechanisms underlying the efficacy of the adjustable gastric band. Surg Obes Relat Dis. 2016;12(4):828–38.
41. Tewari N, Awad S, Lobo DN. Regulation of food intake after surgery and the gut brain axis. Curr Opin Clin Nutr Metab Care. 2013;16(5):569–75.
42. Power ML, Schulkin J. Anticipatory physiological regulation in feeding biology: cephalic phase responses. Appetite. 2008;50:194–206.
43. Kalinowski P, Paluszkiewicz R, Wróblewski T, Remiszewski P, Grodzicki M, Bartoszewicz Z, et al. Ghrelin, leptin, and glycemic control after sleeve gastrectomy versus Roux-en-Y gastric bypass: results of a randomized clinical trial. Surg Obes Relat Dis. 2017;13(2):1818.
44. Karamanakos SN, Vagenas K, Kalfarentzos F, Alexandrides TK. Weight loss, appetite suppression and changes in fasting and postprandial ghrelin and peptide-YY levels after Roux-en-Y gastric bypass and sleeve gastrectomy. A prospective, double blind study. Ann Surg. 2008;247:401–7.
45. Yousseif A, Emmanuel J, Karra E, Millet Q, Elkalaawy M, Jenkinson AD, et al. Differential effects of laparoscopic sleeve gastrectomy and laparoscopic gastric bypass on appetite, circulating acyl-ghrelin, peptide YY3-36 and active GLP-1 levels in non-diabetic humans. Obes Surg. 2014;24:241–52.
46. Miras AD, le Roux CW. Bariatric surgery and taste: novel mechanisms of weight loss. Curr Opin Gastroenterol. 2010;26(2):140–5.
47. Gero D, Steinert RE, le Roux CW, Bueter M. Do food preferences change after bariatric surgery? Curr Atheroscler Rep. 2017;19(9):38.

48. Kapoor N, Al-Najim W, le Roux CW, Docherty NG, Kapoor N. Shifts in food preferences after bariatric surgery: observational reports and proposed mechanisms. Curr Obes Rep. 2017;6(3):246–52.
49. Shoar S, Naderan M, Shoar N, Modukuru VR, Mahmoodzadeh H. Alteration pattern of taste perception after bariatric surgery: a systematic review of four taste domains. Obes Surg. 2019;29(5):1542–50.
50. Tichansky DS, Boughter JD Jr, Madan AK. Taste change after laparoscopic Roux-en-Y gastric bypass and laparoscopic adjustable gastric banding. Surg Obes Relat Dis. 2006;2:440–4.
51. Godlewski AE, Veyrune JL, Nicolas E, Ciangura CA, Chaussain CC, Czernichow S, et al. Effect of dental status on changes in mastication in patients with obesity following bariatric surgery. PLoS One. 2011;6:e22324.
52. Laurenius A, Larsson I, Bueter M, Melanson KJ, Bosaeus I, Forslund HB, et al. Changes in eating behavior and meal pattern following Roux-en-Y gastric bypass. Int J Obes. 2012;36:348–55.
53. Dimitriadis GK, Randeva MS, Miras AD. Potential hormone mechanisms of bariatric surgery. Curr Obes Rep. 2017;6(3):253–65.
54. Ardila-Hani A, Soffer EE. Review article: the impact of bariatric surgery on gastrointestinal motility. Aliment Pharmacol Ther. 2011;34(8):825–31.
55. Deloose E, Janssen P, Lannoo M, Van der Schueren B, Depoortere I, Tack J. Higher plasma motilin levels in obese patients decrease after Roux-en-Y gastric bypass surgery and regulate hunger. Gut. 2016;65(7):1110–8.
56. Sista F, Abruzzese V, Clementi M, Carandina S, Cecilia M, Amicucci G. The effect of sleeve gastrectomy on GLP-1 secretion and gastric emptying: a prospective study. Surg Obes Relat Dis. 2017;13(1):7–14.
57. Ahmad A, Kornrich DB, Krasner H, Eckardt S, Ahmad Z, Braslow A, et al. Prevalence of dumping syndrome after laparoscopic sleeve gastrectomy and comparison with laparoscopic Roux-en-Y gastric bypass. Obes Surg. 2019;29(5):1506–13.
58. Svane MS, Bojsen-Møller KN, Martinussen C, Dirksen C, Madsen JL, Reitelseder S, et al. Postprandial nutrient handling and gastrointestinal hormone secretion after Roux-en-Y gastric bypass vs sleeve gastrectomy. Gastroenterology. 2019;156(6):1627–41.
59. Ramos AC, Marchesini JC, Bastos ELS, Ramos MG, de Souza MD, Campos JM, et al. The role of gastrojejunostomy size on gastric bypass weight loss. Obes Surg. 2017;27(9):2317–23.
60. Farias TMCP, Vasconcelos BCDE, Souto-Maior JR, Lemos CAA, de Moraes SLD, Pellizzer EP. Influence of bariatric surgery on salivary flow: a systematic review and meta-analysis. Obes Surg. 2019;29(5):1675–80.
61. Rehfeld JF. Incretin physiology beyond glucagon-like peptide 1 and glucose-dependent insulinotropic polypeptide: cholecystokinin and gastrin peptides. Acta Physiol. 2011;201:405–11.
62. Grong E, Græslie H, Munkvold B, Arbo IB, Kulseng BE, Waldum HL, et al. Gastrin secretion after bariatric surgery response to a protein-rich mixed meal following Roux-en-Y gastric bypass and sleeve gastrectomy: a pilot study in normoglycemic women. Obes Surg. 2016;26(7):1448–56.
63. Peterli R, Steinert RE, Woelnerhanssen B, Peters T, Christoffel-Courtin C, Gass M, et al. Metabolic and hormonal changes after laparoscopic Roux-en-Y gastric bypass and sleeve gastrectomy: a randomized, prospective trial. Obes Surg. 2012;22:740–8.
64. Billeter AT, Fischer L, Wekerle AL, Senft J, Müller-Stich B. Malabsorption as a therapeutic approach in bariatric surgery. Viszeralmedizin. 2014;30(3):198–204.
65. Müller MK, Räder S, Wildi S, Hauser R, Clavien PA, Weber M. Long-term follow-up of proximal versus distal laparoscopic gastric bypass for morbid obesity. Br J Surg. 2008;95(11):1375–9.
66. Ruiz-Tovar J, Vorwald P, Gonzalez-Ramirez G, Posada M, Salcedo G, Llavero C, et al. Impact of biliopancreatic limb length (70 cm vs 120 cm), with constant 150 cm alimentary limb, on long-term weight loss, remission of comorbidities and supplementation needs after Roux-En-Y gastric bypass: a prospective randomized clinical trial. Obes Surg. 2019;29(8):2367–72 [Epub ahead of print].

67. Via MA, Mechanick JI. Nutritional and micronutrient care of bariatric surgery patients: current evidence update. Curr Obes Rep. 2017;6(3):286–96.
68. Georgiadou D, Sergentanis TN, Nixon A, Diamantis T, Tsigris C, Psaltopoulou T. Efficacy and safety of laparoscopic mini gastric bypass. A systematic review. Surg Obes Relat Dis. 2014;10(5):984–91.
69. Magouliotis DE, Tasiopoulou VS, Tzovaras G. One anastomosis gastric bypass versus Roux-en-Y gastric bypass for morbid obesity: an updated meta-analysis. Obes Surg. 2019;29(9):2721–30 [Epub ahead of print].
70. Antoniewicz A, Kalinowski P, Kotulecka KJ, Kocoń P, Paluszkiewicz R, Remiszewski P, et al. Nutritional deficiencies in patients after Roux-en-Y gastric bypass and sleeve gastrectomy during 12-month follow-up. Obes Surg. 2019; https://doi.org/10.1007/s11695-019-03985-3. [Epub ahead of print]
71. Bal BS, Finelli FC, Shope TR, Koch TR. Nutritional deficiencies after bariatric surgery. Nat Rev Endocrinol. 2012;8(9):544–56.
72. Bloomberg RD, Fleishman A, Nalle JE, Herron DM, Kini S. Nutritional deficiencies following bariatric surgery: what have we learned? Obes Surg. 2005;15(2):145–54.
73. Toh SY, Zarshenas N, Jorgensen J. Prevalence of nutrient deficiencies in bariatric patients. Nutrition. 2009;25(11–12):1150–6.
74. Ziegler O, Sirveaux MA, Brunaud L, Reibel N, Quilliot D. Medical follow up after bariatric surgery: nutritional and drug issues. General recommendations for the prevention and treatment of nutritional deficiencies. Diabetes Metab. 2009;35(6):544–57.
75. Majumder S, Soriano J, Louie Cruz A, Dasanu CA. Vitamin B12 deficiency in patients undergoing bariatric surgery: preventive strategies and key recommendations. Surg Obes Relat Dis. 2013;9(6):1013–9.
76. Ruz M, Carrasco F, Rojas P, Codoceo J, Inostroza J, Basfi-Fer K, et al. Heme- and nonheme-iron absorption and iron status 12 mo after sleeve gastrectomy and Roux-en-Y gastric bypass in morbidly obese women. Am J Clin Nutr. 2012;96:810–7.
77. Steenackers N, Van der Schueren B, Mertens A, Lannoo M, Grauwet T, Augustijns P, et al. Iron deficiency after bariatric surgery: what is the real problem? Proc Nutr Soc. 2018;77(4):445–55.
78. Lakhani SV, Shah HN, Alexander K, Finelli FC, Kirkpatrick JR, Koch TR. Small intestinal bacterial overgrowth and thiamine deficiency after Roux- Y gastric bypass surgery in obese patients. Nutr Res. 2008;28:293–8.
79. Angstadt JD, Bodziner RA. Peripheral polyneuropathy from thiamine deficiency following laparoscopic Roux-en-Y gastric bypass. Obes Surg. 2005;15:890–2.
80. Saab R, El Khoury M, Farhat S. Wernicke's encephalopathy three weeks after sleeve gastrectomy. Surg Obes Relat Dis. 2014;10(5):992–4.
81. Bell TD, Demay MB, Burnett-Bowie SA. The biology and pathology of vitamin D control in bone. J. Cell Biochem. 2010;111:7–11.
82. Liu C, Wu D, Zhang JF, Xu D, Xu WF, Chen Y, et al. Changes in bone metabolism in morbidly obese patients after bariatric surgery: a meta-analysis. Obes Surg. 2016;26(1):91–7.
83. Schafer AL. Vitamin D and intestinal calcium transport after bariatric surgery. J Steroid Biochem Mol Biol. 2017;173:202–10.
84. Ballesteros-Pomar MD, González de Francisco T, Urioste-Fondo A, González-Herraez L, Calleja-Fernández A, Vidal-Casariego A, et al. Biliopancreatic diversion for severe obesity: long-term effectiveness and nutritional complications. Obes Surg. 2016;26(1):38–44.
85. Shoar S, Poliakin L, Rubenstein R, Saber AAA. single anastomosis duodeno-ileal switch (SADIS): a systematic review of efficacy and safety. Obes Surg. 2018;28(1):104–13.
86. Verger EO, Aron-Wisnewsky J, Dao MC, Kayser BD, Oppert JM, Bouillot JL, et al. Micronutrient and protein deficiencies after gastric bypass and sleeve gastrectomy: a 1-year follow-up. Obes Surg. 2016;26(4):785–96.
87. Mahawar KK, Sharples AJ. Contribution of malabsorption to weight loss after Roux-en-Y gastric bypass: a systematic review. Obes Surg. 2017;27(8):2194–206.

88. Elrick H, Stimmler L, Hlad CJ, Arai Y. Plasma insulin response to oral and intravenous glucose administration. J Clin Endocrinol Metab. 1964;24(10):1076–82.
89. Perley MJ, Kipnis DM. Plasma insulin responses to oral and intravenous glucose: studies in normal and diabetic subjects. J Clin Invest. 1967;46(12):1954–62.
90. Holst JJ, Gribble F, Horowitz M, Rayner CK. Roles of the gut in glucose homeostasis. Diabetes Care. 2016;39:884–92.
91. Cavin JB, Bado A, Le Gall M. Intestinal adaptations after bariatric surgery: consequences on glucose homeostasis. Trends Endocrinol Metab. 2017;28(5):354–64.
92. Reimann F, Gribble FM. Mechanisms underlying glucose-dependent insulinotropic polypeptide and glucagon-like peptide-1 secretion. J Diabetes Investig. 2016;7(Suppl 1):13–9.
93. Holst JJ, Madsbad S. Mechanisms of surgical control of type 2 diabetes: GLP-1 is key factor. Surg Obes Relat Dis. 2016;12(6):1236–42.
94. Tsoli M, Chronaiou A, Kehagias I, Kalfarentzos F, Alexandrides TK. Hormone changes and diabetes resolution after biliopancreatic diversion and laparoscopic sleeve gastrectomy: a comparative prospective study. Surg Obes Relat Dis. 2013;9(5):667–77.
95. Korner J, Bessler M, Inabnet W, Taveras C, Holst JJ. Exaggerated glucagon-like peptide-1 and blunted glucose-dependent insulinotropic peptide secretion are associated with Roux-en-Y gastric bypass but not adjustable gastric banding. Surg Obes Relat Dis. 2007;3(6):597–601.
96. Nosso G, Griffo E, Cotugno M, Saldalamacchia G, Lupoli R, Pacini G, et al. Comparative effects of Roux-en-Y gastric bypass and sleeve gastrectomy on glucose homeostasis and incretin hormones in obese type 2 diabetic patients: a one-year prospective study. Horm Metab Res. 2016;48(5):312–7.
97. Maljaars PW, Peters HP, Mela DJ, Masclee AA. Ileal brake: a sensible food target for appetite control. A review. Physiol Behav. 2008;95:271–81.
98. Shah S, Shah P, Todkar J, Gagner M, Sonar S, Solav S. Prospective controlled study of effect of laparoscopic sleeve gastrectomy on small bowel transit time and gastric emptying half-time in morbidly obese patients with type 2 diabetes mellitus. Surg Obes Relat Dis. 2010;6(2):152–7.
99. Cazzo E, Pareja JC, Chaim EA, Geloneze B, Barreto MR, Magro DO. GLP-1 and GLP-2 levels are correlated with satiety regulation after Roux-en-Y gastric bypass: results of an exploratory prospective study. Obes Surg. 2017;27(3):703–8.
100. Laferrère B, Swerdlow N, Bawa B, Arias S, Bose M, Olivan B, et al. Rise of oxyntomodulin in response to oral glucose after gastric bypass surgery in patients with type 2 diabetes. J Clin Endocrinol Metab. 2010;95:4072–6.
101. Chandarana K, Gelegen C, Karra E, Choudhury AI, Drew ME, Fauveau V, et al. Diet and gastrointestinal bypass-induced weight loss: the roles of ghrelin and peptide YY. Diabetes. 2011;60(3):810–8.
102. Olivan B, Teixeira J, Bose M, Bawa B, Chang T, Summe H, et al. Effect of weight loss by diet or gastric bypass surgery on peptide YY3-36 levels. Ann Surg. 2009;249:948–53.
103. Karlsson F, Tremaroli V, Nielsen J, Bäckhed F. Assessing the human gut microbiota in metabolic diseases. Diabetes. 2013;62:3341–9.
104. Turnbaugh PJ, Hamady M, Yatsunenko T, Cantarel BL, Duncan A, Ley RE, et al. A core gut microbiome in obese and lean twins. Nature. 2009;457:480–4.
105. Anhê FF, Varin TV, Schertzer JD, Marette A. The gut microbiota as a mediator of metabolic benefits after bariatric surgery. Can J Diabetes. 2017;41(4):439–47.
106. Murphy R, Tsai P, Jüllig M, Liu A, Plank L, Booth M. Differential changes in gut microbiota after gastric bypass and sleeve gastrectomy bariatric surgery vary according to diabetes remission. Obes Surg. 2017;27(4):917–25.
107. Peat CM, Kleiman SC, Bulik CM, Carroll IM. The intestinal microbiome in bariatric surgery patients. Eur Eat Disord Rev. 2015;23(6):496–503.
108. Ulker İ, Yildiran H. The effects of bariatric surgery on gut microbiota in patients with obesity: a review of the literature. Biosci Microbiota Food Health. 2019;38(1):3–9.

109. Bastos ELS, Liberatore AMA, Tedesco RC, Koh IHJ. Gut microbiota imbalance can be associated with non-malabsorptive small bowel shortening regardless of blind loop. Obes Surg. 2019;29(2):369–75.
110. Eckburg PB, Bik EM, Bernstein CN, Purdom E, Dethlefsen L, Sargent M, et al. Diversity of the human intestinal microbial flora. Science. 2005;308:1635–8.
111. Lozupone CA, Stombaugh JI, Gordon JI, Jansson JK, Knight R. Diversity, stability and resilience of the human gut microbiota. Nature. 2012;489:220–30.
112. Tremaroli V, Karlsson F, Werling M, Stahlman M, Kovatcheva-Datchary P, Olbers T, et al. Roux-en-Y gastric bypass and vertical banded gastroplasty induce long-term changes on the human gut microbiome contributing to fat mass regulation. Cell Metab. 2015;22:228–38.
113. Kong LC, Tap J, Aron-Wisnewsky J, Pelloux V, Basdevant A, Bouillot JL, et al. Gut microbiota after gastric bypass in human obesity: Increased richness and associations of bacterial genera with adipose tissue genes. Am J Clin Nutr. 2013;98:16–24.
114. Palleja A, Kashani A, Allin KH, et al. Roux-en-Y gastric bypass surgery of morbidly obese patients induces swift and persistent changes of the individual gut microbiota. Genome Med 2016;8:67.
115. Cho I, Blaser MJ. The human microbiome: at the interface of health and disease. Nat Rev Genet. 2012;13(4):260–70.
116. Clemente JC, Ursell LK, Parfrey LW, Knight R. The impact of the gut microbiota on human health: An integrative view. Cell. 2012;148(6):1258–70.
117. Le Chatelier E, Nielsen T, Qin J, Prifti E, Hildebrand F, Falony G, et al. Richness of human gut microbiome correlates with metabolic markers. Nature. 2013;500:541–6.
118. De Filippo C, Cavalieri D, Di Paola M, Ramazzotti M, Poullet JB, Massart S, et al. Impact of diet in shaping gut microbiota revealed by a comparative study in children from Europe and rural Africa. Proc Natl Acad Sci USA. 2010;107:14691–6.
119. Furet JP, Kong LC, Tap J, Poitou C, Basdevant A, Bouillot JL, et al. Differential adaptation of human gut microbiota to bariatric surgery-induced weight loss: links with metabolic and low grade inflammation markers. Diabetes. 2010;59:3049–57.
120. Kellerer T, Brandl B, Büttner J, Lagkouvardos I, Hauner H, Skurk T. Impact of laparoscopic sleeve gastrectomy on gut permeability in morbidly obese subjects. Obes Surg. 2019;29(7):2132–43.
121. Kikuchi R, Irie J, Yamada-Goto N, Kikkawa E, Seki Y, Kasama K, et al. The impact of laparoscopic sleeve gastrectomy with duodenojejunal bypass on intestinal microbiota differs from that of laparoscopic sleeve gastrectomy in Japanese patients with obesity. Clin Drug Investig. 2018;38(6):545–52.
122. Ejtahed HS, Angoorani P, Hasani-Ranjbar S, Siadat SD, Ghasemi N, Larijani B, et al. Adaptation of human gut microbiota to bariatric surgeries in morbidly obese patients: A systematic review. Microb Pathog. 2018;116:13–21.
123. Damms-Machado A, Mitra S, Schollenberger AE, Kramer KM, Meile T, Königsrainer A, et al. Effects of surgical and dietary weight loss therapy for obesity on gut microbiota composition and nutrient absorption. Biomed Res Int. 2015;2015:1–11. Article ID 806248.
124. Tabasi M, Ashrafian F, Khezerloo JK, Eshghjoo S, Behrouzi A, Javadinia SA, et al. Changes in gut microbiota and hormones after bariatric surgery: a bench-to-bedside review. Obes Surg. 2019;29(5):1663–74.

Nutritional Deficiencies After Bariatric Surgery

5

Pallawi Priya, Sarfaraz Baig, and Manjari Agarwal

Our Food should be our Medicine & our Medicine should be our Food!

Hippocrates

5.1 Introduction

For about three decades now, bariatric surgery remains the most effective way to achieve sustainable relief from morbid obesity and metabolic syndrome [1].

Because of the proven efficacy and absence of equally effective medical alternatives, number of bariatric and metabolic surgeries are increasing worldwide. According to the IFSO global registry, 634,897 surgeries were performed in the year 2018 [2].

The efficacy of bariatric surgery comes from its restriction and malabsorption components as well as with neurohormonal modulation.

However, the efficacy of bariatric surgery does not come without side effects. Low food intake coupled with the elimination of large portions of the stomach and intestines have the potential to produce multiple nutritional deficiencies. These deficiencies can be minimised with a proper procedure selection, diligent supplementation and strict follow-up with adherence to diet and lifestyle modifications. Therefore, a knowledge of the incidence of deficiencies with different procedures and their treatment is compulsory for any bariatric centre. Additionally, early

P. Priya (✉)
Metabolic and Bariatric Surgery, Belle Vue Clinic, Kolkata, West Bengal, India

S. Baig · M. Agarwal
Department of GI and Minimal Access Surgery, Belle Vue Clinic, Kolkata, West Bengal, India

A. G. Bhasker et al. (eds.), *Management of Nutritional and Metabolic Complications of Bariatric Surgery*,
https://doi.org/10.1007/978-981-33-4702-1_5

identification of the problem as mentioned in the previous chapter is important to reduce the morbidity and financial burden that a sustained and/or progressive deficiency state may lead to.

It needs to be emphasised that bariatric surgery is still an evolving science and much remains to be understood about the physiological changes that happen after different surgeries. While some deficiencies are a direct result of malabsorption due to exclusion of the absorption site, some may have a more indirect mechanism. For example, reduction in intrinsic factor due to stomach resizing leads to decreased absorption of vitamin B 12.

Strict surveillance, data collection, and reporting are important to understand nutritional deficiencies and pave the way for better and clearer guidelines for future patients.

5.2 Mechanism of Deficiency

Most bariatric surgeries involve reduction of stomach volume with or without proximal intestinal bypass. Gastric volume reduction brings about significant caloric reduction. Reduced quantity of food can lead to many deficiencies depending on the quantity and quality of food intake.

Stomach volume reduction is responsible for a decrease in hydrochloric acid and Intrinsic Factor (IF) secretion. This contributes to decreased absorption of iron and vitamin B12.

The proximal intestine is responsible for the absorption of water-soluble vitamins as well as bivalent anions such as Iron, Zinc, Magnesium and Calcium (Fig. 5.1). Exclusion of these areas in malabsorptive procedures like RYGB, OAGB, SADI and BPD-DS leads to deficiencies of minerals like Fe, Ca, Zn, Se, Cu, Mg and water-soluble vitamins like Vitamin B1, B6 and Folate.

Other factor that influences the absorption of micronutrients after bariatric surgery is the alteration of the chemical nature of the chyme. This happens due to:

1. Altered gastric pH—frequently seen after bariatric procedures due to decreased acid-producing gastric surface.
2. Unsatisfactory protein breakdown in the stomach—due to decreased acid and pepsin.

This explains why micronutrients may be malabsorbed even after sleeve gastrectomy where the gastrointestinal continuity is not disturbed.

In addition, studies on sleeve gastrectomy have shown that there is accelerated gastric emptying and small bowel transit which may lead to further malabsorptive effect of the procedure [3].

Water-soluble vitamins are not stored in the body. Therefore, their deficiencies are visible early in the postoperative period unless supplemented. This may be compounded if there is significant vomiting. Of note is vitamin B1 which can be deficient in the early postoperative period and produce neurological complications

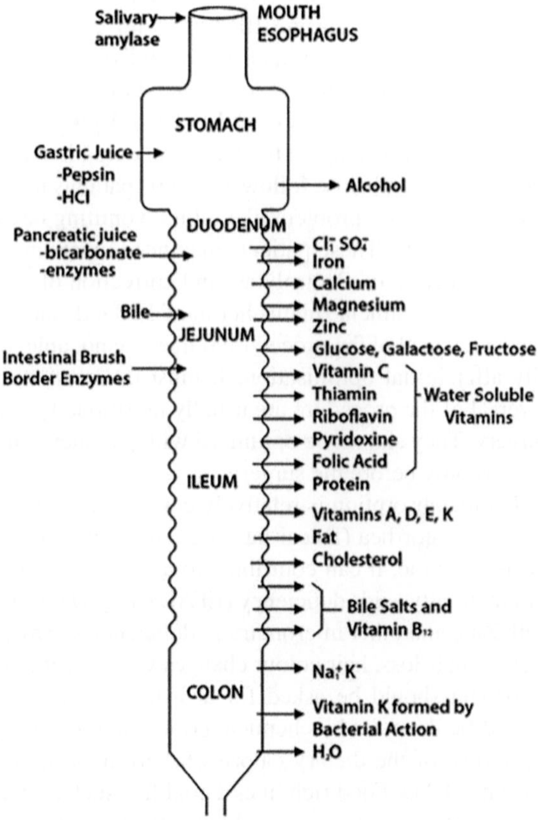

Fig. 5.1 Site of absorption of various micronutrients

as early as a month after bariatric surgery if there is postoperative nausea and vomiting [4].

Deficiencies of fat-soluble vitamins are less pronounced after bariatric surgery since they are stored in the body and are absorbed in the distal intestine as well (not bypassed in most procedures). However, the altered conditions for digestion due to diversion of the proximal intestine and fat malabsorption may lead to their deficiency as well. Clinically, vitamin D and A deficiency states are seen commonly after bariatric surgery. This is particularly important after diversionary procedures like BPD-DS and OAGB. Some patients may develop *de novo* intolerance to meat and lactose further impacting adequate nutritional assimilation.

5.3 Macronutrients

Protein-Energy malnutrition, although not so common, is a real risk in patients who undergo diversionary bariatric procedures. The incidence of severe hypoalbuminemia defined as serum albumin <3 mg/dl has been seen in upto 5.9% in OAGB patients compared to 2.9% in SG and 2.2% in RYGB [5]. Higher rates of PEM have been seen with increasing BP limb with upto 0.6% of patients needing revision surgery for malnutrition in OAGB with BP limb >250 cm [6].

To prevent PEM, it is recommended that patients should be supplemented with at least 60 g of protein/d or at least 1–1.5 g/kg body weight, whichever is higher. While most PEM may be treated on an outpatient basis with increased protein supplementation and close follow-up, some patients may present with an inability to eat due to either a GI problem like reflux, vomiting or extreme malnutrition leading to loss of appetite. These patients may need inpatient treatment with parenteral nutrition, correction of electrolytes, and correction of any anatomical factors amenable to surgical treatment (hiatus hernia, GERD, distal obstruction). Some patients may need a reversal of the procedure if they are not able to maintain their nutrition enterally after initial optimisation. It must be mentioned here that patients needing a reversal of the procedure are usually nutritionally poor and not good candidates for surgery. They should be optimised with parenteral nutrition, a feeding gastrostomy/jejunostomy before the surgery.

Fat malabsorption is relatively common after diversionary procedures and presents as steatorrhea (faecal fat >7 g/day), diarrhoea and increased flatulence. If not treated in time, it can contribute to a deficiency of fat-soluble vitamins as well as essential fatty acids deficiency (EFAD). EFAD presents with symptoms overlapping with Zinc and other micronutrient deficiencies. Any patients coming with scaly dermatitis, hair loss, hair colour changes with or without elevated LFTs, and thrombocytopenia should be asked for a history of steatorrhoea. A triene: tetraene ratio should be done for biochemical confirmation of EFAD. It is recommended that at least 10% of the dietary calories be given as fat and 2–4% from linoleic acid to prevent EFAD. Food rich in essential fats such as nuts should be encouraged.

If a deficiency is diagnosed for patients taking an oral diet, encourage vegetable oils, condiments, nuts and nut butters rich in EFA. For PN-dependent patients, lipid injectable emulsion should be increased [7].

5.4 Micronutrients

Micronutrient deficiencies are relatively more common, (Table 5.1) and therefore need to be actively sought for and screened. Table 5.2 gives the current ASMBS recommendations for micronutrient screening in post-bariatric patients.

The reports prior to 2010 with RYGB, BPD-DS and OAGB with 200 cm or more biliopancreatic limb show a higher rate of deficiencies. Recent reports comparing the outcomes with different BP limb lengths in OAGB have shown that a limb length more than 150 cm does not offer any benefit with weight loss or comorbidity resolution but increases the nutritional deficiencies [6, 8]. Since then, there has been a trend to use lower limb lengths with OAGB including at the authors' centre. Additionally, bariatric surgeons have realised the need for diligent supplementation leading to decreased deficiency rates.

Table 5.1 Commonly observed nutritional deficiencies after different bariatric procedures

Nutrient	LSG (%)	RYGB (%)	OAGB (%)
Thiamine	0	12	–
Folate	10–20	15	–
Pyridoxine	0–15	0	
Cobalamine	10–20	30–50	6.2–29.8
Vitamin A	10–20	10–50	9.4–31.2
Vitamin D	30–70	30–50	6.2–28.1
Vitamin E	0–5	10	–
Vitamin K	0	0	–
Iron	15–45	25–50	12.5–76.7
Zinc	7–15	20–37	–
Copper	10	10	–
Selenium	2%	3–46%	–

Ref:
Via MA, Mechanick JI. Nutritional and Micronutrient Care of Bariatric Surgery Patients: Current Evidence Update. *Curr Obes Rep*. 2017;6(3):286–296
Hassan Zadeh M, Mohammadi Farsani G, Zamaninour N. Selenium Status after Roux-en-Y Gastric Bypass: Interventions and Recommendations. *Obes Surg*. 2019;29(11):3743–3748
Papamargaritis D, Aasheim ET, Sampson B, le Roux CW. Copper, selenium and zinc levels after bariatric surgery in patients recommended to take multivitamin-mineral supplementation. *J Trace Elem Med Biol*. 2015

Table 5.2 Deficiency symptoms and screening recommendations for various micronutrients

Nutrient	Deficiency symptoms	Screening recommendation
Vitamin A	Night blindness, xerophthalmia, developmental defects	Patients should be screened for vitamin A deficiency within the first postoperative year, particularly those who have undergone BPD/DS, regardless of symptoms Vitamin A should be measured in patients who have undergone RYGB and BPD/DS, particularly in those patients with evidence of protein–calorie malnutrition
Vitamin D and calcium	Calcium levels are highly regulated. So no short-term effects. Numbness, tingling of hands and fingers, muscle cramps, convulsions, osteopenia	Routine post-BMS screening of vitamin D status is recommended for all patients
Vitamin E	Loss of coordination, muscle weakness, generalized feeling of unwellness, vision problems, hair and skin changes	Screen if symptomatic
Vitamin K	Coagulation defects	Screen if symptomatic

(continued)

Table 5.2 (continued)

Nutrient	Deficiency symptoms	Screening recommendation
Thiamine (B1)	Beriberi, enlarged heart, neurological dysfunction (confusion, irritability, loss of memory), muscular weakness and GI tract affected. Anorexia, weight loss	Routine screening is recommended in high-risk patients such as those with postoperative nausea/vomiting, African Americans, poor follow-up, females, SIBO, concomitant illnesses such as cardiomyopathy If signs and symptoms or risk factors are present in post-BMS patients, thiamine status should be assessed at least during the first 6 months, then every 3–6 months until symptoms resolve
Folate	Neural tube development impaired and perhaps other birth defects. Megaloblastic anaemia, fatigue, difficulty in concentration, heart palpitations, shortness of breath, neural tube defect	Routine post-BMS screening of folate status is recommended in all patients. Special attention in women of childbearing age
Vitamin B12 (Cobalamin)	Megaloblastic anaemia, fatigue, neurological disorders (numbness, tingling), weakness	Routine post-BMS screening of vitamin B12 status is recommended for all patients More frequent screening (e.g. every 3 months) is recommended in the first post-BMS year, and then at least annually or as clinically indicated for the at-risk patient (patients on nitrous oxide, neomycin, metformin, colchicine, PPIs, and seizure medications)
Iron	Impaired physical work performance, especially in endurance exercises Anaemia	Routine post-BMS screening of iron status is recommended within 3 months after surgery, and then every 3–6 months until 12 months, and annually for all patients
Zinc	Growth retardation, loss of appetite, impaired immune function. Hair loss, diarrhoea, impotence, taste abnormalities, mental lethargy	Post-RYGB and post-BPD/DS patients should be screened at least annually for zinc deficiency Screen if anaemia without iron deficiency or in the presence of chronic diarrhoea Screen if any of the deficiency symptoms are present
Copper	Normocytic, hypochromic anaemia, leukopenia, and neutropenia, osteoporosis, neurologic and psychiatric defects, motor defects, heart enlargement, skin changes	Screen if symptomatic
Selenium	Keshan disease (cardiomyopathy), Kashin-Beck disease (endemic osteoarthropathy), cretinism, immune system dysfunction, infertility in men, hypercholesterolemia	Screen if symptomatic

Apart from restriction and diversion, Small intestinal bacterial overgrowth (SIBO) and food intolerance can alter the absorption of nutrients. They should be suspected if there are complaints of persistent foul-smelling diarrhoea and bloating. Patients should be treated with antibiotics, pancreatic enzyme supplementation and probiotics. A hydrogen breath test may be useful to diagnose SIBO.

Little is known about the deficiency rates after relatively newer bariatric procedures like SADI, SADI-S, Ileal transposition.

Early results have shown deficiencies of Vitamin A (7.3–44%), Vitamin D (48.4–50%), B12 (0–8%) and ferritin (17.5%) at 1 year after SADI-S [9, 10].

5.5 Clinical Manifestation

Clinical examination and manifestation of micronutrient deficiency have been covered comprehensively in the previous chapter. Table 5.2 gives a summary of clinical symptoms and screening recommendations for different nutrients.

The symptoms and signs of nutritional deficiencies are often vague and overlapping. Deficiency of one nutrient can indicate a poor diet, absorption or compliance and can be a surrogate marker for multiple deficiencies. Therefore, for any suspicion of deficiency a comprehensive panel of the investigations as mentioned in Table 5.3 should be done.

Table 5.3 Various tests to measure micronutrient deficiencies

Nutrient	Routine tests	Additional parameters
Vitamin D	Total Serum 25-hydroxyvitamin D level	Decreased serum phosphorus, increased alkaline phosphatase, increased serum PTH, decreased urinary calcium
Thiamine (B1)	Whole blood (erythrocyte) levels of Thiamine diphosphate	Decreased RBC transketolase, increased pyruvate
Folate	Serum levels below 3 ng/ml. Erythrocyte folate levels below 140 ng/ml	Urinary FIGLU (formiminoglutamic acid), normal serum and urinary MMA, increased serum total Homocysteine
Vitamin B12 (Cobalamin)	Plasma/serum B12. Serum homocysteine >13 µmol/L	Increased serum and urinary MMA (methylmalonic acid), increased serum total Homocysteine
Calcium	Serum calcium is not a good indicator of its deficiency since its value is tightly controlled	Screen with tests described in panel for vitamin D
Iron	Ferritin <20 ng/ml, Serum iron <50 mcg/dl, TIBC >450 mcg/dl, Transferrin saturation <20%, peripheral smear	Decreased serum iron, higher TIBC
Copper	Serum blood copper levels (<70 mcg/dl), 24 h urine copper (<15 U), blood ceruloplasmin (<22.9 mg/dl)	Erythrocyte superoxide dismutase activity

5.6 Lab Tests

ASMBS recommendations for routine screening of nutrients and frequency of screening are mentioned in Table 5.2. The surveillance is more frequent in the first 2 years with all bariatric procedures and follow-up is usually good till this time. However, after 2 years, a significant number of patients start falling out of the follow-up loop. Therefore, it is important to actively follow-up with these patients to prevent accruing deficiencies.

Important points to remember regarding the interpretation of lab tests:

1. Serum thiamine responds to dietary supplementation but is a poor indicator of body stores. RBC transketolase is a better indicator of its deficiency.
2. Serum vitamin B6 values may be altered in diabetes. Consider checking B6 levels in unresponsive anaemia.
3. Serum B12 levels may miss deficiencies in 25–30% of cases. Consider testing for methylmalonic acid (MMA) and homocysteine if there is a suspicion of deficiency and serum B12 levels are low normal.
4. Serum folate is representative of dietary intake more than body stores. RBC folate is a more sensitive marker of deficiency. Also, excessive folate supplementation can mask vitamin B12 deficiency while the neurological symptoms persist.
5. Haemoglobin and haematocrit levels may be normal with low body stores of iron and low levels signifying stage 3 or 4 anaemia. Ferritin is an acute-phase reactant and its levels may be elevated in the presence of infection or inflammatory state.
6. To assess for vitamin D deficiency state—a complete panel including serum phosphorus (reduced), alkaline phosphatase (increased), PTH (increased) should be done. Of note is the fact that serum calcium levels can be low or normal in the presence of vitamin D deficiency.
7. As vitamin A levels are routinely not done, it is important to actively look for ocular and skin findings. Levels should be checked at the earliest suspicion.
8. Although vitamin E deficiencies are uncommon, serum levels alone may not be representative of the deficiency states. Plasma α-tocopherol to plasma lipids (0.8 mg/g total lipid) should be used in the presence of hyperlipidaemia.
9. No reliable tests exist to determine zinc status and serum zinc levels are most commonly used. Serum zinc levels should be interpreted in accordance with serum albumin levels since albumin is the primary binding protein for zinc. Zinc supplementation can precipitate copper deficiency and therefore copper should be supplemented along with zinc.

5.7 Supplementation

The supplementation doses [11] are mentioned in Table 5.4.

It may be easy to underestimate the nutritional deficiencies after LSG. However, many studies have confirmed the malabsorptive nature of the procedure [12] and

Table 5.4 Prophylactic and therapeutic doses of various micronutrient

Nutrient (vitamin/mineral)	Post-BMS supplementation	
	Prevention	Repletion
Vitamin B1	12 mg/day At Risk: 50–100 mg/day	Oral: 100 mg until resolution IV: 200–500 mg/3–5 days; followed by 250 mg/3–5 days; followed by 100 mg/day orally till resolution IM: 250 mg/3–5 days or 100–250 mg/month *Simultaneous administration of phosphorous, potassium and magnesium
Vitamin B12	Oral: 350–500 mcg Nasal spray: As directed Parenteral (IM/SQ):1000 mcg/month	Patients with B12 deficiency: 1000 mcg/day to achieve normal levels
Folate	Oral: 400–800 mcg/day from MV For childbearing women: 800–1000 mcg	Patients with folate deficiency: 1000 mcg/day Above 1 mg/day doses are not recommended
Calcium	LAGB/LSG/RYGB: 1200–1500 mg/day BPD/DS: 1800–2400 mg/day	LAGB/LSG/RYGB: 1200–1500 mg/day BPD/DS: 1800–2400 mg/day
Vitamin A	LAGB: 5000 IU/day LSG/ RYGB: 5000–10,000 IU/day BPD/DS: 10,000 IU/day	Without corneal changes, oral dose: 10,000–25,000 IU/day, until improvement With corneal changes, IM dose: 50,000–100,000 IU/day for 3 days followed by 50,000 IU/day for 2 weeks *also evaluate for iron and copper deficiency
Vitamin E	15 mg/day	100–400 IU/day
Vitamin K	LAGB/LSG/RYGB:90–120 μg/day BPD/DS: 300 μg/day	Acute malabsorption, parenteral dose: 10 mg/day Chronic malabsorption: Oral dose:1–2 mg/day and Parenteral dose:1–2 mg/week
Vitamin D	D3 dose: 3000 IU/day to maintain D, 25OH levels >30 ng/ml	D3 dose: 2000–6000 IU/day or D2 dose: 50,000 IU/1–3 times/week *D3 is more potent than D2
Iron	LAGB/LSG:18 mg/day from MV RYGB/BPD/DS and menstruating women: 45–60 mg/day (all sources)	Oral: 150–200 mg/day to 300 mg/2–3 times/day of elemental iron *Divided doses separate from calcium supplements, acid-reducing medicines and phytates/polyphenols *IV infusion if not responded to oral therapy
Zinc	LAGB/LSG: 8–11 mg/day RYGB: 8–11 mg to 16–22 mg/day BPD/DS: 16–22 mg/day *To minimise copper deficiency: supplement with 1 mg of copper/8–15 mg zinc	60 mg/day (needs further evaluation) *Repletion doses should not precipitate copper deficiency

(continued)

Table 5.4 (continued)

Nutrient (vitamin/mineral)	Post-BMS supplementation	
	Prevention	Repletion
Copper	LAGB/LSG: 1 mg/day RYGB: 1–2 mg/day BPD/DS: 2 mg/day *Copper Gluconate/Copper Sulphate supplement sources recommended	Mild to moderate deficiency with low haematological indices, Oral dose: 3–8 mg/day (copper gluconate/copper sulphate) until the normal index Severe deficiency, IV: 2–4 mg/day for 6 days until normal serum level

Adapted from: Parrott J et al. ASMBS Integrated Health Nutritional Guidelines For The Surgical Weight Loss Patient- 2016 Update: Micronutrients

significant nutritional deficiencies have been noted. Additionally, a reduced intake can produce a deficiency of almost any nutrient in the absence of a balanced diet.

Although intestinal adaptation takes place over a period of approximately 2 years after the bariatric surgery, it is often insufficient. It cannot be stressed enough that all bariatric patients should be counselled preoperatively regarding the requirement for lifelong nutritional supplementation in addition to a nutritious diet.

It should be noted that even with therapeutic doses, deficiencies are difficult to correct in the postoperative period. Additionally, many pre-existing deficiencies exacerbate in the postoperative period [13]. This is probably because it is difficult to correct deficiencies after bariatric surgery which reduces the ingestive and absorptive potential of the gut. Therefore, potential bariatric patients should not only be screened for pre-existing deficiencies but also corrected religiously before surgery.

Although there exists a recommendation for prophylactic supplementation doses for widely performed bariatric procedures, the repletion doses have to be tailored to the deficiency status, and efficiency of enteral supplementation. Frequently, parenteral supplementation is needed as the oral supplementation is inadequate due to poor absorption from the GI tract.

In the absence of adequate data about the less commonly performed procedures like SADI, SADI-S, ileal interposition, it is difficult to make nutritional recommendations for the same. According to the authors, it may be safe to supplement these patients according to the recommendation for diversionary procedures [11] (Table 5.4) until the time more is known on the subject.

Key Points

- *Bariatric surgery by its very nature of alteration of GI anatomy induces nutritional complications, both macronutrients (protein and fat mainly) and micronutrients (vitamins and minerals).*
- *The mechanism of deficiencies is multifactorial—restricted calorie intake, decreased absorption and biological.*
- *All bariatric procedures produce nutritional complications but diversionary procedures such as RYGB, OAGB, BPD-DS, SADI-S create more pronounced effects.*
- *Lifelong surveillance in terms of clinical evaluation and laboratory tests is critical to prevent and treat nutritional deficiencies.*

- *Clinical evaluation is important to pick-up subtle signs and symptoms of deficiencies and prevent complications.*
- *Lab tests should be interpreted carefully and serum markers of deficiencies alone cannot be accepted as evidence of normalcy.*
- *One nutrient deficiency should be seen as a surrogate marker of widespread malnutrition.*
- *Supplementation is lifelong and multivitamin–multimineral tablets should be checked for adequacy based on current guidelines. Protein intake is frequently suboptimal and effort should be made to improve its intake especially in the early postoperative period.*
- *Once a deficiency is detected in the follow-up, it should be corrected aggressively and promptly by therapeutic doses to prevent dangerous complications such as PEM and neurological complications. Other conditions that contribute to malnutrition such as SIBO, surgical complications (stenosis, obstruction, hernia) should be excluded. Eating behaviour can also be influenced by reflux, vomiting and alteration of taste and bowel habit, and should be addressed simultaneously.*

5.8 Case Reports

5.8.1 Case 1

A 55/F with BMI 45 and hypertension had a sleeve gastrectomy 3 weeks back. She presented with recurrent vomiting and dysphagia to the clinic. She was feeling weak and complained of dribbling of saliva. On examination, she was confused and had diplopia.

How would you approach the case?

Answer

The Differential diagnoses are:

1. *Cerebrovascular accident*
2. *Mechanical obstruction due to incisural stenosis/torsion*
3. *Thiamine deficiency*

Check:

1. *MRI brain*
2. *CECT with oral contrast/barium series to exclude incisural stenosis*
3. *Upper GI endoscopy*
4. *Serum thiamine*

Serum thiamine 12.2 ng/ml (reference range 10–64 ng/ml) MRI, CECT and UGE normal.

What is the diagnosis?

Answer

Wernicke's encephalopathy

How do you treat the case?

Inj Thiamine 100–300 mg/day IV once daily till the patient shows improvement. At the time of discharge, oral thiamine 600 mg/day is administered till the patient recovers fully.

5.8.2 Case 2

A 38-year-old lady with BMI 62 had an OAGB-MGB done a year ago complaining of weakness.

She gives a history of breathlessness on exertion. A hemogram advised by her family physician showed a haemoglobin of 7.8 g/dl.

How would you approach the case?

Answer

Anaemia can be multifactorial in a post-bariatric patient. We follow the following protocol for a workup and treatment of anaemia (Fig. 5.2)

There was no history of any GI bleed. Investigations revealed low haemoglobin. Peripheral smear showed microcytic hypochromic cells. On further probing, the patient agreed to stopping iron tablets due to constipation and metallic taste. How would you treat this patient?

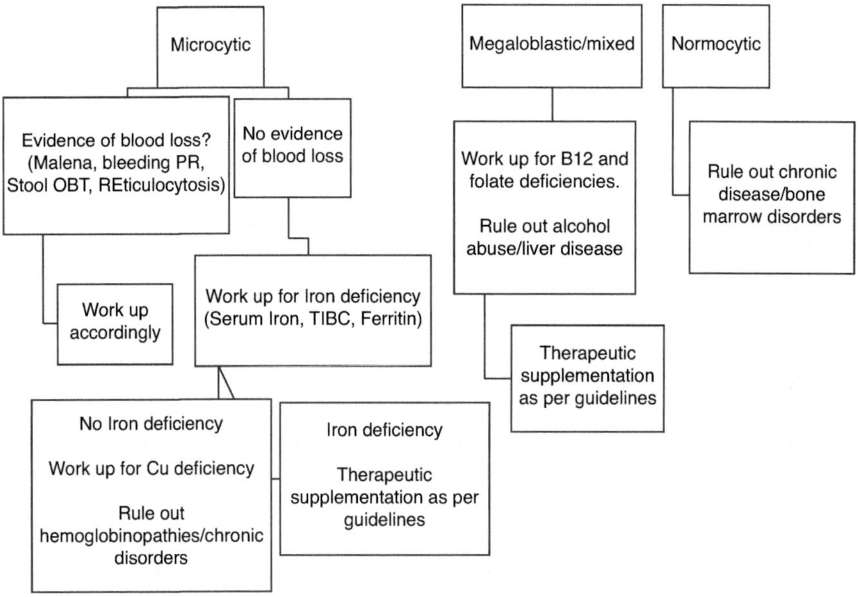

Fig. 5.2 Flowchart for diagnosis and management of anaemia in a post-bariatric patient

Answer

This patient has an intolerance to oral iron. She needs to be supplemented with 1 g of IV iron supplementation. In patients who can tolerate oral iron, 150–200 mg of elemental iron daily and up 300 mg 2–3 times a day can be prescribed. These patients need to be monitored every 3 months for their iron states as described earlier.

Is there a need for folic acid and vitamin B12 supplementation along with iron if the serum values of the above nutrients are normal?

Answer

Yes. Rapid hemopoiesis may precipitate the deficiency of these nutrients.

References

1. Azagury D, Papasavas P, Hamdallah I, Gagner M, Kim J. ASMBS Position Statement on medium- and long-term durability of weight loss and diabetic outcomes after conventional stapled bariatric procedures. Surg Obes Relat Dis. 2018;14(10):1425–41.
2. Himpens J et al. The IFSO Global Registry IFSO Global Registry Report 2018.
3. Melissas J, et al. Alterations of global gastrointestinal motility after sleeve gastrectomy: a prospective study. Ann Surg. 2013;258(6):976–82.
4. Samanta D. Dry beriberi preceded Wernicke's encephalopathy: Thiamine deficiency after laparoscopic sleeve gastrectomy. J Pediatr Neurosci. 2015;10(3):297.
5. Baig SJ, Priya P, Mahawar KK, Shah S. Weight regain after bariatric surgery—a multicentre study of 9617 patients from Indian Bariatric Surgery Outcome Reporting Group. Obes Surg. 2019;29(5):1583–92.
6. Mahawar K, Parmar C, Carr WJ, Jennings N, Schroeder N, Small P. Impact of biliopancreatic limb length on severe protein–calorie malnutrition requiring revisional surgery after one anastomosis (mini) gastric bypass. J Minim Access Surg. 2018;14(1):37.
7. Mogensen, Kris. (2017). Essential Fatty Acid Deficiency. Practical gastroenterology.
8. Ahuja A, et al. MGB-OAGB: effect of biliopancreatic limb length on nutritional deficiency, weight loss, and comorbidity resolution. Obes Surg. 2018;28(11):3439–45.
9. Moon RC, Kirkpatrick V, Gaskins L, Teixeira AF, Jawad MA. Safety and effectiveness of single- versus double-anastomosis duodenal switch at a single institution. Surg Obes Relat Dis. 2019;15(2):245–52.
10. Sánchez-Pernaute A, Rubio MÁ, Cabrerizo L, Ramos-Levi A, Pérez-Aguirre E, Torres A. Single-anastomosis duodenoileal bypass with sleeve gastrectomy (SADI-S) for obese diabetic patients. Surg Obes Relat Dis. 2015;11(5):1092–8.
11. Parrott J, Frank L, Rabena R, Craggs-Dino L, Isom KA, Greiman L. American Society for Metabolic and Bariatric Surgery Integrated Health Nutritional Guidelines for the Surgical Weight Loss Patient 2016 Update: Micronutrients. Surg Obes Relat Dis. 2017;13(5):727–41.
12. Emile SH, Elfeki H. Nutritional deficiency after sleeve gastrectomy: a comprehensive literature review. Eur Med J. 2017 [Online]. Available: https://www.emjreviews.com/gastroenterology/article/nutritional-deficiency-after-sleeve-gastrectomy-a-comprehensive-literature-review/. Accessed 30 Oct 2019.
13. Xanthakos SA. Nutritional deficiencies in obesity and after bariatric surgery. Pediatr Clin N Am. 2009;56(5):1105–21.

Clinical Examination of a Post-bariatric Surgery Patient

6

Sarfaraz Baig, Pallawi Priya, and Manjari Agarwal

Listen to your patient. He is telling you the diagnosis!

—William Osler

6.1 Introduction

Bariatrics is an evolving science and by nature of the surgery itself, patients are at risk of developing several nutritional, metabolic and psychosocial problems. Most of them, if not caught and treated on time, may have the potential to lead to irreversible damage [1, 2]. Hence, early diagnosis is of paramount importance.

Outpatient follow-ups are a great opportunity to closely examine the patient. A thorough history and physical examination can help us to diagnose most complications in their early stages.

Although there are guidelines available on how to examine patients before and after bariatric surgery [3], the need for a protocol-based clinical pathway remains unfulfilled. The purpose of this chapter is to provide a sample protocol for the clinical evaluation of a patient who has undergone bariatric/metabolic surgery. The purpose of such an evaluation is to assess the response to surgery and look for signs of any nutritional, metabolic or psychosocial issues.

The clinical evaluation comprises of history, examination, and laboratory tests. The following provides a general overview of the history and examination of a bariatric patient. Laboratory tests have been covered in another chapter and therefore, will not be discussed here.

S. Baig (✉) · M. Agarwal
Department of GI and Minimal Access Surgery, Belle Vue Clinic, Kolkata, West Bengal, India

P. Priya
Metabolic and Bariatric Surgery, Belle Vue Clinic, Kolkata, West Bengal, India

A. G. Bhasker et al. (eds.), *Management of Nutritional and Metabolic Complications of Bariatric Surgery*,
https://doi.org/10.1007/978-981-33-4702-1_6

6.2 History

History of a patient before bariatric and metabolic surgery (BMS) focuses on the evaluation of eating behaviour, motivation for a lifestyle change, associated comorbidities, weight loss attempts, substance abuse and activity levels. In comparison, evaluation after surgery focuses on weight loss, adaptation to new diet and lifestyle, gastrointestinal symptoms, symptoms of nutritional deficiencies/metabolic complications, changes in effect as well as changes in pre-existing comorbidities.

Table 6.1 describes the salient points in history taking in a patient after bariatric surgery.

History starts by noting the weight loss of the patient. Weight loss, if more than expected, can be a warning signal regarding possible protein–energy malnutrition (PEM). This is particularly important in case of malabsorptive procedures like OAGB, BPD-DS and SADI-S.

Table 6.1 Salient points in history taking of bariatric patients

Diet		
Food recall	Food diary/24 or 72-h recall	Assessment of nutritional adequacy of diet Assessment of eating patterns
Food tolerance		Intolerance to supplements, especially protein supplements and meat may be problematic
Eating disorders	Binge eating/ grazing/ loss of control	Continued psychological counselling may be needed to overcome eating disorders which may prevent achievement of the lifestyle and weight loss goals
Surgical problems		
Wounds	Healing/discharge/lump	
GI symptoms	Nausea/vomiting/reflux/dumping/ diarrhoea/steatorrhoea/anorexia	
Comorbidities		
	History of change in medication requirement, well-being, and achievement of near-physiological parameters	Comment on no change, resolution, remission, relapse
Social		
Stress	Stress producing factors which may come in the way of lifestyle goals	
Knowledge	Problems with food preparation/ cultural or social misconceptions	
Financial	Problems with the purchase of required food, supplements	
Others		
Substance abuse	Smoking/alcohol/other addictions	
Activity	Activity level	
Mood		

Dietary history starts with a recall that indicates the quality and quantity of food intake with special emphasis on protein intake. Patients are asked if they are eating quickly or taking water with food. Any food intolerances are noted. Frequently, bariatric patients may have meat or lactose intolerance that may hamper the protein intake. Binge eating, grazing, mindless eating and emotional eating are assessed preferably by the psychologist. Sometimes, the relatives of the patient may help to answer these questions as some patients lack insight into their own behaviour.

Many comorbidities improve after surgery leading to a change in medications. For example, many patients will be off medications for diabetes immediately after surgery. Some may require a reduction of medications. It is important to note the blood glucose trends after surgery so that the physician can appropriately titrate the dose of anti-diabetic medications. Diseases such as dyslipidaemia, chronic liver disease, chronic renal disease, obstructive sleep apnea, cardiac conditions and arthritis may also need a change in the treatment protocol. History should be focused on the same. We ask the patients to maintain a chart of their comorbidity-related manifestations (fasting blood glucose, blood pressure, pain, reflux) to make the necessary adjustments in medications.

There is literature to suggest that addictions or substance abuse may increase after bariatric surgery [4]. Hence, it is important to note the consumption of alcohol and status of other addictions after surgery. There is increasing awareness regarding food addiction, especially sugar-sweetened beverages (SSBs) and should be looked for. Behaviour is one of the most important reasons for weight regain and therefore incorporating a psychologist in the team may go a long way in assessing and managing the patient.

Some studies have noted a higher incidence of suicides in bariatric patients [5]. Hence, the assessment of mental health is important. Patients who have a pre-existing history of depression, anxiety and other mental health issues should be monitored more closely. Psychologists and psychiatrists should be a part of a bariatric team and their help should be sought whenever appropriate.

People who routinely do some physical activity have been found to experience less weight regain [6] compared to sedentary people. It is important to encourage exercise, sports and other physical activities with the understanding that different patients have different levels of performance.

Some patients may complain of various gastrointestinal symptoms. Many of them may signify a problem that needs early evaluation and intervention.

Table 6.2 on signs and symptoms of deficiencies of micronutrients is useful to remember and gives an overview of what to look for specifically in a patient from the nutritional perspective after bariatric surgery.

Table 6.3 provides a list of symptoms to be asked for and their potential causes. From a clinical application point of view, Table 6.3 is more important than Table 6.2. It is important to understand what issue a particular symptom represents rather than learning the deficiency signs alone.

Nausea and vomiting are common post-operative issues in gastrointestinal surgery. It is of special importance in bariatrics, as prolonged and untreated vomiting

Table 6.2 Symptoms of various nutritional deficiencies after bariatric surgery

Thiamine (B1)	Neuropsychiatric: aggression, hallucination, confusion, ataxia, nystagmus, paralysis of motor nerves of eyes
Riboflavin (B2)	Anaemia, dermatitis, stomatitis, glossitis
Niacin (B3)	Diarrhoea, confusion, dermatitis, ataxia
Pantothenic acid (B5)	Depression, infections, orthostatic hypotension, paraesthesia, foot drop, gait disorders
Pyridoxine (B6)	Dermatitis, neuropathy, confusion
Folic acid (B9)	Weakness, weight loss, anorexia
Cobalamine (B12)	Depression, malaise, ataxia, paraesthesia
Ascorbic acid (C)	Malaise, myalgia, gum disease, petechiae
Biotin (B7)	Loss of taste, seizure, hypotonia, ataxia, dermatitis, hair loss
Vitamin A	Night blindness, itching, dry hair
Vitamin D and calcium	Arthralgias, depression, fasciculation, myalgia
Vitamin E	Anaemia, ataxia, motor speech disorder, muscle weakness
Vitamin K	Bleeding disorder
Iron	Fatigue, shortness of breath, chest pain, anaemia, hair loss, koilonychia
Zinc	Skin lesions, nail dystrophy, alopecia, glossitis
Copper	Anaemia
Selenium	Dyspnea, fatigue, leg swelling, cardiomyopathy

Table 6.3 Clinical significance of common symptoms after bariatric surgery

Symptoms	Significance
Nausea/vomiting	Poor eating behaviour, nutritional deficiencies, surgical complications (stenosis/internal hernia/ulcer/reflux)
Diarrhoea	Malabsorption, SIBO (small intestinal bacterial growth), dumping
Steatorrhoea	Malabsorption, poor dietary choice
Bloating	Poor food choice, obstruction
Black stools	Stapler line bleed, anastomotic ulcer
Abdominal pain	Stones, ulcers, obstruction, internal hernia
Heartburn and reflux	May induce anorexia, check for consumption of smoking/alcohol
Giddiness and falls	Dehydration, nutritional deficiencies, neuropathy, dumping, postural hypotension, hypoglycemia
Constipation	Lack of dietary fibre
Hair loss	Nutritional deficiencies (protein, iron, zinc, Biotin, EFA)
Taste alteration	Biotin
Weakness	Exclude dehydration, dumping, anaemia, autonomic deficiency, micronutrient deficiency, psychological reasons, protein–energy malnutrition and neurological cause (DAMPEN—see below)
Dribbling of saliva/double vision/gait issues/paraesthesia	Neuropathy—deficiencies of Thiamine, copper, B12, Guillain-Barre syndrome
Knee/back and ankle pain	Osteopenia, vitamin D and calcium

may lead to potentially serious complications. Untreated, it can precipitate dehydration, acute renal failure, thiamine deficiency and neuropathy. Effort should be made to ascertain if this is due to surgical complications such as stenosis or obstruction. The quantity and nature of vomitus, eating behaviour (eating too fast, overeating, inadequate chewing, eating and drinking together) and the precipitating factor may point to the aetiology.

Reflux may be a pre-existing problem or can develop de novo after surgery. It has been commonly associated with fried food, caffeine, smoking, alcohol and inadequate chewing. Higher incidence of reflux has been reported with sleeve gastrectomy [7]. Reflux can be distressing and influences eating behaviour and therefore, weight loss. It is important to elicit this history and plan treatment for the same.

Patients may develop diarrhoea or steatorrhoea after bariatric surgery. History on the quality of stools should identify and differentiate between the two since the implications and management of the two are different (Fig. 6.1). Prompt addressal is crucial to prevent nutrition and electrolyte disturbances. Constipation is also seen

Fig. 6.1 Evaluation of diarrhoea in a post-bariatric patient

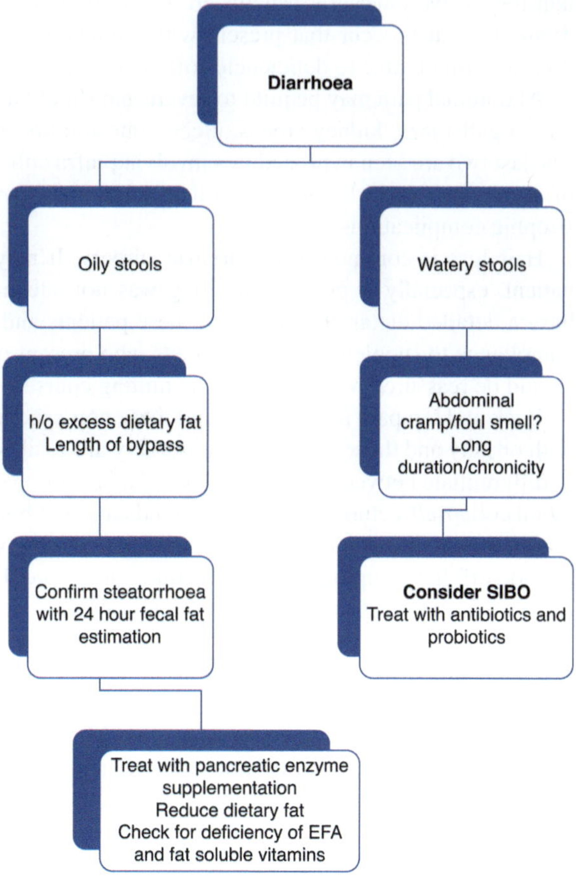

frequently and may be due to lack of fibre in diet or nutritional deficiencies such as vitamin D and Thiamine.

Giddiness can be because of dumping syndrome, orthostatic intolerance, dehydration or malnutrition. Careful history regarding the precipitating factors (food, position or decreased water intake) may indicate the cause of the symptom. If the symptom is precipitated by high carbohydrate food, dumping syndrome is a strong possibility. If it is brought about by standing from a lying down position, orthostatic intolerance should be suspected.

Other neurological symptoms such as double vision, abnormal gait, paraesthesia, dribbling of saliva, stuttering speech and confusion may indicate an impending neurological complication. Early diagnosis and treatment make a huge difference to the outcome as with time some neurological damages become irreversible. The timing of the neurological symptoms guides to the diagnosis. Early presentations are usually due to pressure on the nerves during surgery. Meralgia paresthetica is an example of the same. Wernicke's encephalopathy and Beri-Beri are also seen in the early post-operative course since thiamine is not stored in the body and a history of early non-responsive emesis is usually present in these cases. Guillain-Barre-like syndrome may also occur that present with paraparesis. Late neurological complications are usually due to deficiencies of copper, vitamin B12, vitamin E and folate.

Abdominal pain may be mild to severe and should not be neglected. This may be due to gallstones, kidney stones, ulcers, intestinal obstruction and internal hernia. The last two are seen in procedures involving infra colic compartment. A high index of suspicion should be present to detect internal hernia in time to prevent catastrophic complications.

Hair loss is common after bariatric surgery. It may be very distressing to the patient, especially if prior counselling was not adequate. The nutritionist should have a detailed dietary history from these patients and must be sure regarding the compliance to supplementation. Patients who present in the first year after surgery should be reassured regarding its self-limiting course.

Back and hip pain are common and these non-specific complaints in the patients with obesity and those after bariatric surgery are easily overlooked. Clinicians need to differentiate between back pain due to bad posture versus a back pain due to vertebral collapse/fracture. The latter is an indication of bone loss and is usually a silent complication with some patients presenting suddenly with hip and spine fractures [8]. Identifying symptoms of cord compression—problems in evacuating urine and stool—is important to identify the critical patients.

Weakness is a very important symptom and at some point in time, many patients complain about it after having bariatric surgery. They may call it "weakness", "fatigue" or "not feeling well". It is important to take a detailed history to exclude an organic cause. We use the mnemonic "DAMPEN" in our centre to remember the causes and to ask relevant questions to ascertain it.

- **D**ehydration
- **D**umping
- **A**naemia
- **A**utonomic insufficiency

- **M**icronutrient deficiency
- **P**sychological
- **P**rotein–**E**nergy malnutrition
- **N**eurological

With any bariatric surgery, food intake becomes drastically low and raises doubts in the patient and their family members about the adequacy of nutritional fulfilment. These patients may sometimes complain of weakness, which may be psychological and need reassurance.

Somatic neuropathy is a significant cause of weakness. The typical history is of post-surgery emesis that led to weakness, dribbling of saliva, poor gait and double vision.

Autonomic insufficiency [9] is increasingly recognized as a potential cause of orthostatic intolerance in patients after bariatric surgery, which is interpreted as weakness. These patients also complain of giddiness on standing up from a sitting position.

Many patients with dumping syndrome who experience post-prandial giddiness report it as weakness. Elaboration of the symptoms brought on by sugary food/drinks, can clarify the diagnosis in these cases.

Deficiencies such as vitamin D, iron, folate and B12 are also important nutritional causes of weakness that need clinical and laboratory evaluations for confirmation.

It is recommended that each centre creates its own checklists and protocols to make a note of these points. Tables 6.1 and 6.3 are the standard proformas followed at our centre.

6.2.1 Scoring Systems

Although not a part of any guidelines, scoring systems help track the outcomes in an objective way. BAROS, BQLI, and GIQLI are commonly used scoring systems to assess the outcomes of bariatric surgery. We suggest that any of these scores be used routinely for ease of audit, outcome assessment and comparison. In addition, pre-operative scores like ABCD and DiaRem may help in the assessment of comorbidity resolution.

6.3 Examination

The purpose of the examination of post-bariatric surgery patients is to know the response to the surgery and to find out any postsurgical complications. While BMI and anthropometry are important at each follow-up, a complete head-to-toe examination as well as a complete systemic examination is essential and should not be omitted. Table 6.4 gives a comprehensive view of the examination of a post-bariatric patient.

Table 6.4 Points to note in clinical examination of a post-bariatric patient

Anthropometry		
Height		
Weight		
BMI		
Waist circumference		
Hip circumference		
WHR		
BCA (Body composition analysis)		
Head-to-toe examination		
Examination	*To look for*	*Significance*
Hair	Texture, alopecia	May indicate deficiencies of protein, iron, zinc, EFA
Eyes	Xerophthalmia Bitot's spots	Vitamin A deficiency
Tongue	Glossitis Angular cheilitis	May indicate deficiencies of B complex vitamins
Gums	Ulcers Bleeding	
Oral mucosa	Aphthous ulcers Aphthous stomatitis	B complex deficiency
Nails	Brittle nails Koilonychia Poikilonychia	Iron deficiency
Skin	Acanthosis Hyperkeratosis plantaris Striae Intertrigo Chicken skin Xerosis Phrynoderma Acrodermatitis enteropathica Leg ulcers and abscesses Hyperpigmentation Necrotic dermatitis Erythema nodosum like lesions	These may be pre-existent in a patient suffering from obesity May indicate deficiencies of B12, A, D, C, zinc, selenium, iron Altered skin immunity with deposition of immune complexes
Limbs	Oedema Phrynoderma Lipodermatosclerosis	Protein, selenium deficiency May indicate deficiencies of vitamin A, B complex, E, EFA
Cardiovascular examination		
Heart sounds		
Orthostatic hypotension		Autonomic insufficiency
Neurological examination		
Sensations—touch, vibration, proprioception Motor power Tendon jerks Eye movements		Neuropathy (deficiency of B12, B1, copper), Guillain-Barre syndrome

Table 6.4 (continued)

Abdomen		
Skin redundancy		May indicate the need for abdominoplasty. Can interfere with gait
Hepatomegaly		
Splenomegaly		May indicate portal hypertension
Ascites		Can indicate worsening liver disease, malnutrition

Anthropometric evaluation requires a measuring tape and a weighing scale suitable for obese patients. For measuring the waist-hip ratio, it is important to note that the waist is measured at the midpoint between the lower margin of the last palpable ribs and top of the iliac crest and the hip is measured around the widest portion of the buttocks.

Body composition analyser is a good add-on to assess the fat, muscle and skeletal mass of the patient. These may be helpful for prognostication and comparison during follow-up. Fat loss is more important to assess than weight loss since muscle loss is a disadvantage after bariatric surgery—also known as sarcopenia. Sarcopenic obesity is known to increase after bariatric surgery and carries higher morbidity and mortality [10]. Preservation of fat-free mass has also been shown to be beneficial in preventing weight regain [11]. Therefore, it is important to know the ratio of fat loss vs muscle loss after BMS as a part of the follow-up and fat-free mass loss, which is excessive or protracted. Dagan et al. [12] studied patients who underwent sleeve gastrectomy and showed progressive fat-free mass loss after the first 6 months (following which it stabilizes) should warn the clinician to take action. Bariatric centres should have a Body Composition Analysis (BCA) machine and measure fat mass and fat-free mass and not rely entirely on body weight as an outcome parameter.

Having a plan for doing a general examination helps. We prefer going from head to toe to keep from missing any important findings.

We look for alopecia in the scalp. Some authors have reported impetigo-like lesions in the scalp [13] that may signify malnutrition.

Eyes are inspected for xerophthalmia and Bitot's spots that indicate vitamin A deficiency. Oral cavity examination may show glossitis, cheilitis, stomatitis, aphthous ulcers all of which may signify vitamin B deficiencies. Nails may show brittleness, ridges, spoon shape and may indicate iron deficiency. Face and neck are examined for skin lesions such as acanthosis.

Upper limb examination involves examination of nails, looking for skin lesions and blood pressure measurement. Blood pressure should be measured both in the erect and supine position to pick up orthostatic intolerance. Enough time should be given before measuring blood pressure at these positions to allow for hemodynamic equilibrium.

Examination of legs can give valuable information. Many patients with obesity have oedema that may be due to weight-related poor circulation, right heart failure or protein deficiency. Lipodermatosclerosis is a specific condition seen typically in patients with obesity due to venous hypertension and stasis. There is a combination of swelling, pigmentation and induration of legs and is frequently misunderstood as cellulitis. Usually, with bariatric surgery, this condition resolves and it should be noted in the follow-up visits. Deep venous thrombosis (DVT) is a sinister complication and may present with calf swelling and tenderness.

Nutritional deficiencies produce an array of skin lesions and a general dermatological examination offers an excellent opportunity to detect these. The common skin lesions that have been reported in the literature are xerosis, phrynoderma, acanthosis, acrodermatitis enteropathica, leg ulcers and abscesses, hyperpigmentation, necrotic dermatitis and erythema nodosum-like lesions. The last two are manifestations of altered skin immunity. Figures 6.2, 6.3, 6.4 and 6.5 show examples of various skin lesions that may present after bariatric surgery.

It is important for clinicians dealing with post bariatric surgery patients to examine all parts of the body and diagnose these skin lesions. It is also crucial to have complete exposure on examination since skin lesions such as phrynoderma are hidden behind the elbows.

There are many skin lesions that are present in patients with obesity and it is vital to know them and not confuse them with post-bariatric dermatological complications.

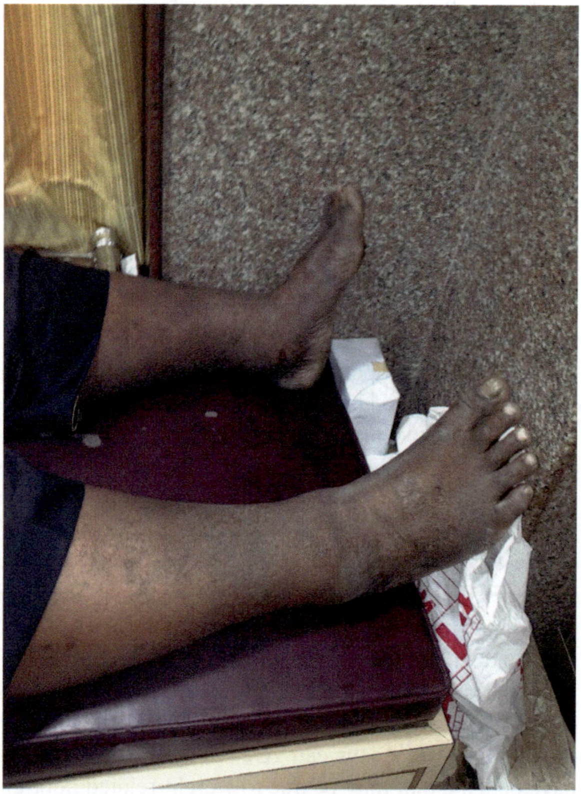

Fig. 6.2 Lipodermatosclerosis

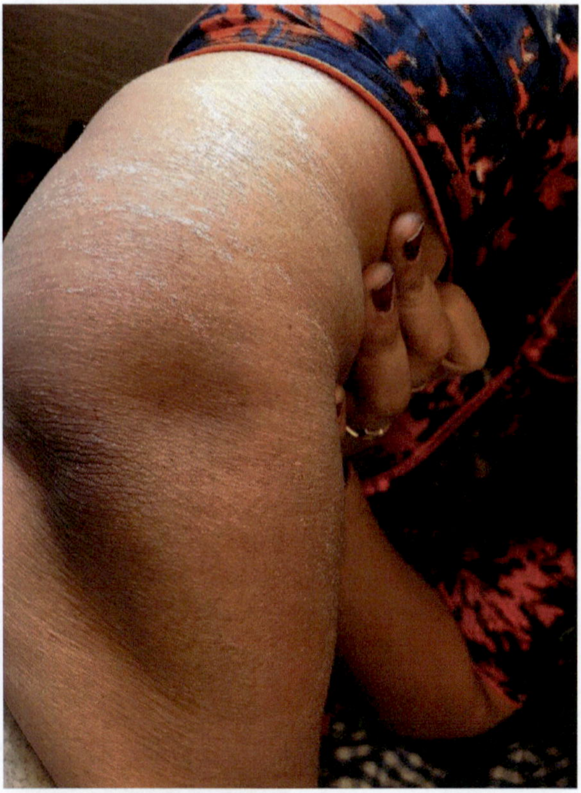

Fig. 6.3 Xerosis

They are acanthosis, hyperkeratosis plantaris, striae, intertrigo and chicken skin. Amongst these, acanthosis usually improves after bariatric surgery in the majority.

Psoriasis, a skin disease, has been shown to be associated with obesity [14] and most patients show resolution of these lesions after surgery although some aggravation has also been reported [15]. It is useful to remember that zinc deficiency can lead to skin eruptions in the form of psoriasiform dermatitis [16]. As we can appreciate, a bariatrician needs to diagnose a wide array of skin lesions and seek the help of a dermatologist wherever necessary.

Abdomen is checked superficially for any port site hernias, pre-existing paraumbilical and incisional hernia, intertrigo, lower abdominal cellulitis and distended abdominal veins. Deep palpation is done to detect any hepatomegaly, splenomegaly or tenderness. Many of these findings pre-exist in patients with obesity undergoing bariatric surgery and should be observed for resolution or non-response.

The respiratory system is assessed by noting the rate of breathing, orthopnea and lung sounds. Many post bariatric surgery patients have obstructive sleep apnea preoperatively and their assessment should be a part of examination at each visit. These patients are also prone to pneumonia and pulmonary embolism, something that can be picked up by chest auscultation.

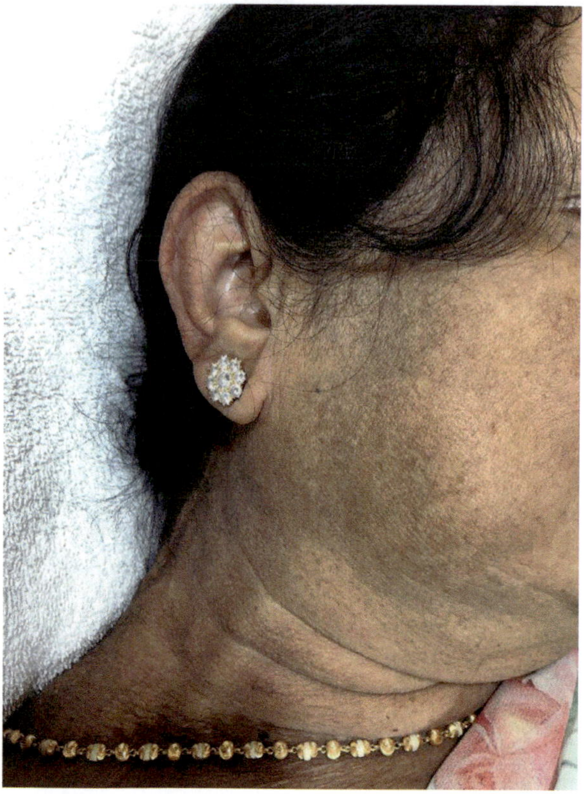

Fig. 6.4 Acanthosis nigricans

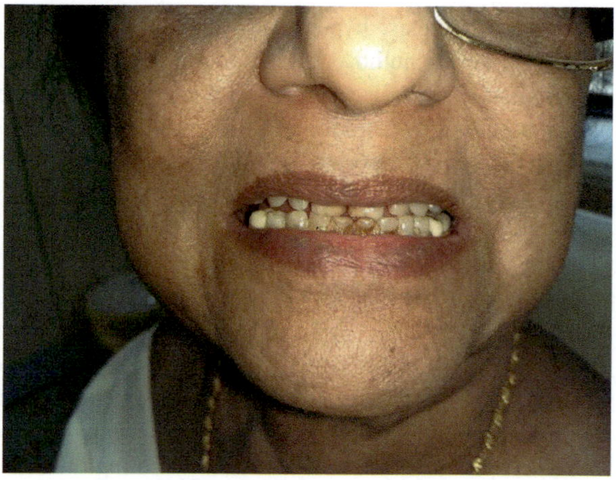

Fig. 6.5 Iron stains in teeth

The awareness for neurological examination needs to be stressed. There is increasing evidence suggesting that the neurological complications after bariatric surgery are not as uncommon as thought earlier [17]. The examination should involve evaluation of mental status, sensorimotor functions, position and vibration sense and eye movements to pick up optic neuropathy, encephalopathy, radiculopathy, myelopathy, peripheral neuropathy, and myopathy. This also implies that the kit to perform a neurological examination should be available in the bariatric OPD. Picking up the subtle signs and early referral/treatment should be the goal rather than waiting for full-blown neuropathies that take weeks to months to reverse, with frequent permanent residual damages.

Key Points

- *Follow-up visits are the appropriate station for picking up post-bariatric nutritional and metabolic problems. A clinician (bariatric surgeon, nutritionist, psychologist, and a physician) must have the necessary knowledge to enable him or her to look for the relevant symptoms and signs.*
- *Clinical evaluation should include detailed history regarding weight loss, comorbidity resolution, gastrointestinal symptoms, neurological symptoms, pain and weakness. Examination should be head to toe. Anthropometric examination should include body composition analysis. Blood pressure measurement should be in both supine and erect positions. Neurological examination should include a complete sensorimotor and cranial nerve evaluation. Therefore, a neurological examination kit should always be available in a bariatric clinic.*
- *Many problems cannot be confirmed biochemically in the lab, therefore the importance of clinical examination cannot be overemphasized.*
- *Complications can be prevented if we can pick up and treat the subtle signs before their full-blown clinical state sets in. Centres should have their own standard checklists for clinical evaluation.*
- *Rarely, some cases of neuropathy, refractory anaemia, fractures, leg drop, cardiomyopathy, liver failure, skin lesions, pigmentation, psychiatric disturbances remain unexplained signifying the lack of knowledge on the subject. A complete clinical evaluation and documentation should be the appropriate starting point to take this science forward.*

Case Examples

Case 1a

A 22-year-old girl with BMI 48 and no other coexisting comorbidities apart from a feeling of low self-esteem, presents 6 months after bariatric surgery with hair loss from the scalp that is very worrisome to her. How would you approach the case? (Fig. 6.6).

Answer

- *Reassurance*
- *Ensure compliance to diet and supplements*

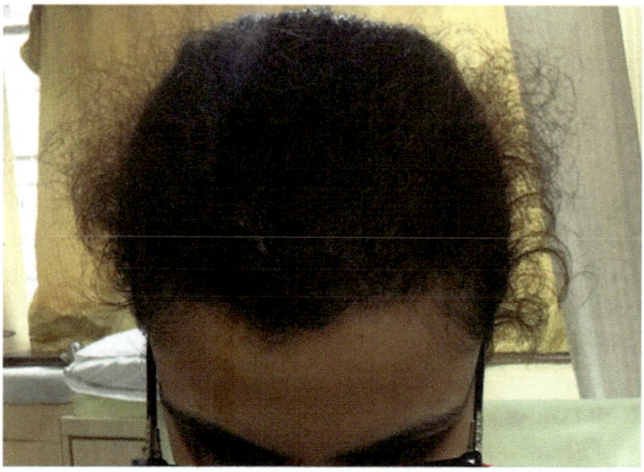

Fig. 6.6 Alopecia

Comments

Alopecia after bariatric surgery is common and parallels the weight loss curve. It is usually observed between 3 and 9 months after surgery following which the hair fall usually stops and returns to normal within months.

However, it is important to ensure compliance with a high protein diet and nutritional supplements during this period.

Case 1b

The same patient returns at 2 years with persistent alopecia. What will you do now?

Answer

Ask for

1. *Dietary recall*
2. *Compliance with supplements*

Check

1. *Albumin*
2. *Iron, ferritin, transferrin, TSAT*
3. *Zinc*

Give

1. *Iron and zinc supplements*
2. *Protein supplements—whey/casein*
3. *Essential fatty acids—nuts/supplements*

Comments

Alopecia at 2 years is a matter of concern. Patients are distressed and are unhappy with the situation. Protein and iron deficiencies are the commonest known causes of the condition. Evidence in the literature suggests that there is an association between low iron+zinc levels with alopecia but not with individual levels [16].

Biotin, though a popular supplement used for the condition, does not have any convincing evidence in its favour [17].

Prevention seems to be the most important management strategy. Ensuring compliance with a good diet and supplements, especially in the initial phase of follow-up after bariatric surgery is vital.

Case 2

A 45-year-old lady with a history of RYGB done 7 years ago presented with a sudden onset back pain after having to lift a vacuum cleaner from her closet. AP and lateral radiographs advised by the family physician showed a compressed fracture at L2 (Fig. 6.7). On asking further, she gave the history of stopping her multivitamin supplements after taking them irregularly for 3 years.

How would you approach the case?

Answer

The differential diagnoses are:

1. *Bone loss secondary to vitamin D and calcium deficiency*
2. Spinal disease such as *Tuberculosis*

Check

1. *Urinary calcium*
2. *Serum Vitamin D*
3. *Alkaline phosphatase*
4. *Serum PTH*
5. *DEXA scan*

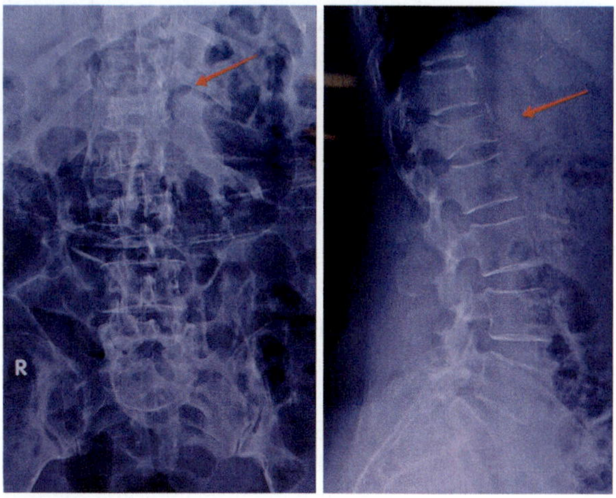

Fig. 6.7 Compression fracture due to osteoporosis (Pic credits: Dr. Keshav Goel, Sr. Consultant, Dept. of Orthopaedics, Park Hospital Karnal)

Bone density test revealed a spine T score of −2.63 and hip T score of −2.09. Serum PTH levels, urinary calcium levels and bone alkaline phosphatase were raised. Serum vitamin D was 4.63 ng/dL.

What is the diagnosis?

Answer

It is an osteoporotic fracture secondary to calcium and vitamin D deficiency compounded by perimenopausal status and non-compliance to recommended supplementation.

Would you do serum calcium levels?

Answer

Serum calcium level, although an indicator, is a poor indicator of total body calcium and a poor predictor of bone health.

How would you treat this patient?

Answer

Orthopaedic referral

Vitamin D supplementation up to 6000 IU/day, or 50,000 IU 1–3 times a week till levels become normal.

1200–1500 mg/day of calcium supplementation

Case 3

A 60-year-old gentleman who had a BPD-DS done 2.5 years ago presents in the OPD. He has lost 80 kg from his preoperative 150 kg weight and is still losing (Fig. 6.8). The nutritionist had seen him at 2 years and was happy with the progress and the fact that he had reached his ideal body weight. At 2.5 years, he presented to the clinic with weakness, inability to walk, swollen legs, exertional breathlessness and passing foul-smelling, oily stools. How would you approach the case?

Answer

This is a case of protein–energy malnutrition post-bariatric surgery. The alarm should have been raised when the patient showed 100% EWL or muscle mass was more than 20% of weight loss in the follow-up. The patient should be admitted, nutritional parameters assessed and replacement to be instituted immediately. The

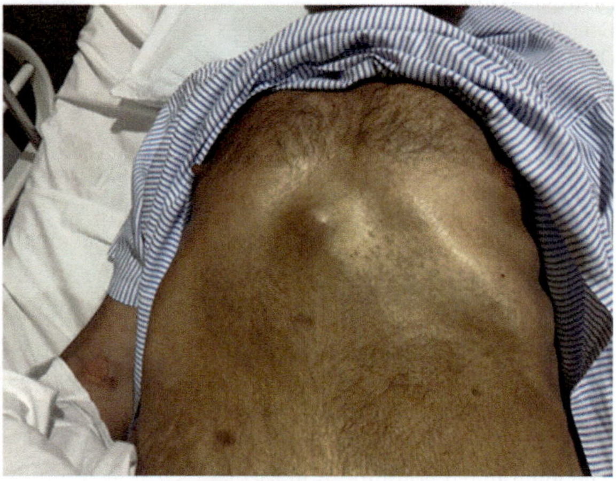

Fig. 6.8 Cachexia in a malnourished post-bariatric patient

patient may require hydration, electrolyte correction, blood transfusion, enteral and parenteral nutritional supplementation and multivitamin infusion. This should be monitored till the patient shows signs of recovery. A bariatric surgeon should be consulted for considering a reversal of the procedure and restoration of normal gastrointestinal anatomy.

The patient was actively treated with nutritional support. He developed acute respiratory distress, neurological symptoms and cardiac arrhythmia at the end of the second week. What may be the cause of the condition?

Answer

This may be a case of Refeeding syndrome. This happens if the calorie replacement is too rapid in a malnourished patient. In order to create ATP, certain minerals like potassium, phosphate and magnesium can decrease substantially in the serum leading to cardiorespiratory and neurological symptoms.

The treatment is to increase the caloric replacement slowly with the monitoring and correction of these electrolytes.

Case 4

A 32-year-old vegetarian, lady with BMI 42 Kg/m^2 and infertility underwent a Roux en Y Gastric Bypass. She became pregnant a year later against medical advice. She was not compliant with nutritional supplementation.

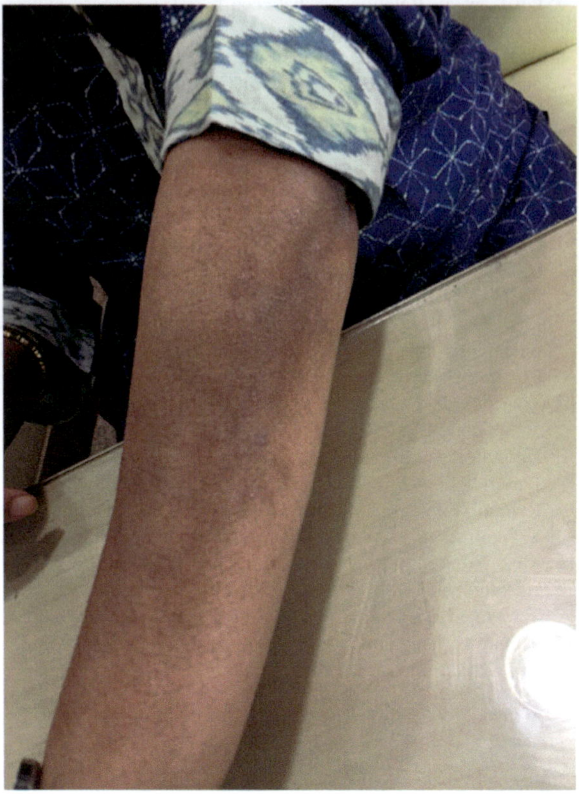

Fig. 6.9 Phrynoderma

Three months after childbirth, she presented with weakness. On examination, she had this skin lesion (Fig. 6.9). What is this?

Answer

This is phrynoderma, a hyperkeratotic papular skin lesion usually observed in the extensor aspect of limbs, shoulders and buttocks. It represents severe malnutrition with a strong association with deficiencies of vitamins E, B, A and essential fatty acids. These patients need aggressive nutritional supplementation.

References

1. Lammers WJ, van Tilburg AJ, Apers JA, Wiebolt J. Liver failure caused by prolonged state of malnutrition following bariatric surgery. World J Hepatol. 2018;10(3):396–9.
2. Goodman JC. Neurological complications of bariatric surgery. Curr Neurol Neurosci Rep. 2015;15(12):79.
3. Aills L, Blankenship J, Buffington C, Furtado M, Parrott J. ASMBS Allied Health Nutritional Guidelines for the surgical weight loss patient. Surg Obes Relat Dis. 2008;4(5 Suppl):S73–108.
4. King WC, et al. Alcohol and other substance use after bariatric surgery: prospective evidence from a U.S. multicenter cohort study. Surg Obes Relat Dis. 2017;13(8):1392–402.
5. Müller A, Hase C, Pommnitz M, de Zwaan M. Depression and suicide after bariatric surgery. Curr Psychiatry Rep. 2019;21(9). Current Medicine Group LLC 1.
6. Thivel D, Brakonieki K, Duche P, Béatrice M, Yves B, Laferrère B. Surgical weight loss: impact on energy expenditure. Obes Surg. 2013;23(2):255–66.
7. Gu L, et al. Relationship between bariatric surgery and gastroesophageal reflux disease: a systematic review and meta-analysis. Obes Surg. 2019;29:4105–13.
8. Ablett AD, Boyle BR, Avenell A. Fractures in adults after weight loss from bariatric surgery and weight management programs for obesity: systematic review and meta-analysis. Obes Surg. 2019;29(4):1327–42.
9. Billakanty SR, et al. New-onset orthostatic intolerance following bariatric surgery. Pacing Clin Electrophysiol. 2008;31(7):884–8.
10. Voican CS, et al. Predictive score of sarcopenia occurrence one year after bariatric surgery in severely obese patients. PLoS One. 2018;13(5).
11. Cardeal MA, Faria SL, Faria OP, Facundes M, Ito MK. Diet-induced thermogenesis in postoperative Roux-en-Y gastric bypass patients with weight regain. Surg Obes Relat Dis. 2016;12(5):1098–107.
12. Sherf Dagan S, Tovim TB, Keidar A, Raziel A, Shibolet O, Zelber-Sagi S. Inadequate protein intake after laparoscopic sleeve gastrectomy surgery is associated with a greater fat free mass loss. Surg Obes Relat Dis. 2017;13(1):101–9.
13. Zouridaki E, Papafragkaki D-K, Papafragkakis H, Aroni K, Stavropoulos P. Dermatological complications after bariatric surgery: report of two cases and review of the literature. Dermatology. 2014;228(1):5–9.
14. Jensen P, Skov L. Psoriasis and obesity. Dermatology. 2017;232(6):633–9.
15. Romero-Talamás H, Aminian A, Corcelles R, Fernandez AP, Schauer PR, Brethauer S. Psoriasis improvement after bariatric surgery. Surg Obes Relat Dis. 2014;10(6):1155–9.
16. Ruiz-Tovar J, et al. Hair loss in females after sleeve gastrectomy: predictive value of serum zinc and iron levels. Am Surg. 2014;80(5):466–71.
17. Soleymani T, Lo Sicco K, Shapiro J. The infatuation with biotin supplementation: is there truth behind its rising popularity? A comparative analysis of clinical efficacy versus social popularity. J Drugs Dermatol. 2017;16(5):496–500.

Gastrointestinal Complications of Bariatric Surgery

7

Sandeep Agarwal, Vitish Singla, Devender Singh, Amit Bhambri, and Prasanna Ramana Arumugasamy

The stomach is a slave that must accept everything that is given to it, but which avenges wrongs as slyly as does the slave.

—Émile Souvestre

7.1 Introduction

Prevalence of bariatric surgery is on increasing trend all over the globe due to sustainable weight loss, improvement in quality of life, and comorbidity resolution. Therapies for obesity can be divided broadly into four groups: behavioural (primarily diet and exercise), drugs, devices (intragastric balloon), and surgery. The complications of bariatric surgery include gastrointestinal complications, venous thromboembolism, and nutritional complications. The overall complication rate is low ranging from 0.29% to 0.78% [1], which is similar to most elective abdominal operations like cholecystectomy. The reported common early complications include leak, bleeding, obstruction, venous thromboembolism while the late complications include internal hernias, dumping, nutritional deficiencies, and gastro-oesophageal reflux. In this chapter, we will discuss the common metabolic GI complications specific to each procedure. Hormonal and physiological changes following bariatric surgery are covered in another chapter and therefore, will not be discussed here. The delayed and long-term surgical complications like Internal hernia, obstruction, stenosis etc. will also not be discussed as the focus of the book is on metabolic complications. Additionally, liver complications, nesidioblastosis, and nutritional complications have been discussed in other chapters and will not be discussed.

S. Agarwal (✉) · V. Singla · D. Singh · A. Bhambri · P. R. Arumugasamy
Department of Surgical Disciplines, All India Institute of Medical Sciences (AIIMS), New Delhi, India

A. G. Bhasker et al. (eds.), *Management of Nutritional and Metabolic Complications of Bariatric Surgery*,
https://doi.org/10.1007/978-981-33-4702-1_7

Table 7.1 Gastrointestinal and Metabolic complications of Bariatric surgical procedures

	AGB	SG	RYGB	OAGB
Nutritional complications	+	+	+	+
Reflux	+	+	–	+
Nausea	+	+	+	+
Vomiting	+	+	+	+
Marginal ulcers	–	–	+	+
Oesophagitis	+	+	+	–
Barrett's oesophagus	+	+	+	–
Diarrhoea	–	+	+	+
Steatorrhoea	–	–	+	+
Constipation	+	+	+	+
Early dumping syndrome	–	+	+	+
Late dumping	–	–	+	+
SIBO	–	–	+	+
Liver dysfunction	–	–	+	+
Gallstones	+	+	+	+
Alteration in taste	–	+	+	+
De novo food intolerance	–	+	+	+
Nesidioblastosis	–	–	+	+

AGB Adjustable Gastric Banding, *SG* Sleeve Gastrectomy, *RYGB* Roux-en-Y Gastric Bypass, *OAGB* One Anastamoses Gastric Bypass, *SIBO* small intestinal bacterial over-growth

The metabolic GI complications after bariatric surgery are summarised in Table 7.1.

Table 7.1 shows the commonly seen metabolic complications after various bariatric surgeries.

7.2 Reflux

The prevalence of gastroesophageal reflux disease (GERD) is 10–20% in normal population as compared to 37–72% in patients with obesity [2]. In general, weight loss brings about a decrease in intra-abdominal pressure leading to a decrease in GERD. However, after bariatric surgery, depending on the procedure patients can be at an increased or decreased risk of GERD.

7.2.1 Adjustable Gastric Band

Functional or anatomical obstruction due to band can lead to oesophageal dilatation and ineffective motility. This can happen either because of overtight bands or large bites of food being stuck up in the pouch above the band. Patients with oesophageal dilatation present with reflux-like symptoms [3]. These symptoms require band deflation/band removal and conversion to a sleeve gastrectomy or a Roux en Y gastric bypass (RYGB) to maintain weight loss.

7.2.2 Laparoscopic Sleeve Gastrectomy (SG)

GERD is known to decrease following RYGB, but its incidence after SG is controversial. In a systematic review, four studies showed an increase in incidence of GERD and seven studies found a decrease in GERD postoperatively [4]. At our institute, we found that GERD improved following SG as assessed by symptom questionnaire as well as endoscopy. De novo GERD was seen in some patients on scintigraphy, however, that might not be pathologically significant because of a reduction in total acid amount after sleeve [5]. Some patients have an improvement in their reflux symptoms. Possible mechanisms include accelerated gastric emptying, decreased total acid production, and reduced intrabdominal pressure due to weight loss. In a recent metanalysis, there was a slight trend towards an increase in GERD but a definitive conclusion could not be made. The results of oesophageal function tests and 24 h pH monitoring also yielded conflicting results in different studies [2]. There are various mechanisms that might be responsible for de novo GERD after SG. In a single centre study a triphasic response to GERD after SG was observed [6]. In the first year after SG, reflux increased probably due to disruption of angle of His, incompetence of sling fibres at cardia (these fibres are transacted during LSG), decreased tone of lower oesophageal sphincter, decreased distensibility of stomach, and increased intragastric pressure. Second year onwards, the reflux is decreased due to weight loss and a decrease in intra-abdominal pressure. In another paper, the same authors have [7] demonstrated a 22% incidence of post-SG GERD after 1 year, which came down to 3% after 3 years. However, with time, a neofundus is formed. Neo fundus occurs when a part of fundus is left behind at the level of left crus, which results in a conical sleeve with narrowing at mid-body region leading to weight regain and a mid-stomach functional stenosis leading to a second peak in GERD [6]. This can predispose the patients undergoing SG to develop GERD [8]. Other anatomical factors like twisting of sleeve causing a functional obstruction as well as incisural stenosis can cause reflux. We strongly believe that a missed hiatal hernia might be an important factor for persistence/development of symptoms of GERD (Fig. 7.1).

Despite this, not all patients develop GERD following sleeve. A common notion that sleeve leads to worsening of reflux should be considered with caution. Precautions such as avoiding narrowing at incisura, not leaving any fundus behind the left crus, and selecting proper bougie size should be undertaken during surgery. A low threshold should be maintained for dissection of hiatus on suspicion during laparoscopy and for repairing any concomitant hiatal hernia. There is also a need to standardize the technique of sleeve gastrectomy to decrease the incidence of GERD following it.

Most patients who develop GERD can be managed by dietary modification, proton pump inhibitors (PPIs), and prokinetics. Endoscopy and a contrast study should be done to rule out mechanical causes or a missed hiatal hernia. Patients with symptoms unresponsive to medical management as well as severe nocturnal symptoms require conversion to RYGB. In our experience post-SG, we have encountered

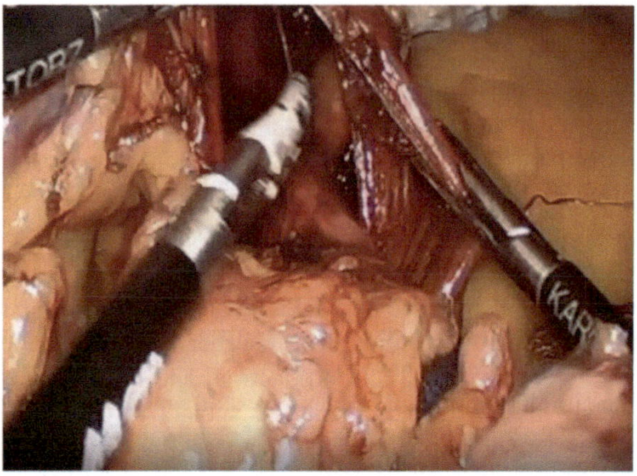

Fig. 7.1 Hiatal hernia after dissection which was missed initially

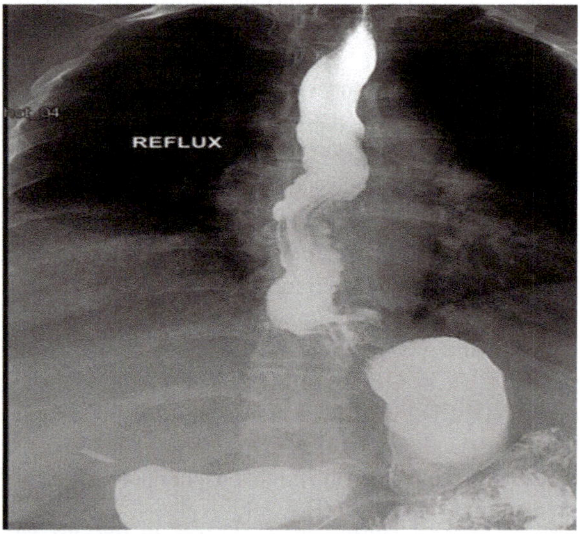

Fig. 7.2 Reflux after LSG

GERD (Fig. 7.2) due to remnant fundus which got twisted, twisting of sleeve in mid-part due to dense adhesions with the left lobe, and hiatus hernia with excessive posterior fundus. All these patients were converted to RYGB.

7.2.3 One Anastomosis Gastric Bypass (OAGB)

One anastomosis gastric bypass is usually associated with biliary reflux. It is defined as the presence of bile in the gastric pouch and into the oesophagus with/without symptoms of gastroesophageal reflux disease (GERD). The occurrence of GERD correlates with a gastric pouch shorter than 9 cm in length and with the presence of preoperative GERD [9]. Usually, 10–12 cm length of the gastric pouch is recommended [9]. It can be identified by clinical findings through validated questionnaires [10]. In a study by Tolone et al., 15 patients underwent oesophagogastric junction function evaluation by endoscopy, 24 h pH-impedance monitoring, and high-resolution impedance manometry performed both preoperatively and 1 year after surgery. No patient reported heartburn or de novo regurgitation postoperatively. On endoscopy at 1 year no patient had oesophagitis or biliary gastritis. There was no difference in manometric features and patterns after surgery, whereas gastroesophageal pressure gradient (GEPG) and intragastric pressures (IGP) were statistically diminished [11]. On the contrary, laparoscopic sleeve gastrectomy (SG) showed a high-pressure gastric pouch with gastroesophageal reflux [12].

The correct anatomical configuration including creating a long and narrow pouch without any twist at gastrojejunostomy site is necessary. In addition, we take an anti-reflux stitch at top of gastrojejunostomy site to align anastomosis vertically and hence preventing bile reflux. Gastric and/or oesophageal symptomatic bile reflux is quite rare (0–0.7%) in OAGB [13, 14]. Chevallier et al. had reported that seven patients following OAGB presented with intractable biliary reflux. They were re-operated after a mean of 23 months when the mean BMI was 25.7 kg/m^2. All patients got cured of intractable bile reflux after conversion to a Roux en Y gastric bypass [13].

Dietary and lifestyle modifications, PPIs (40 mg twice a day for 6 months), and sucralfate (1 g before every meal and before bedtime for 3 months, followed by 1 g before bedtime for another 3 months) [15]. If conservative treatment fails, a revisional surgery is advised with conversion to either RYGB or Braun side-to-side anastomosis between the afferent and the efferent limb about 15–20 cm beyond the gastro-jejunal anastomosis [16].

7.3 Barret's Oesophagus and Adenocarcinoma

Reflux can further complicate the long-term course of sleeve gastrectomy patients as it can predispose to Barrett's oesophagus (BE). Limited literature is available in regard to the incidence of BE in post-sleeve gastrectomy patients. The incidence of BE has been reported with a wide range, varying from 1.2% to 17.2% in recent studies [17–19]. However, the authors did not follow the strict criteria to take a biopsy at least 1 cm above the gastro-oesophageal junction, which might have resulted in a falsely positive Barrett's. A biopsy within 1 cm of he gastroesophageal junction can have normal gastric mucosa, which is misinterpreted as BE [20].

Since BE is a known premalignant condition, it is imperative that adequate studies should be performed to formulate guidelines for its screening and treatment. There have been three case reports of oesophageal adenocarcinoma following SG. However, preoperative endoscopy was performed only in one of them. [21–23]. In another case report oesophageal adenocarcinoma developed on a pre-existing BE (diagnosed on preoperative endoscopy), 3 years after SG [24]. These are rare case reports in literature considering the number of sleeve gastrectomies performed all over the globe. Moreover, preoperative endoscopy was done only in one patient and other two cases might already have an underlying dysplasia. De novo/worsening of GERD may be avoided by proper preoperative evaluation of reflux symptoms and intraoperative precautions, keeping in mind that the benefits of sleeve gastrectomy far outweigh its potential complications.

After OAGB, there are serious concerns not only regarding the symptomatic biliary reflux (BR) into the stomach and the oesophagus [25, 26], but also the increased risk of malignancy after OAGB [27, 28]. BR is known to cause histological changes in oesophagus and gastric pouch, secondary to acute and chronic inflammatory changes in oesophageal and gastric mucosa. These changes might progress to premalignant condition, Barrett's oesophagus [29]. Under the influence of constant BR, Barrett's oesophagus can progress to an incomplete intestinal metaplasia (type III) instead of complete intestinal metaplasia (type I), which has a higher risk of gastro-oesophageal cancer development [30]. We recently reported probably the first case of adenocarcinoma of oesophagus involving gastro-oesophageal junction following OAGB within 2 years of surgery [31] (Fig. 7.3).

7.4 Nausea and Vomiting

Nausea and vomiting after SG can be due to anatomical or functional causes. The most common site for anatomical stenosis after SG is at the incisura angularis. The common causes being inappropriate placement of bougie and oversewing of staple line, especially when it is done without a bougie in place. Functional stenosis can also occur due to a twist in the sleeve. Twisting usually occurs due to excessive traction on anterior/posterior wall of the stomach when firing the stapler. The twist can be localized at an area between body and antrum or along the full length of sleeve resulting in a spiral sleeve. Diagnosis of anatomical stenosis can be made by endoscopy; however, the diagnosis of functional stenosis is difficult as the endoscope can easily negotiate the twist. CT scan with three-dimensional reconstruction is best to diagnose spiral sleeve [32]. Endoscopic balloon dilatation is the first line of

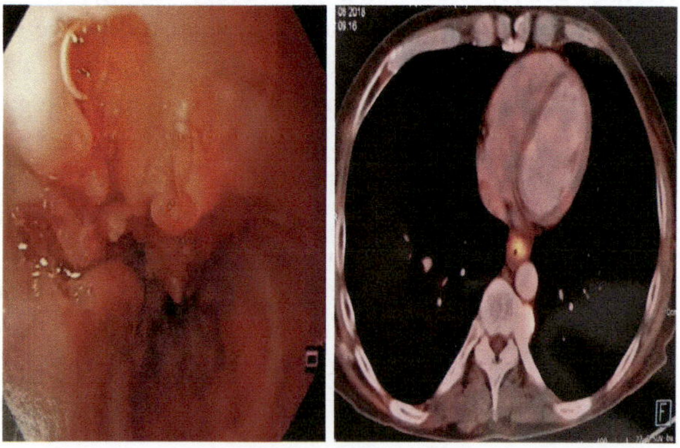

Fig. 7.3 Endoscopic image of growth in lower oesophagus (left) and Positron Emission Tomography (PET) showing increased uptake in lower oesophageal growth (right)

Table 7.2 Grades of anastomotic stricture on the basis of endoscopy

Grade: I	Mild stenosis, which allows a 10.5-mm endoscope to pass
Grade: II	Moderate stenosis, which allows an 8.5-mm paediatric endoscope to pass
Grade: III	Severe stenosis, which allows only guide-wire to pass
Grade: IV	Complete obstruction, which is non-traversable

treatment requiring multiple sessions over several weeks. Patients are kept on a liquid diet, ensuring adequate calorie intake and nutritional supplementation. Failure of endoscopic treatment and long segment stricture requires conversion to RYGB, which is considered the gold standard for this complication.

Anastomotic Stricture An anastomotic stricture post-RYGB can happen due to anastomotic tension, ischemia, and subclinical leaks. Patients with stricture usually present with dysphagia, nausea, vomiting, and painless post-prandial regurgitation. Upper gastro-intestinal endoscopy (UGIE) is required for confirmation of diagnosis. Table 7.2 gives a classification for the degree of anastomotic stricture.

Treatment includes endoscopic balloon dilatation to at least 15 mm in the first sitting to decrease the recurrence rate by the use of through-the-scope (TTS) balloon catheters [33]. They lead to circumferential dilatation and gradual expansion of stenosis and thus prevent excess pain and minimizes the risk of perforation. In 95% of cases, obstruction is relieved by two separate sessions of dilatation [34], however, re-stenosis may occur in 3% of these patients [35]. Patients not responding to endoscopic therapy even after four sessions of balloon dilatation are candidates for surgical revision of Gastro-jejunal (G-J) anastomosis, which is required in less than 0.4% cases [36].

To prevent stenosis after OAGB, an anastomotic size of ≥2.5 cm is highly recommended. We perform an anastomotic size of 5–6 cm. This complication can be managed by pneumatic endoscopic dilations successfully or conversion to laparoscopic Roux en Y gastric bypass if endoscopic dilatations fail.

7.5 Marginal Ulcers

Marginal ulcer is characterized by the development of mucosal erosion at the gastrojejunal (G-J) anastomosis, usually on the jejunal side as it does not have the acid buffering capacity of the duodenum and hence becomes vulnerable to ulcer formation [37]. Reported incidence of marginal ulcers is variable, ranging from 0.6 to 16% [38, 39] after RYGB. Marginal ulcer rate is lower following OAGB (0.5–4%) [40]. In a systematic review of 11 studies (1 RCT, 5 prospective, 5 retrospectives) were analyzed; of which 1174 patients underwent RYGB and 767 patients underwent MGB-OAGB. Marginal ulcer was reported in 7/362 (1.9%) of RYGB and 15/523 (2.86%) of MGB-OAGB patients [41]. In our own experience, marginal ulcer was detected in 4/46 (13.04%) of OAGB patients all of them being asymptomatic. So routine surveillance by endoscopy may be recommended in all OAGB patients. Marginal ulcer rates and need for surgical revisions after OAGB in some large series and long-term follow-up papers are shown in Table 7.3.

The actual incidence is much higher than reported, as documented ulcers represent only those that are diagnosed on endoscopy, but many are treated medically based on symptoms without undergoing any endoscopic evaluation. Risk factors for development of marginal ulcer include smoking (causes mucosal ischaemia), use of NSAIDS (causes mucosal breakdown) and risk decreases with the use of proton pump inhibitors. The exact aetiology of marginal ulcers is not clear, but the possible mechanisms proposed are increased acid production in an oversized pouch, ischaemia of the pouch due to tension on roux limb, presence of *Helicobacter pylori* infection, staple line disruption, and presence of suture material within the pouch [42]. The use of absorbable suture instead of permanent suture was found to significantly reduce the incidence of postoperative marginal ulcers [43] (Fig. 7.4).

7.5.1 Diagnosis

Patients with marginal ulcers usually present with abdominal pain (especially post prandial), nausea and vomiting, and in extreme cases with haematemesis or malena

Table 7.3 Incidence of marginal ulcers after OAGB

OAGB series	Percentage of marginal ulcer reported (%)	Surgical revisions
Musella et al. n-974	1.43%	4
Carbajo et al. n-1200	0.5%	0
Chevallier et al. n-1000	2%	2
Lee et al. n-1163	NA	7
Kular et al. n-1054	0.47%	0

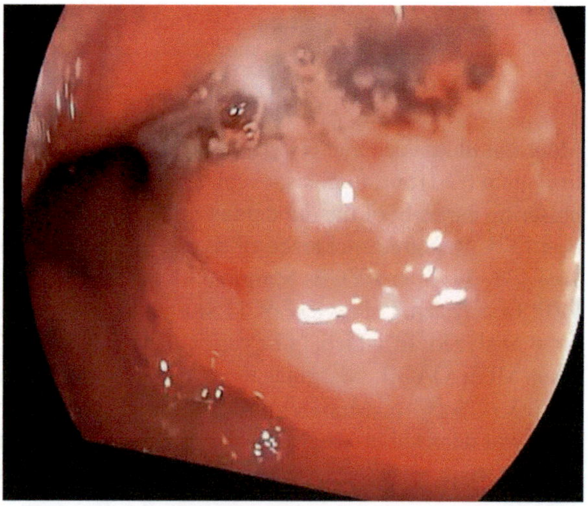

Fig. 7.4 Endoscopic image of marginal ulcer after 1 year of RYGB. Ulcer is at 2 o'clock position

or even perforation [44]. Patel et al. reported abdominal pain (66.6%) as the most common presentation of marginal ulcers [45]. Upper GI endoscopy is the diagnostic study of choice and biopsies should be taken to evaluate for *H. pylori* during same sitting [46].

7.5.2 Management

Treatment depends on the aetiology of marginal ulcer (Fig. 7.5). For smokers, smoking cessation is imperative and in patients on NSAIDs, they should be stopped. The use of proton pump inhibitors in the immediate post-operative period, for the first 3–6 months, is critical from a prophylactic perspective. However, there is no consensus about the exact duration of usage. In the literature duration of post-operative PPI, administration ranges from 30 days to 2 years [47]. In our practice, we prescribe PPI for 3 months and then subsequently on the basis of symptoms. For a patient with documented marginal ulcer either by symptoms or on endoscopy, initial treatment includes the use of proton pump inhibitor and sucralfate suspension (1 g oral liquid/6 h) for a period of 3–6 months. For comprehensive therapy, urea breath test, serology, or endoscopic biopsies should be performed for *H. pylori* and if found to be positive medical eradication should be considered using two antibiotics and a proton pump inhibitor popularly known as triple regimen [48]. If ulcer is left untreated or persists despite medical treatment, it may lead to stricture formation and ultimately gastric outlet obstruction, which may require multiple endoscopic dilatations [49]. Thus, it is of utmost importance to assess whether the ulcer is responding to medical treatment and has evidence of healing on repeat endoscopy.

Surgical intervention is required in case of failure of medical management or if ulcer leads to perforation. The operative approach includes excision of the ulcer and revision of the gastrojejunal (G-J) anastomosis, reduction in the size of gastric pouch if it is oversized. If the ulcer is associated with suture material, it should be

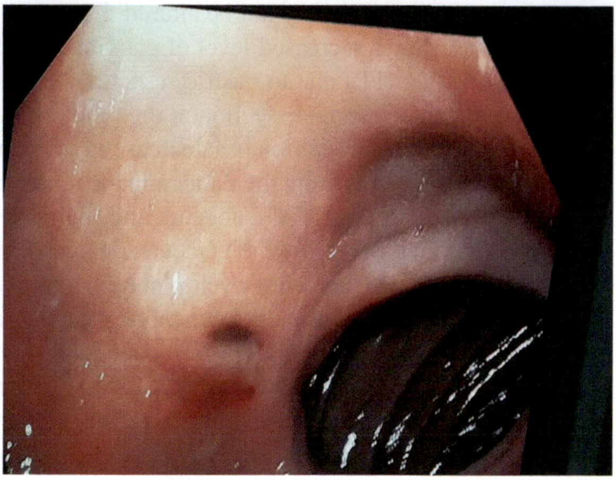

Fig. 7.5 Marginal ulcer in a female, non-smoker asymptomatic post MGB-OAGB patient

removed and the roux limb should be mobilized if there is excess tension leading to mucosal ischaemia [50].

7.6 Diarrhoea

Up to 75% of patients report a change in bowel habits after bariatric surgery. Diarrhoea is more common after bypass procedures and is more predominant when there is a short common absorptive channel. This accounts for the more predominance of diarrhoea in distal RYGB as compared to proximal RYGB and Bilio-Pancreatic Diversion (BPD) with a short common absorptive channel.

Diarrhoea can be secondary to many causes—decreased intestinal transit time, dumping syndrome, and small intestinal bacterial over-growth (SIBO.) Rare cases of gastro-colic fistulas have also been implicated in diarrhoea.

Most bypass patients report episodes of 3–4 bowel motions 2–3 times a year. Most of these episodes subside with diet alteration, fibre supplements, and anti-motility medications. If associated with steatorrhoea, pancreatic enzyme supplementation should be given. Associated symptoms like palpitation, dizziness, fainting should prompt for evaluation of dumping syndrome and should be treated with small non-sugary meals with a high-fibre content and avoidance of water with food. Non-responding foul-smelling diarrhoea should arise the suspicion of SIBO and should be treated accordingly.

7.7 Steatorrhoea and Pancreatic Exocrine Insufficiency

Steatorrhoea can occur both after SG and bypass surgeries. The prevalence after proximal and distal RYGB is around 19% and 48%, respectively. The causes include changes in the food and caloric content, an altered pancreatic response to the food, shorter time of contact of chyme with food due to bypass, degradation of the enzymes in Bilio-Pancreatic (BP) limb due to absence of food. The actual secretion from the pancreas may or may not be altered. Factors primarily decreasing the pancreatic output include decreased level of gastrin, cholecystokinin (CCK), and pancreatic polypeptide (PP) due to gastric resection, exclusion of the duodenum, and vagal nerve damage during dissection at the time of pouch formation. The primary stimulus for pancreatic secretion is a decrease in duodenal pH post meals. Decrease in the amount of acid reaching the duodenum de to decreased stomach volume (SG) and bypass of duodenum (RYGB) occurs after bariatric surgery. Additionally, ileal infusion of nutrients as in distal RYGB can decrease the pancreatic enzyme secretion. Rarely, some patients who develop non-insulinoma pancreatic hypersecretion (nesidioblastosis) and are forced to undergo pancreatectomy can develop primary pancreatic insufficiency. Symptoms of pancreatic insufficiency include steatorrhoea, borborygmi post meals, and weight loss. However, these symptoms are non-specific in a post-bariatric patient. Pancreatic insufficiency is defined by symptoms and faecal pancreatic elastase-1 (PE-1) <200 μg/g stool or a faecal PE-1 between 200 and 500 μg/g stool and the patient has benefited from pancreatic enzyme replacement [51]. Direct stimulation testing can be done by intubating the duodenum and measuring the pancreatic response to CCK or secretin. This is technically not feasible in RYGB patients. Measurement of faecal elastase is easier, however, patients with a normal value can still suffer from pancreatic insufficiency due to indirect factors discussed above. Regardless, pancreatic enzyme replacement therapy is the treatment of choice. It is important to remove the acid protective coating over the supplements for better absorption as the acid levels in stomach post-bariatric surgery are usually lower [52].

7.8 Constipation

Bowel habits after bariatric surgery is an important issue for the patient and affect their quality of life. Many obese individuals have a pre-existing bowel disturbance. In a systematic review, it was observed that the rates of faecal incontinence and diarrhoea were higher in obese patients compared with non-obese patients. Constipation rates were similar [53].

Bariatric and metabolic surgeries have been claimed to have a diverse effect on bowel habits. Some authors have reported higher prevalence of diarrhoea after RYGB and Bilio-Pancreatic Diversion-Duodenal Switch (BPD-DS) and constipation after adjustable gastric band (AGB) and sleeve gastrectomy [54, 55].

Other authors on the other hand have reported resolution of loose stools after RYGB [56].

These contrasting findings may be the result of heterogeneity of patient cohort, food habits, assessment tools, and procedure variations. Afshar et al. [57] studied bariatric patients prior and after their surgery with a validated food frequency questionnaire and 7 day Bristol Stool Form Scale that has been validated and found to correlate with whole gut transit time. RYGB, sleeve gastrectomy, and intra-gastric balloon were assessed. They found that the frequency of stool decreased and stools were more formed at a median follow-up of 6.4 months after surgery.

This increased rate of constipation after bariatric surgery may be explained by the decrease in dietary fibre [57] and increase in GI hormones such as Glucagon-Like Peptide-1 (GLP-1) and Polypeptide YY (PYY) seen as an effect after surgery. Based on the literature and our own experience, we may opine that constipation is a frequent complaint of the bariatric patient. Clinicians involved in the care of bariatric patients should be aware of these findings and treat constipation as and when required with laxatives. They should also encourage patients to increase the fibre content in the diet. Paying attention to these details may go a long way in improving the quality of life of these patients.

7.9 Dumping Syndrome

Dumping syndrome was first described by Hertz in 1913, correlating the symptoms with accelerated gastric emptying and the term "dumping" was coined by Mix in 1922 [58]. It is the most common syndrome that may occur after any form of gastrectomy or damage to vagus nerve during upper gastrointestinal (GI) surgeries. Dumping may occur in sleeve gastrectomy but is more common after gastric bypass surgery and may cause both gastrointestinal and autonomic symptoms. It occurs when hyperosmolar undigested food gets directly "dumped" from stomach pouch into the small intestine without being properly digested. Post RYGB, the prevalence of dumping syndrome is around 13% with a median follow-up of 4.5 years and is more commonly found in young females [59]. There are two types of dumping syndrome: Early and Late.

Early dumping occurs 10–30 min after a meal and is characterized by gastrointestinal symptoms such as nausea, vomiting, bloating, cramping abdominal pain, diarrhoea, dizziness, and fatigue. It is caused by shift of osmotically driven fluid from the blood vessels to the gastrointestinal lumen. Late dumping occurs 1–3 h after a meal and is characterized by autonomic symptoms like weakness, sweating, and dizziness due to rebound hypoglycaemia when insulin surge overcompensates for the glucose load delivered to the portal circulation, and the blood glucose level falls precipitously. Dumping syndrome leads to desired behaviour modification post RYGB that prevents individuals from consuming calorie-dense foods and thereby contributes to weight loss [60].

7.9.1 Diagnosis

a) History and clinical examination: Importance of proper history and evaluation of signs and symptoms cannot be overlooked and it gives the first clue to the diagnosis.
b) Oral glucose tolerance test: 50 g of glucose is given in water. Blood sugar, haematocrit, and the pulse are then recorded at 30 min intervals for 3 h. The diagnosis is confirmed if there is initial hyperglycaemia followed by hypoglycaemia (<60 g/dl or 3.33 mmol/l) [61].
c) Gastric emptying test: A radiotracer material is added to food to assess how quickly food moves through the stomach.
d) Diagnostic Questionnaires: Sigstad Score Scale (Table 7.4) and the Arts Dumping Questionnaire can be used to identify clinically significant symptoms. Sigstad scores ≥7, after glucose intake, is considered diagnostic of dumping syndrome [62].

Treatment of dumping syndrome is based on delaying the gastric emptying time. The symptoms of early dumping are likely to resolve on its own in three months but if they are troublesome and affecting the quality of life then treatment includes:

1. Lifestyle and dietary modification such as:
    - Eating smaller meals—Try to eat five or six small meals a day instead of three large meals.
    - Avoiding fluids with meals—Drink liquids either 30 min before meals or 30 min after meals.
    - Dietary changes—Eat more protein and complex carbohydrates rather than simple sugars. Limit high-sugar foods, such as candy, table sugar, syrup, sodas, and juices.

Table 7.4 Sigstad score

Pre-shock or shock	+5
Loss of consciousness, fainting	+4
Will lie down or sit	+4
Dyspnoea	+3
Physical fatigue, exhaustion	+3
Sleep, listlessness, blurred vision	+3
Palpitation	+3
Restlessness, agitation	+2
Dizziness, vertigo	+2
Headache	+1
Feeling hot, sweating, pallor, clammy skin	+1
Nausea	+1
Abdominal distension	+1
Borborygmi	+1
Eructation	−1
Vomiting	−4

A score of >7 is suggestive of dumping syndrome. A score less than <4 is suggestive of an alternate diagnosis

- Increasing fibre intake—Psyllium husk, guar gum, and pectin in food delay the absorption of carbohydrates in the small intestine and also prolongs gastric emptying time.

2. Pharmacological management:
   - Acarbose (alpha-glucosidase inhibitor)—Can be used to delay the digestion of carbohydrates, but its use is limited due to lack of efficacy and occurrence of side effects such as flatulence and diarrhoea.
   - Octreotide (somatostatin analogues)—Acts by slowing the emptying of food into the intestine. It can be administered subcutaneously (three times daily) for early symptoms or intramuscularly every 2 or 4 weeks for late symptoms. Possible side effects include nausea, vomiting, and stomach upset [61].
3. Surgical management:
   - Surgical treatment is reserved only for severely affected patients, with intense and disabling symptoms, not resolved by the above measures. Possible options include reconstruction of a gastric reservoir, adding restrictive intervention like band, insertion of a short anti-peristaltic loop. The last resort is the reversal of the operation [63].

7.10 Small Intestinal Bacterial Overgrowth

Small intestinal bacterial overgrowth (SIBO) is defined as an excessive number of bacteria (>10^5 CFU/ml) in the small bowel. The incidence is 2.5% in a healthy population; however, it increases up to 41% in patients with obesity due to impaired small intestinal motility. SIBO can also occur in patients post-gastric bypass sugery [51]. SIBO is associated with bypass procedures and is not related to weight loss as the rate of bacterial overgrowth is similar both before and after the restrictive procedures. The symptoms may be diarrhoea, malabsorption, pain abdomen, obstruction, or extra -digestive complaints (arthritis, dermatologic abnormalities). Studies have shown bacterial overgrowth in both the pouch and the remnant stomach after RYGB. Hypotheses for development of SIBO after gastric bypass are alteration of the anatomy, influence of proton pump inhibitors, modifications in the caloric intake, and dietary composition. The commonly used tests for the diagnosis of SIBO include hydrogen breath test with the gold standard being endoscopic sampling of the bowel yielding bacterial count >10^5 CFU/ml. In the breath test, the patient is given lactulose that is fermented and the hydrogen in breath is used as a marker. In post-gastric bypass patients, breath test is unreliable due to exclusion of the part of a bowel from normal pathway. Routine endoscopy is technically not feasible in the bypassed bowel making aspiration and culture difficult. Moreover, the consequences of SIBO in post-bariatric patients are of questionable value. RYGB patients with and without SIBO report a similar percentage of digestive symptoms making the clinical significance of SIBO uncertain. The nutrients which escape digestion in the bowel due to SIBO can get fermented to a short- and medium-chain fatty acids in the colon and can theoretically increase the caloric uptake. However, studies have failed to prove such hypothesis.

An infection of clinical significance is *Clostridium difficile*-associated colitis. It might present in the form of protein-losing enteropathy without any signs of inflammation. The diagnosis requires measurement of *C. difficile* toxin in the stool samples. These tests need to be evaluated carefully taking into consideration the patients' symptoms to avoid treating asymptomatic carriers. The first line of treatment is probiotics with oral metronidazole. Oral treatment can be suspect in post RYGB patients due to altered anatomy and a high percentage of absorption of metronidazole in the small intestine. Intravenous metronidazole or vancomycin might be used in cases of fulminant colitis. Faecal microbiota transplant is a new treatment option but is not usually practiced.

7.11 Gallstones

The incidence of hepatobiliary complications after bariatric surgery is around 5.5 cases/1000 patient years, with biliary colic amounting to three cases/100 patient years. Rapid weight loss (>25% of original weight) following bariatric surgery is one of the main factors responsible for the formation of gall stones as it results in higher biliary cholesterol levels. Other factors include gallbladder stasis, increased production of calcium, and arachidonic acid derivative with the disturbed enterohepatic circulation. Patients can thus present with gall stones and their complications including common bile duct stones, which can be difficult to manage via ERCP due to altered anatomy (RYGB).

Prophylactic concomitant cholecystectomy could reduce the incidence of such complications; however, it has been seen that concomitant surgery increases the perioperative morbidity as compared to bariatric surgery alone. A concomitant procedure also poses a diagnostic dilemma in case a complication such as a leak is suspected in the bariatric surgery. Moreover, it is technically difficult due to visceral obesity, large liver size, torque, and different port placement. Overall a concomitant procedure has a higher rate of post-operative minor complications with a similar rate of severe post-operative complications (Clavien Dindo ≥IIIa) and increases the operative time. Prophylactic cholecystectomy should be avoided given the lower rate of biliary symptoms after bariatric surgery. Moreover, many of the patients who develop gall stones remain asymptomatic and do not require treatment. Prophylaxis with ursodiol at a dose of 600 mg/day for 6 months can further reduce the incidence with the effect lasting until 1 year [64, 65].

7.12 Taste Alteration

The taste preferences have also been found to be altered post-operatively after bariatric surgery. It has been seen in a systematic review that there is decreased mesolimbic activation to high energy foods and decreased preference for sweet and fatty stimuli. The taste sensitivity to sweet stimuli increases resulting in a lesser intake of sweets, which might also help in persistent weight loss after bariatric surgery [66].

7.13 De Novo Food Intolerance

There are reports of development of intolerance to certain food products after bariatric surgery. In a study by Boerlage et al. [67] patients reported de novo intolerance to a median of four food items after surgery. The most commonly reported items were fried products, carbonated drinks, and cakes. Intolerance to meat was usually associated with dysphagia. Nicoletti et al. [68] have also reported red meat intolerance after gastric bypass. The patients usually present with other commonly reported GI symptoms like nausea, vomiting, and diarrhoea. No significant impacts of these alterations have been noted on the nutritional profile.

7.14 Nesidioblastosis

Nesidioblastosis, also known as non-insulinoma pancreatic hypersecretion is due to increased beta cell–trophic polypeptides or incretins, such as glucagon-like peptide 1, PYY, GIP, and Oxyntomodulin. The increased levels of these hormones lead to the hypertrophy of pancreatic beta cells. The details of this are discussed in the chapter on endocrine complications.

7.14.1 Portal and Mesenteric Vein Thrombosis

Although portal and mesenteric vein thrombosis are early complications after bariatric surgery, there have been reports of delayed portal vein thrombosis (PVT) and mesenteric vein thrombosis (MVT) [69]. A hypercoagulable state with protein C and protein S deficiencies, oral contraceptive pill (OCP) intake, smoking, as well as chronic dehydration have been implicated. Postoperative abdominal pain associated with nausea, vomiting, fever, and leucocytosis should arouse suspicion for venous thrombosis. Treatment have been attempted with unfractionated heparin, vitamin K antagonists, low molecular weight heparin, and thrombolytics. Bowel resection and/ or splenectomy may be required.

7.14.1.1 Bile Acid Malabsorption

Bile acids play an important role in the metabolic improvement post surgery. Farsenoid X receptor (FXR) and the G protein-coupled bile acid receptor (Gpbar1/ TGR5) are the targets through which bile acids suppress hyperphagia and improve glucose metabolism. It has been shown that the amount of circulating bile acids increases after SG and RYGB due to diversion of bile to mid-jejunum resulting in increased secretion of GLP-1. The action of bile acids through FXR allows many diabetic patients to stop oral hypoglycaemic drugs just after surgery even when there is hardly any weight loss. Improved circulation of bile acids also results in a change in the gut microbiome.

However, bile acid malabsorption also can occur due to altered enterohepatic cycle and bile acid production. Majority of the bile acids are absorbed in the ileum. Malabsorption can stem from a variety of causes including ileal dysfunction, such as after resection, ileal dysmotility, SIBO, post cholecystectomy, change in microbiota, or changes in food consumption. It can be idiopathic also and can result in irritable bowel syndrome—diarrhoeal type as seen sometimes in post-cholecystectomy patients. Many patients with obesity also undergo cholecystectomy concomitantly or afterwards due to gall stones. Bile acid malabsorption might be more common in patients with short common channel (distal RYGB or BPD), however, studies to support this are lacking. The diagnostic tests include faecal bile acid determination, radiolabelled Selenium homotaurocholic acid or the serum-C4-concentration measurement. These are expensive tests and difficult to apply in clinical practice. Treatment is relatively simpler with cholestyramine—a raisin that binds bile acids with up to 95% response rate [51].

7.14.1.2 Short Bowel Syndrome

Short bowel syndrome (SBS) is defined by lack of absorptive surface resulting in failure of intestine to absorb macro- and micronutrients to fulfil the demands of the body. In the most commonly performed RYGB with alimentary limb (AL) of 100–150 cm and a Bilio-Pancreatic (BP) limb of 40–80 cm, the common channel is not measured. In OAGB also the common channel is not measured generally. Moreover, there is a constant debate regarding optimal limb lengths. The major causes of SBS post-bariatric surgery include intestinal herniation through the mesenteric defect and mesenteric thrombosis. There is no consensus on the routine closure of the mesenteric defect. There should be a high index of suspicion (pain out of proportion to the expected) for intestinal herniation and a low threshold for diagnostic laparoscopy in such cases. Mesenteric venous thrombosis is a rare cause with suspected etiologies being splanchnic blood flow alteration during bariatric surgery and reverse Trendelenberg position. Routine anticoagulation is usually advised post-bariatric surgery. Overall, SBS occurs in up to 4% of the patients post-bariatric surgery [70]. This might be averted by routine measurement of whole of the bowel length, but this also predisposes to the risk of iatrogenic bowel injury. Nonetheless, the initial treatment consists of conservative measures including parentral nutrition; surgical options are lengthening of the common channel, enteral nutrition via gastrostomy tube in the remnant stomach, and the last resort is restoration of normal anatomy or intestinal transplantation. Such patients also might have associated liver disease and require a liver inclusive intestinal transplant. The waiting list mortality for isolated intestinal transplant is lower as compared to combined transplant due to absence of liver disease in the former group. Isolated liver is another option in patients whom intestinal failure is reversible, and the transplant is required for liver disease. To summarize, SBS is a devastating complication requiring multidisciplinary approach. The initial treatment includes medical and surgical techniques to lengthen the bowel. Transplantation is a last resort in such patients.

Key Points

- The late GI complications after bariatric surgery are related to altered motility, bile flow alteration, reduction of gastric size, anatomical gut rearrangement and altered flow of nutrients, vagal manipulation, and enteric and adipose hormones modulation.
- Commonly seen complications are Reflux, Esophagitis, Barrett's oesophagus, Nausea, Vomiting, Marginal ulcers, Diarrhoea, Steatorrhoea, Constipation, Early Dumping syndrome, Late dumping, SIBO, Liver dysfunction, Gallstones, Alteration in taste, de novo food intolerance, and Nesidioblastosis.
- Most complications are mild and respond to changes in diet and pharmacotherapy. Some like reflux, esophagitis, gallstones, and nesidioblastosis may require surgical intervention.

References

1. Ma IT, Madura JA. Gastrointestinal complications after bariatric surgery. Gastroenterol Hepatol (N Y). 2015;11:526–35.
2. Oor JE, Roks DJ, Ünlü Ç, Hazebroek EJ. Laparoscopic sleeve gastrectomy and gastroesophageal reflux disease: a systematic review and meta-analysis. Am J Surg. 2016;211:250–67.
3. Suter M, Giusti V, Worreth M, Héraief E, Calmes J-M. Laparoscopic gastric banding: a prospective, randomized study comparing the Lapband and the SAGB: early results. Ann Surg. 2005;241:55–62.
4. Chiu S, Birch DW, Shi X, Sharma AM, Karmali S. Effect of sleeve gastrectomy on gastroesophageal reflux disease: a systematic review. Surg Obes Relat Dis. 2011;7:510–5.
5. Sharma A, Aggarwal S, Ahuja V, Bal C. Evaluation of gastroesophageal reflux before and after sleeve gastrectomy using symptom scoring, scintigraphy, and endoscopy. Surg Obes Relat Dis. 2014;10:600–5.
6. Himpens J, Dobbeleir J, Peeters G. Long-term results of laparoscopic sleeve gastrectomy for obesity. Ann Surg. 2010;252(2):319–24.
7. Himpens J, Dapri G, Cadiere GB. A prospective randomized study between laparoscopic gastric banding and laparoscopic isolated sleeve gastrectomy: results after 1 and 3 years. Obes Surg. 2006;16:1450–6.

8. Nahata M, Muto S, Oridate N, Ohnishi S, Nakagawa K, Sadakane C, et al. Impaired ghrelin signaling is associated with gastrointestinal dysmotility in rats with gastroesophageal reflux disease. Am J Physiol Gastrointest Liver Physiol. 2012;303:G42–53.
9. Rutledge R. The mini-gastric bypass: experience with the first 1,274 cases. Obes Surg. 2001;11:276–80.
10. Vakil N, van Zanten SV, Kahrilas P, Dent J, Jones R, Global Consensus Group. The Montreal definition and classification of gastroesophageal reflux disease: a global evidence-based consensus. Am J Gastroenterol. 2006;101:1900–20; quiz 1943
11. Tolone S, Cristiano S, Savarino E, Lucido FS, Fico DI, Docimo L. Effects of omega-loop bypass on esophagogastric junction function. Surg Obes Relat Dis. 2016;12:62–9.
12. Mion F, Tolone S, Garros A, Savarino E, Pelascini E, Robert M, et al. High-resolution impedance manometry after sleeve gastrectomy: increased intragastric pressure and reflux are frequent events. Obes Surg. 2016;26:2449–56.
13. Chevallier JM, Arman GA, Guenzi M, Rau C, Bruzzi M, Beaupel N, et al. One thousand single anastomosis (omega loop) gastric bypasses to treat morbid obesity in a 7-year period: outcomes show few complications and good efficacy. Obes Surg. 2015;25:951–8.
14. Conversion of one-anastomosis gastric bypass (OAGB) is rarely needed if standard operative techniques are performed. https://www.ncbi.nlm.nih.gov/pubmed/27067910. Accessed 30 Jun 2019.
15. Carbajo MA, Luque-de-León E, Jiménez JM, Ortiz-de-Solórzano J, Pérez-Miranda M, Castro-Alija MJ. Laparoscopic one-anastomosis gastric bypass: technique, results, and long-term follow-up in 1200 patients. Obes Surg. 2017;27:1153–67.
16. Complications following the mini/one anastomosis gastric bypass (MGB/OAGB): a multi-institutional survey on 2678 patients with a mid-term (5 years). https://www.ncbi.nlm.nih.gov/pubmed/28569357. Accessed 30 Jun 2019.
17. Brethauer SA, Hammel JP, Schauer PR. Systematic review of sleeve gastrectomy as staging and primary bariatric procedure. Surg Obes Relat Dis. 2009;5:469–75.
18. Genco A, Soricelli E, Casella G, Maselli R, Castagneto-Gissey L, Di Lorenzo N, et al. Gastroesophageal reflux disease and Barrett's esophagus after laparoscopic sleeve gastrectomy: a possible, underestimated long-term complication. Surg Obes Relat Dis. 2017;13:568–74.
19. Felsenreich DM, Kefurt R, Schermann M, Beckerhinn P, Kristo I, Krebs M, et al. Reflux, sleeve dilation, and Barrett's esophagus after laparoscopic sleeve gastrectomy: long-term follow-up. Obes Surg. 2017;27:3092–101.
20. Mahawar KK, Carr WRJ, Borg C-M, Aminian A. Does Sleeve Gastrectomy Cause Barrett's Oesophagus? Obes Surg. 2018;28:4049–50.
21. Sohn S, Fischer J, Booth M. Adenocarcinoma of the gastro-oesophageal junction after sleeve gastrectomy: a case report. ANZ J Surg. 2017;87:E163–4.
22. Scheepers AF, Schoon EJ, Nienhuijs SW. Esophageal carcinoma after sleeve gastrectomy. Surg Obes Relat Dis. 2011;7:e11–2.
23. Wright FG, Duro A, Medici JR, Lenzi S, Beskow AF, Cavadas D. Esophageal adenocarcinoma five years after laparoscopic sleeve gastrectomy. A case report. Int J Surg Case Rep. 2017;32:47–50.
24. El Khoury L, Benvenga R, Romero R, Cohen R, Roussel J, Catheline J-M. Esophageal adenocarcinoma in Barrett's esophagus after sleeve gastrectomy: case report and literature review. Int J Surg Case Rep. 2018;52:132–6.
25. Johnson WH, Fernanadez AZ, Farrell TM, Macdonald KG, Grant JP, McMahon RL, et al. Surgical revision of loop ("mini") gastric bypass procedure: multicenter review of complications and conversions to Roux-en-Y gastric bypass. Surg Obes Relat Dis. 2007;3:37–41.
26. Mahawar KK, Carr WRJ, Balupuri S, Small PK. Controversy surrounding "mini" gastric bypass. Obes Surg. 2014;24:324–33.
27. One thousand consecutive mini-gastric bypass: short- and long-term outcome. https://www.ncbi.nlm.nih.gov/pubmed/22411569. Accessed 29 Jun 2019.

28. Musella M, Milone M. Still "controversies" about the mini gastric bypass? Obes Surg. 2014;24:643–4.
29. Dixon MF, Neville PM, Mapstone NP, Moayyedi P, Axon AT. Bile reflux gastritis and Barrett's oesophagus: further evidence of a role for duodenogastro-oesophageal reflux? Gut. 2001;49:359–63.
30. Filipe MI, Muñoz N, Matko I, Kato I, Pompe-Kirn V, Jutersek A, et al. Intestinal metaplasia types and the risk of gastric cancer: a cohort study in Slovenia. Int J Cancer. 1994;57:324–9.
31. Aggarwal S, Bhambri A, Singla V, Dash NR, Sharma A. Adenocarcinoma of oesophagus involving gastro-oesophageal junction following mini-gastric bypass/one anastomosis gastric bypass. J Minim Access Surg. 2019.
32. Iannelli A, Treacy P, Sebastianelli L, Schiavo L, Martini F. Perioperative complications of sleeve gastrectomy: review of the literature. J Minim Access Surg. 2019;15:1–7.
33. Huang CS, Forse RA, Jacobson BC, Farraye FA. Endoscopic findings and their clinical correlations in patients with symptoms after gastric bypass surgery. Gastrointest Endosc. 2003;58:859–66.
34. Go MR, Muscarella P, Needleman BJ, Cook CH, Melvin WS. Endoscopic management of stomal stenosis after Roux-en-Y gastric bypass. Surg Endosc. 2004;18:56–9.
35. Ahmad J, Martin J, Ikramuddin S, Schauer P, Slivka A. Endoscopic balloon dilation of gastroenteric anastomotic stricture after laparoscopic gastric bypass. Endoscopy. 2003;35:725–8.
36. Rosenthal RJ. Dilating the stenotic gastrojejunostomy after laparoscopic Roux-en-Y gastric bypass for morbid obesity: when things go wrong. J Gastrointest Surg. 2009;13:1561–3.
37. Gumbs AA, Duffy AJ, Bell RL. Incidence and management of marginal ulceration after laparoscopic Roux-Y gastric bypass. Surg Obes Relat Dis. 2006;2:460–3.
38. Sapala JA, Wood MH, Sapala MA, Flake TM. Marginal ulcer after gastric bypass: a prospective 3-year study of 173 patients. Obes Surg. 1998;8:505–16.
39. Sverdén E, Mattsson F, Sondén A, Leinsköld T, Tao W, Lu Y, et al. Risk factors for marginal ulcer after gastric bypass surgery for obesity: a population-based cohort study. Ann Surg. 2016;263:733–7.
40. Georgiadou D, Sergentanis TN, Nixon A, Diamantis T, Tsigris C, Psaltopoulou T. Efficacy and safety of laparoscopic mini gastric bypass. A systematic review. Surg Obes Relat Dis. 2014;10:984–91.
41. Chaar ME, Stoltzfus J, Elias B, Claos L. Laparoscopic Roux-en-Y gastric bypass vs. mini gastric bypass: a systematic review of the literature. Surg Obes Relat Dis. 2017;13:S192.
42. MacLean LD, Rhode BM, Nohr C, Katz S, McLean AP. Stomal ulcer after gastric bypass. J Am Coll Surg. 1997;185:1–7.
43. Capella JF, Capella RF. Gastro-gastric fistulas and marginal ulcers in gastric bypass procedures for weight reduction. Obes Surg. 1999;9:22–7; discussion 28
44. Marginal ulcers after Roux-en-Y gastric bypass: pain for the patient…pain for the surgeon. Bariatric Times [Internet]. http://bariatrictimes.com/marginal-ulcers-after-roux-en-y-gastric-bypass-pain-for-the-patientpain-for-the-surgeon/. Accessed 2 Jun 2019.
45. Patel RA, Brolin RE, Gandhi A. Revisional operations for marginal ulcer after Roux-en-Y gastric bypass. Surg Obes Relat Dis. 2009;5:317–22.
46. Lee JK, Van Dam J, Morton JM, Curet M, Banerjee S. Endoscopy is accurate, safe, and effective in the assessment and management of complications following gastric bypass surgery. Am J Gastroenterol. 2009;104:575–82. quiz 583
47. Kang X, Zurita-Macias L, Hong D, Cadeddu M, Anvari M, Gmora S. A comparison of 30-day versus 90-day proton pump inhibitor therapy in prevention of marginal ulcers after laparoscopic Roux-en-Y gastric bypass. Surg Obes Relat Dis. 2016;12:1003–7.
48. Nguyen NT, Hinojosa MW, Gray J, Fayad C. Reoperation for marginal ulceration. Surg Endosc. 2007;21:1919–21.
49. Schirmer B, Erenoglu C, Miller A. Flexible endoscopy in the management of patients undergoing Roux-en-Y gastric bypass. Obes Surg. 2002;12:634–8.

50. Frezza EE, Herbert H, Ford R, Wachtel MS. Endoscopic suture removal at gastrojejunal anastomosis after Roux-en-Y gastric bypass to prevent marginal ulceration. Surg Obes Relat Dis. 2007;3:619–22.
51. Borbély YM, Osterwalder A, Kröll D, Nett PC, Inglin RA. Diarrhea after bariatric procedures: diagnosis and therapy. World J Gastroenterol. 2017;23:4689–700.
52. Borbély Y, Plebani A, Kröll D, Ghisla S, Nett PC. Exocrine pancreatic insufficiency after Roux-en-Y gastric bypass. Surg Obes Relat Dis. 2016;12:790–4.
53. Poylin V, Serrot FJ, Madoff RD, et al. Obesity and bariatric surgery: a systematic review of associations with defecatory dysfunction. Color Dis. 2011;13(6):e92–e103. https://doi.org/10.1111/j.1463-1318.2011.02584.x.
54. Potoczna N, Harfmann S, Steffen R, et al. Bowel habits after bariatric surgery. Obes Surg. 2008;18(10):1287–96. https://doi.org/10.1007/s11695-008-9456-4.
55. El Labban S, Safadi B, Olabi A. The effect of Roux-en-Y gastric bypass and sleeve gastrectomy surgery on dietary intake, food preferences, and gastrointestinal symptoms in post-surgical morbidly obese Lebanese subjects: a cross-sectional pilot study. Obes Surg. 2015.
56. Foster A, Laws HL, Gonzalez QH, et al. Gastrointestinal symptomatic outcome after laparoscopic Roux-en-Y gastric bypass. J Gastrointest Surg. 2003;7(6):750–3. https://doi.org/10.1016/S1091-255X(03)00092-1.
57. Afshar S, Kelly SB, Seymour K, Woodcock S, Werner A-D, Mathers JC. The effects of bariatric procedures on bowel habit. Obes Surg. 2016;26(10):2348–54.
58. Chaves YS, Destefani AC. Pathophysiology, diagnosis and treatmentof dumping syndrome and its relation to bariatric surgery. ABCD, Arq Bras Cir Dig. 2016;29:116–9.
59. Nielsen JB, Pedersen AM, Gribsholt SB, Svensson E, Richelsen B. Prevalence, severity, and predictors of symptoms of dumping and hypoglycemia after Roux-en-Y gastric bypass. Surg Obes Relat Dis. 2016;12:1562–8.
60. Banerjee A, Ding Y, Mikami DJ, Needleman BJ. The role of dumping syndrome in weight loss after gastric bypass surgery. Surg Endosc. 2013;27:1573–8.
61. Tack J, Deloose E. Complications of bariatric surgery: dumping syndrome, reflux and vitamin deficiencies. Best Pract Res Clin Gastroenterol. 2014;28:741–9.
62. Sigstad H. A clinical diagnostic index in the diagnosis of the dumping syndrome. Changes in plasma volume and blood sugar after a test meal. Acta Med Scand. 1970;188:479–86.
63. Lamers CB, Bijlstra AM, Harris AG. Octreotide, a long-acting somatostatin analog, in the management of postoperative dumping syndrome. An update. Dig Dis Sci. 1993;38:359–64.
64. Karadeniz M, Görgün M, Kara C. The evaluation of gallstone formation in patients undergoing Roux-en-Y gastric bypass due to morbid obesity. Ulus Cerrahi Derg. 2014;30:76–9.
65. Quesada BM, Kohan G, Roff HE, Canullán CM, Porras LTC. Management of gallstones and gallbladder disease in patients undergoing gastric bypass. World J Gastroenterol. 2010;16:2075–9.
66. Ahmed K, Penney N, Darzi A, Purkayastha S. Taste changes after bariatric surgery: a systematic review. Obes Surg. 2018;28:3321–32.
67. Boerlage TC, van de Laar AW, Westerlaken S, Gerdes VE, Brandjes DP. Gastrointestinal symptoms and food intolerance 2 years after laparoscopic Roux-en-Y gastric bypass for morbid obesity. Br J Surg. 2017;104(4):393–400. https://doi.org/10.1002/bjs.10419.
68. Nicoletti CF, de Oliveira BA, Barbin R, Marchini JS, Salgado Junior W, Nonino CB. Red meat intolerance in patients submitted to gastric bypass: a 4-year follow-up study. Surg Obes Relat Dis. 2015;11(4):842–6.
69. Shoar S, Saber AA, Rubenstein R, et al. Portomesentric and splenic vein thrombosis (PMSVT) after bariatric surgery: a systematic review of 110 patients. Surg Obes Relat Dis. 2018;14(1):47–59.
70. McBride CL, Petersen A, Sudan D, Thompson J. Short bowel syndrome following bariatric surgical procedures. Am J Surg. 2006;192:828–32.

Pulmonary Complications After Bariatric Surgery

8

Pradeep Chowbey, Rajesh Khullar, Anil Sharma, Vandana Soni, Manish Baijal, and Mudassir Shahdhar

Just breathing can be such a luxury at times.

—Unknown

8.1 Introduction

Bariatric surgery is a proven treatment for sustained long-term weight loss in patients suffering from morbid obesity. Along with a sustained weight loss, it leads to improvement in many obesity-related illnesses [1–4].

Adiposopathy is associated with pathophysiological effects on almost every system in the human body including. Obesity is known to impair pulmonary function, which in turn increases the risk of complications after bariatric surgery. Major pulmonary complications could be life threatening or extremely morbid in the long term. In addition, pre-existing obstructive sleep apnea (OSA) may increase morbidity and mortality from respiratory complications in patients with obesity. Complications like sputum retention, atelectasis, bronchopulmonary infections, and pulmonary embolism may cause significant postoperative morbidity and mortality after an elective surgery.

The recognition and management of these conditions prior to bariatric surgery is important to minimize the risk of postoperative complications. Although the focus of the book is on metabolic or chronic complications after bariatric surgery, there are very few reports in the bariatric literature about the long-term complications and most of them are sequelae of surgical complications like fistulae, etc. In this chapter, we will discuss the effect of obesity on pulmonary functions, and various pulmonary complications after bariatric surgery.

P. Chowbey (✉) · R. Khullar · A. Sharma · V. Soni · M. Baijal · M. Shahdhar
Max Institute of Minimal Access, Metabolic and Bariatric Surgery, Saket, Delhi, India

A. G. Bhasker et al. (eds.), *Management of Nutritional and Metabolic Complications of Bariatric Surgery*,
https://doi.org/10.1007/978-981-33-4702-1_8

8.1.1 Etiology and Pathophysiology of Pulmonary Complication in Obese

Obesity has a wide spectrum of effects on pulmonary function. Spirometry is usually normal in mild obesity. A restrictive effect is seen with increasing body mass index (BMI), with proportional reductions in both the forced expiratory volume in 1 s (FEV1) and the forced vital capacity (FVC). FEV1-to-FVC ratio is either normal or increased [5]. Total respiratory system compliance is reduced, mainly due to a decrease in chest wall compliance, and due to excess fat accumulation around the chest and abdomen as well as increased intraabdominal pressure reducing the diaphragmatic movements [6].

In the morbidly obese, additional reductions in mid-expiratory flow rates have been observed, which may represent true airflow obstruction due to early small airway collapse as a result of breathing at low lung volumes [7]. Respiratory rate is usually increased in order to compensate for the normally depressing tidal volumes. Reduced expiratory reserve volume (ERV) is the most common lung function abnormality seen in obesity [8].

The work and energy cost of breathing is elevated in obesity. When compared to normal controls, patients with morbid obesity spend a disproportionately higher percentage of their oxygen consumption (VO_2) on respiratory work during quiet breathing [9]. This increase in energy expenditure suggests a limited energy reserve and could predispose these individuals to respiratory failure in the face of an acute pulmonary or systemic illness.

It is unclear if obesity is an independent risk factor for asthma [10, 11] though obesity decreases lung volumes and increases airway resistance, which could mimic asthma. Obesity is also associated with increased asthma severity, increased symptoms of asthma, and an increase in gastrooesophageal reflux, which may exacerbate asthma.

8.2 Obstructive Sleep Apnea and Obesity Hypoventilation Syndrome

Obesity also increases the risk of OSA. Possible mechanisms include increased upper airway collapsibility during sleep, increased upper airway fat deposits, narrow pharyngeal caliber, increased upper airway resistance and negative intrathoracic pressure and the development of central obesity. All these factors increase the work of breathing during sleep, increasing the risk of nocturnal hypoventilation. The combination of all these factors predisposes to upper airway collapse during sleep and anesthesia [12, 13].

Because of the high prevalence of OSA in the obese, all patients presenting for bariatric surgery should be assessed for OSA. Assessment of the patient includes a history, examination, and testing. Screening questionnaires may be helpful in identifying those likely to have OSA. The Berlin questionnaire includes 11 questions in three categories and has been recently validated in the surgical population with a sensitivity ranging from 68.9% to 87.2% depending on the severity of OSA [14]. The STOP-BANG questionnaire (an eight-question screening questionnaire related to snoring, tiredness during daytime, observed apnea, high blood pressure, BMI, age, neck, and gender) has frequently been used as a screening tool preoperatively in the obese. It is easy to use and score. The sensitivities of the STOP-BANG questionnaire at apnea/hypopnea index (AHI) cut-offs of 5, >15, and >30 are 83.6%, 92.9%, and 100%, respectively [15].

Obesity Hypoventilation Syndrome (OHS) refers to the combination of awake hypercapnia $PaCO_2$ >45 mm Hg in the obese patient (BMI > 30 kg/m^2) after other causes of hypoventilation have been excluded. Sustained low baseline oxygen saturation during sleep suggests the presence of nocturnal or rapid eye movement hypoventilation and is probably a precursor to awake hypercapnia. To formally monitor nocturnal hypoventilation, transcutaneous CO_2 ($TcCO_2$) is recommended though careful calibration is required and the majority of sleep laboratories do not routinely monitor Tc CO_2.

Weight loss after bariatric surgery has been shown to be associated with improvements in OSA, with a 10% reduction in weight shown to be associated with a reduction of 26% in AHI, and a 20% reduction in weight associated with a reduction of 48% in AHI [16]. Despite surgical weight loss and a mean reduction of 17.9 kg/m^2 in BMI and reductions of AHI of up to 71%, it is rare for sleep apnea to completely resolve. Majority of patients have at least ongoing moderate OSA with a mean residual AHI of 15.8 events per hour of sleep.

Ongoing treatment of sleep apnea with nasal CPAP is required in the majority of patients, though CPAP pressure requirements may fall with weight loss. Patients should be informed about what is likely to occur with weight loss, with explanation of possible symptoms if CPAP requirements fall. If ongoing CPAP levels are too high, this may affect sleep quality, symptoms, and reduce compliance with CPAP. Regular 3-monthly visits to the sleep physician are required to supervise CPAP requirements and ongoing treatment adjustments.

Surgical interventions such as uvulopalatopharyngoplasty (UVPP) are available to treat OSA but are generally not recommended as first-line therapy as they can interfere with the acclimatization and long-term adherence to CPAP therapy, which has demonstrably superior outcomes. In patients with mild OSA, or those intolerant of CPAP, mandibular advancement splints can be considered, although they are less effective in reducing the AHI when compared to CPAP. Positional sleep apnea, especially in the supine position is quite common in patients with mild OSA and can be managed by avoiding supine position during sleep using the "tennis ball technique" [17], or newer position monitoring and supine alarm devices [18].

8.3 Aspiration of Gastric Acid

Patients with morbid obesity have increased risk of gastric acid aspiration. The risk factors contributing toward aspiration pneumonitis include presence of hiatal hernia, gastroesophageal reflux, increased intra-abdominal pressure, high volume of gastric contents, and low pH gastric contents after fasting. Aspiration can in turn cause transient pneumonitis progressing to severe acute lung injury and acute respiratory distress syndrome. Therefore, potential bariatric surgical patients should be carefully evaluated preoperatively to rule out any GERD or hiatus hernia.

8.4 Venous Thromboembolism

This is composed of two clinical entities: deep vein thrombosis (DVT) and pulmonary embolism. DVT is the formation of blood clots in deep veins of pelvis or legs. Pulmonary embolism occurs if this clot gets dislodged and travels to pulmonary arteries and can be fatal.

The incidence of venous thromboembolism (VTE) including deep vein thrombosis (DVT) and pulmonary embolism (PE) after bariatric surgery has been reported to be around 0.3–2.2% [26–31]. The occurrence of VTE is noted to be 0.88% during hospitalization, which increases to 2.17% at 1 month and 2.99% at 6 months post-bariatric surgery [32].

All patients should be evaluated for the risk of VTE after surgery. Patient-related risk factors include: male sex, increasing age [31, 33, 34], smoking [35, 36] previous history of DVT, preoperative weight, and BMI. Finks et al. [31] have demonstrated that previous history of VTE was associated with four times the risk of postoperative VTE and every 10 units increment in BMI was associated with a 37% increase in VTE risk. Procedure-related risk factors for VTE include operative time [31, 37], procedure type, postoperative complications, and open technique [33, 34]. Masoomi et al. [38] have found that gastric bypass procedures carry a higher risk compared to other types of bariatric procedures.

Pulmonary embolism is one of the major causes of morbidity and mortality after bariatric surgery. There are numerous prospective studies that have shown obesity to be a significant risk factor for venous thromboembolism (VTE) [19, 20]. There are multiple factors contributing toward increased incidence of VTE in obese patients. These factors are increased blood viscosity, decreased concentration of antithrombin III, increased concentrations of fibrinogen, and plasminogen activator inhibitor-1 produced by adipose tissue [20–22]. In recent studies, it has been found that hospitalized patients as well as recently discharged patients are at high risk for VTE [23].

The risk of venous thromboembolism (VTE) in obesity is reported to be twice that of normal-weight subjects [24]. Despite the routine use of pre- and postoperative coagulation prophylaxis, pulmonary embolism continues to be one of the leading causes of death following bariatric surgery. The reported incidence is between 0.84 and 0.95%, with over a third of cases being diagnosed only after discharge and up to 30 days postoperatively [25]. A hypercoagulable state exists in obesity and is thought to be related to a combination of increased coagulation cascade activity, decreased fibrinolysis, and endothelial dysfunction [24]. Additional factors such as increased intra-abdominal pressure impairing venous circulation from legs and venous stasis caused by the artificial pneumoperitoneum induced during bariatric surgery, also increase the risk of postoperative deep vein thrombosis and pulmonary embolism.

8.4.1 Prevention of VTE post bariatric surgery

I. *Early Ambulation*—Early ambulation reduces venous stasis and DVT.

II. *Lower extremity compression (LEC)*—LEC methods are mainly by elastic stockings such as graduated compression stockings or by intermittent pneumatic compression (IPC) as with sequential compression devices. Sachdeva et al. [39] have reported a 65% reduction in risk of VTE events postoperatively with graduated compression stockings. In a metanalysis, IPC with prophylaxis reduced the DVT risk by 60% [40]. The drawbacks of using LEC include occasional ulcers, blisters, and skin necrosis [41]. However, these complications are too rare and mild to be prohibitive.

III. *Prophylaxis*—There is a debate on the use of Unfractionated Heparin (UFH) and low molecular weight heparin (LMWH). UFH in doses of 5000–7500 IU subcutaneously is given 2–3 times a day [42]. However, due to an exaggerated response in people who are obese, the pharmacokinetics remains variable. The doses need to be tailored as per the patient's partial thromboplastin time [43]. LMWHs are preferred chemoprophylactic agents and have several advantages of higher bioavailability, longer half-life, more predictable anticoagulant response, and lower risk of heparin-induced thrombocytopenia (HIT). Scholten et al. have compared two dosages of Enoxaparin—30 mg twice daily and 40 mg twice daily. The study concluded that the incidence of DVT was higher (5.4%) in the low dose group as compared to 0.6% in high dose group [44]. In the EFFORT trial, a randomized double-blind pilot trial comparing enoxaparin with fondaparinux in bariatric surgical patients, adequate anti-factor Xa levels were more frequent with fondaparinux (74.2%) than with enoxaparin (32.4%), although DVT incidence was similar in both groups [45]. The HAT Committee of the UK Clinical Pharmacy Association suggests a body weight-based dosage of 40 mg once a day for an individual <100 kg, a dosage of 40 mg twice a day for >100 kg, and a dosage of 60 mg twice a day for >150 kg in the NHS practice guidelines for doses of thromboprophylaxis.

IV. *Oral Anticoagulants for VTE prophylaxis*
There is limited literature on the usage of oral anticoagulants for VTE prophylaxis after bariatric surgery. Bariatric procedures alter the absorption, distribution, metabolism, or elimination (disposition) of orally administered drugs via changes in the gastrointestinal tract anatomy, body weight, and adipose tissue composition. The drug disposition is unpredictable and needs individual independent monitoring. Currently available literature recommends avoiding direct thrombin inhibitors in favor of Vitamin K antagonists, which can be easily monitored, and dose adjusted. Therapeutic anticoagulation after bariatric sur-

gery suggests lower dose requirements of warfarin within the first month after surgery, with rising requirements as time from surgery increases [46].

Duration of Thromboprophylaxis AACE/TOS/ASMBS guidelines state that thromboprophylaxis should be started within 24 h of surgery [47]. The suggested VTE prevention strategies are summarized in the table below [48].

Level of risk	Patients characteristics	Suggested prevention strategies
Moderate risk	All bariatric surgical patients without additional risk factors	• Early and aggressive postoperative mobilization. • Intermittent pneumatic compression • In hospital pharmacoprophylaxis[a,b]
High risk	A calculated post-discharge VTE risk >0.4%[c] Past history of DVT Congenital or acquired hypercoagulable conditions Significant chronic venous insufficiency	• Early and aggressive postoperative mobilization • Intermittent pneumatic compression • In hospital pharmacoprophylaxis[a,b] • Extend post-discharge prophylaxis for 2 weeks[b]
Very high risk	A calculated post-discharge VTE risk >1%[d]	• Early and aggressive postoperative mobilization • Intermittent pneumatic compression • In hospital pharmacoprophylaxis • Extended post-discharge prophylaxis for 4 weeks[b] • Consider LMWH dose adjustment based on anti X a level[e] • Consider DVT screening with a duplex scan

BMI body mass index, *DVT* deep vein thrombosis, *LMWH* low molecular weight heparin, *PE* pulmonary embolism, *SC* subcutaneous, *VTE* venous thromboembolism

[a]In the absence of major risk or concern for ongoing postoperative bleeding requiring serial monitoring and/or treatment

[b]Dose adjustment can be based on body weight. At Cleveland Clinic, the institutional practice is to adjust the postoperative prophylactic dose of Enoxaparin based on the BMI (40 mg SC q12h for BMI < 50 kg/m^2 vs. 60 mg for BMI > 50 kg/m^2) [30]

[c]VTE risk of 0.4% was chosen as a cut off-point representing a high combined sensitivity and specificity; this cut off-point included 20% of our study population

[d]VTE risk of 1% chosen as a cut off-point included 2.5% of the study population

[e]Target Anti-Xa level: Peak concentration (4 h after subcutaneous injection of LMWH) of 0.2–0.4 IU/mL [49]

V. *Inferior vena cava filters*

The use of Inferior vena cava (IVC) filters in bariatric surgery is controversial due to complications such as filter migration and thrombosis of vena cava. There are studies that have suggested longer hospital stay, higher rate of DVT as well as mortality with the use of IVC filters [50]. Bariatric Outcomes Longitudinal Database data has also shown similar results [33]. There are also studies in favor of using prophylactic IVC decreasing risk of PE [51–53]. Overall, the available literature does not support the placement of IVC filter as prophylaxis in bariatric surgery. The risks of placement of IVC filters need to be balanced against the favorable outcomes.

8.4.2 Diagnosis

The most common clinical signs and symptoms of pulmonary embolism are sudden onset dyspnea, chest pain, fainting, syncope, hemoptysis, cough, unilateral painful swelling of lower or upper extremity, tachycardia or bradycardia, cyanosis, hypotension, and fever greater than 38 °C. There are various clinical prediction systems to rule out pulmonary embolism. The goal is early detection and management to minimize the morbid consequences. Characteristically ECG shows a new complete or incomplete right bundle branch block with ST elevation or depression. However, the most common changes seen are sinus tachycardia and non-specific ST-T changes suggestive of right ventricular strain. Elevation of D-dimer and BNP (Brain Natriuretic Peptide), Troponin I and T are suggestive of PE. Compression Ultrasonography is a bedside procedure to diagnose DVT and is highly predictive of PE with sensitivity of 39% and specificity of 99% [54]. Computed tomographic pulmonary angiography (CT-PA), Pulmonary Angiography (PA), and Ventilation Perfusion scan (VQ) are all highly sensitive. However, pulmonary angiography is the gold standard test with almost 100% sensitivity [54].

Various recommendations for prevention of VTE are recommended in Table 8.1.

8.4.3 Management

Patients with suspected acute PE should be immediately started on anticoagulants during ongoing diagnostic workup. Initial treatment with unfractionated heparin, LMWH, or fondaparinux should be continued for at least 5 days. Vitamin K antagonists can be started 5 days after surgery and UFH, LMWH, or fondaparinux are stopped only when INR levels >2 are achieved [54]. In acute pulmonary embolism, thrombolytic therapy is effective in thromboembolic obstruction. Streptokinase, urokinase, and alteplase are approved for use in PE.

8.5 Postoperative Respiratory Complications in Bariatric Population

Postoperative pulmonary complications (PRC) are one of the major causes of perioperative morbidity and mortality. The incidence reported in literature is around 3–7.9% in general surgery [55, 56] and higher rates reported in lung surgery [57]. Pulmonary complications after bariatric surgery are reported to be as high as 8% [58]. The complications can be broadly categorized under:

- Atelectasis
- Pneumonia
- Acute respiratory distress syndrome

Table 8.1 Recommendations and Guidelines for prevention of VTE

Guidelines	Early ambulation	Lower extremity compression	Pharmacologic prophylaxis	Post discharge pharmacologic prophylaxis	Prophylactic vena cava filter	Other recommendations
American Association of Clinical Endocrinologists/ American Society for Metabolic and Bariatric Surgery (2013)	R	R—SCD	SC UFH or LMWH is given within 24 h of surgery Dose not specified	Consider for high-risk patients (history of DVT)	Risks may exceed benefits	Discontinue estrogen therapy preoperatively Patients with history of DVT or Cor Pulmonale should undergo evaluation for DVT
American Society for Metabolic and Bariatric Surgery (2013)	R	R—for all	Combination of chemoprophylaxis should be considered based on clinical judgment and risk of bleeding. Conflicting data—Data suggest LMWH over UFH	Consider but insufficient data to recommend specific dose or duration	VCF is only method not recommended. Consider addition of VCF in high-risk patients where VTE risk >risk of filter-related complications	None
Interdisciplinary European Guidelines on Metabolic and Bariatric Surgery (2013)	R	R—ES and IPC	SC LMWH. Dose not specified	Not mentioned	Not mentioned	None

R recommended, *NR* not recommended, *SCD* Sequential Compression Device, *ES* elastic stocking, *IPC* Intermittent pneumatic compression

PRCs contribute to increase hospital stay, financial burden, and mortality [59–62]. Furthermore, postoperative reintubation, pulmonary edema, and atelectasis are predictors of adverse discharge disposition—defined as in-hospital mortality or discharge to a nursing home [59].

Pulmonary edema can lead to unanticipated inpatient stays, the need for ICU admission, reintubation, and increased costs [63, 64].

8.5.1 Prevention of PRC After Bariatric Surgery

Preoperative Screening

A careful preoperative screening is essential to anticipate any adverse event and minimize postoperative respiratory complications. Awake intubation should be discussed by the anesthetist. Preoperative CPAP therapy for OSA patients aids in better ventilation and during induction of anesthesia. Non-invasive ventilation (NIV) may be required in patients with OHS in whom CPAP therapy alone is inadequate to control nocturnal hypoventilation and daytime hypercapnia, rarely supplementary oxygen is required in order to achieve acceptable control of sleep-disordered breathing [65]. The components of preoperative screening are as follows:

- Careful history taking
- Evaluation of medical records
- Physical examination
  - Airway assessment
  - Neck circumference
  - Tongue size
  - Extended Mallampati Score
  - Screening pertaining to OSA (STOPBANG/Berlin questionnaire)

Preoperative assessment is vital to identify the high risk for postoperative respiratory failure and to be equipped to manage the PRC.

Intraoperative Preventive Strategies

Obesity may cause difficult mask ventilation during induction of anesthesia [66]. Optimizing airway management with upright posture may be prudent in some patients in the preinduction stage to optimize mask ventilation [67].

After the induction of general endotracheal anesthesia, lung protective mechanical ventilation strategies are used to avoid derecruitment without overdistension of alveoli. It is done by keeping transpulmonary pressures in the range to keep the lung tissue in the linear part of its local pressure–volume curve. This strategy has gained widespread acceptance in ICUs following large studies showing that it decreases morbidity and mortality in the setting of acute lung injury [68, 69]. There are studies that have shown protective ventilation is associated with decreased PRCs, with PEEP (positive end expiratory pressure) at least 5 cm H_2O and a median plateau pressure of 16 cm H_2O or less having the lowest risk of PRCs [70].

Although high FiO_2 may improve tissue oxygenation, it can impair pulmonary function. High FiO_2 (mean of 0.79) compared with low FiO_2 (mean of 0.31) was associated with significant, dose-dependent increases in rates of PRCs, and 30-day mortality in one study [71]. A laparoscopic surgical approach is beneficial for postoperative respiratory outcomes compared to open surgery [72].

In OSA, the upper airway is more collapsible [73], and supine positioning promotes upper airway collapse and doubles the AHI index compared with the lateral position [74]. Sitting position significantly improves the cross-sectional area of the retropalatal and retroglossal airways and decreases the closing pressure (indicating a more patent airway) compared with supine position [75].

Postoperative Preventive Strategies

Prolonged postoperative hypoxemia can occur during recovery from surgery [76]. Patients receiving opioids for postoperative analgesia are particularly at risk of experiencing desaturation due to opioid-induced respiratory depression [77]. A pharmacophysiologic interaction trial showed that continuous positive airway pressure compared with atmospheric pressure applied through an oronasal mask improved sleep-disordered breathing and ameliorated the respiratory-depressant effects of opioids postoperatively [78]. Proper monitoring in the PACU can decrease the number of ICU transfers and improves patients' outcomes by detecting early signs of respiratory complications [79].

In the postoperative period, CPAP, NIV, or oxygen therapy may be required to minimize complications such as atelectasis and respiratory failure. Patients are therefore usually advised to bring their own CPAP machine and mask to hospital when attending surgery, so that the equipment is readily available for use in the postoperative period [80].

8.5.2 Management of PRC After Bariatric Surgery

Atelectasis

Atelectasis is common during anesthesia and is frequently noted in critically ill patients with different underlying etiologies and pathophysiology [81]. Atelectasis is the loss of lung volume, either a part or all of a lung with or without mediastinal shift. General anesthesia in patients with morbid obesity causes atelectasis with a higher frequency and severity than in non-obese. Moreover, while atelectasis disappears in non-obese, it persists for at least 24 h in patients with obesity. There are studies that suggest decreased functional residual capacity, increased alveolar–arterial oxygenation gradient, high intrabdominal pressure, and ventilation–perfusion mismatch in patients with obesity [82–84].

The clinical presentation is small and slowly developing areas of collapse, which may be asymptomatic or present as a nonproductive cough. Rapidly developing large-scale atelectasis can present with features of hypoxia and respiratory failure. Physical examination reveals decreased movement in the affected lung area, dullness on percussion, absent breath sounds, and deviation of the trachea to the affected site.

X-rays, CT scans, and ultrasound are the investigation tools used to access and evaluate the degree of atelectasis. X-rays present with radiological signs of entire lung collapse as complete opacification of hemithorax (white out) with mediastinal displacement to the side of collapse. CT scans help in identification and localization of endobronchial lesions and differentiation of obstructive lesions from other forms of atelectasis. Atelectasis on ultrasound shows area of low homogeneity.

Management

Postoperative pain interferes with spontaneous deep breathing and coughing resulting in decreases in FRC, leading to atelectasis. Atelectasis is managed in postoperative period by a variety of lung expansion exercises including chest physical therapy, deep breathing exercises, incentive spirometry, intermittent positive pressure breathing, and CPAP. CPAP is useful for the management of spontaneously breathing patients with nonobstructive atelectasis, who are unable to breathe deeply. The aim is to open up collapsed alveoli to reduce shunt and improve ventilation–perfusion homogeneity, hence reversing hypoxemia [81].

PEEP is a core component of artificial ventilation to prevent recollapse of the lung, but the level of PEEP required depends on the clinical condition of the patient. The airway pressure above PEEP is responsible for alveolar recruitment. Early diagnosis and management are crucial for a good outcome.

Pneumonia

Recurrent aspiration pneumonia is an unusual and less commonly reported complication of Laparoscopic Adjustable Gastric Banding (LAGB). An observational study of 749 patients by Parikh et al. reported a 0.8% incidence of aspiration pneumonia [85]. A recent retrospective cohort study by Avriel et al. looked at major respiratory adverse events after LAGB [86]. In their study of 2100 patients who underwent LAGB, the most commonly reported major respiratory complications included aspiration pneumonia (19 patients) and pulmonary abscess (4 patients). The factors contributing to developing aspirations include obstructive sleep apnea, presence of extra-thoracic restriction, exertional dyspnea, hypoventilation syndrome, and GERD. While there is no established tool to help risk-stratify patients, a review of literature suggests that abnormal preoperative pH monitoring, pre-existing esophageal dysmotility, and an esophageal caliber >35 mm are risk factors, and a preceding history of GERD, or hiatal hernias are inconsistent predictors [87, 88]. Patients who develop respiratory symptoms such as chronic cough, nocturnal cough, nocturnal wheeze, or symptoms of aspiration should have additional investigations including chest X-ray, and when necessary, high-resolution chest CT. In some cases, bronchoscopy with bronchoalveolar lavage and, rarely, lung biopsy may be necessary to rule out interstitial lung disease and malignancy. Ideally, when patients develop respiratory symptoms, the band should be loosened. The diameter of the stoma can be adjusted by injecting or aspirating the band contents via the connected port to inflate or deflate the band. Removal or partial deflation of the band leads to symptom resolution in most patients. However, there can be irreversible complications. Aspiration pneumonia is less reported but can be fatal.

Acute Respiratory Distress Syndrome

The incidence of acute respiratory distress syndrome (ARDS) is increased in obese patients [89, 90]. Evaluation of the efficacy and safety of mechanical ventilation settings and treatments is a cornerstone of the early phase of the management of ARDS patients. The settings of ventilation parameters, such as PEEP, are based on their efficacy and tolerance. Moreover, the indication for some treatments depends on the severity of ARDS and these treatments will only be implemented when there is insufficient response to first-line treatments.

The treatment includes optimization of mechanical ventilation as the first step of management. Early evaluation of efficacy based on the PaO_2/FiO_2 ratio is necessary in order to discuss the relevance of neuromuscular blocking agents and of prone position.

8.6 Chronic Pulmonary Complications After Bariatric Surgery

Pancreatic fistula (PF) is a rare complication and mostly develops after pancreatic disorders or as a result of surgical trauma, or percutaneous radiologic procedures [91]. Pleuropulmonary complications of pancreatitis are rare but have been reported. Pancreaticopleuralfistula (PPF) could be a consequence of pancreatitis in post-bariatric patients.

Gastropleural Fistula

Gastropleural fistula (GPF) is a rare condition where there is a pathological communication between stomach and pleural cavity and is usually a sequela of chronic leak. The first case of gastropleural fistula was described by Markowttz and Herter in 1960 [92]. It is a newer complication that should be considered in patients with unexplained pleural effusion after Laparoscopic Sleeve Gastrectomy (LSG).

Gastropleural fistula after bariatric surgery is infrequent. There have been some case reports after gastric band placement, LSG, and Laparoscopic Roux-en-Y Gastric Bypass (LRYGB) [93–96]. The patient usually presents with late respiratory complications like persistent cough, sometimes associated with liquid or food ingestion, hemoptysis, wheezing, pleuritic pain, and findings consistent with left pleural effusion or lung consolidation. Fever, leukocytosis, hypoxemia, or frank sepsis may be present. The proposed mechanism is suggestive of secondary to post-operative leak that leads to abscess formation and subsequent creation of a tract between the stomach and the pleural cavity in GPF and a bronchus in GBF [97]. Diagnostic investigations include contrast swallow studies, computed tomography (CT), endoscopy, and bronchoscopy.

There is a debate in the literature on the management of patients with gastropleural fistulas due to the absence of guidelines and scarcity of case reports. Most reports show that a laparoscopic approach might yield good outcomes [8]. Conservative management with antibiotics, parenteral nutrition, percutaneous drainage of collections, and endoscopic therapies have been tried varying results [98, 99].

High index of suspicion is required to identify patients with this gastropleural fistula and the diagnosis should be considered in patients presenting with recurrent respiratory infections. The patients are usually treated conservatively for recurrent lung infections. Surgical repair is usually required for treatment. Endoscopic closures have been reported to be successful in some cases.

Key Points

1. *Pulmonary respiratory complications are as high as 8% after bariatric surgery.*
2. *Postoperative atelectasis is less amenable to spontaneous resolution in patients with obesity.*
3. *Pulmonary embolism is one of the major causes of morbidity and mortality after bariatric surgery.*
4. *VTE is a life-threatening complication and correct duration of thromboprophylaxis post-surgery is vital in the high-risk category.*
5. *The most commonly reported major respiratory complications after LAGB include aspiration pneumonia and pulmonary abscess.*
6. *Perioperative and postoperative control of medical comorbidities, particularly respiratory disease, and OSA are essential for optimal outcomes.*
7. *Rare cases of pleuropulmonary fistula has been reported as a sequelae of chronic leak.*

Acknowledgment I am thankful to Dr. Rajesh Sardana, Medical Writer, Max Institute of Minimal Access, Metabolic and Bariatric Surgery for compiling the content.

References

1. Buchwald H, Avidor Y, Braunwald E, et al. Bariatric surgery: a systematic review and meta-analysis. JAMA. 2004;292(14):1724–37.
2. Picot J, Jones J, Colquitt JL, et al. The clinical effectiveness and cost-effectiveness of bariatric (weight loss) surgery for obesity: a systematic review and economic evaluation. Health Technol Assess. 2009;13(41):1–190, 215–357, iii–iv
3. Gloy VL, Briel M, Bhatt DL, et al. Bariatric surgery versus non-surgical treatment for obesity: a systematic review and meta-analysis of randomised controlled trials. BMJ. 2013;347:f5934.
4. Arterburn DE, Courcoulas AP. Bariatric surgery for obesity and metabolic conditions in adults. BMJ. 2014;349:g3961.
5. Koenig SM. Pulmonary complications of obesity. Am J Med Sci. 2001;321(4):249–79.
6. Naimark A, Cherniack RM. Compliance of the respiratory system and its components in health and obesity. J Appl Physiol. 1960;15:377–82.
7. Biring MS, Lewis MI, Liu JT, Mohsenifar Z. Pulmonary physiologic changes of morbid obesity. Am J Med Sci. 1999;318(5):293–7.
8. Ray CS, Sue DY, Bray G, Hansen JE, Wasserman K. Effects of obesity on respiratory function. Am Rev Respir Dis. 1983;128(3):501–6.
9. Kress JP, Pohlman AS, Alverdy J, Hall JB. The impact of morbid obesity on oxygen cost of breathing (VO(2RESP)) at rest. Am J Respir Crit Care Med. 1999;160(3):883–6.
10. Eneli IU, Skybo T, Camargo CA Jr. Weight loss and asthma: a systematic review. Thorax. 2008;63:671–6.
11. Sin DD, Sutherland ER. Obesity and the lung: 4. Obesity and asthma. Thorax. 2008;63:1018–23.

12. Benumof JL. Obstructive sleep apnea in the adult obese patient: implications for airway management. Anesthesiol Clin N Am. 2002;20:789–811.
13. Isono S. Obstructive sleep apnea of obese adults: pathophysiology and perioperative airway management. Anesthesiology. 2009;110:908–21.
14. Chung F, Yegneswaran B, Liao P, et al. Validation of the Berlin questionnaire and American Society of Anesthesiologists checklist as screening tools for obstructive sleep apnea in surgical patients. Anesthesiology. 2008;108:822–30.
15. Silva GE, Vana KD, Goodwin JL, et al. Identification of patients with sleep disordered breathing: comparing the four-variable screening tool, STOP, STOP-Bang, and Epworth Sleepiness Scales. J Clin Sleep Med. 2011;7:467–72.
16. Peppard PE, Young T, Palta M, et al. Longitudinal study of moderate weight change and sleep-disordered breathing. JAMA. 2000;284:3015–21.
17. Bignold JJ, Deans-Costi G, Goldsworthy MR, Robertson CA, McEvoy D, Catcheside PG, Mercer JD. Poor long-term patient compliance with the tennis ball technique for treating positional obstructive sleep apnea. J Clin Sleep Med. 2009;5(5):428–30
18. Bignold JJ, Mercer JD, Antic NA, McEvoy RD, Catcheside PG. Accurate position monitoring and improved supine-dependent obstructive sleep apnea with a new position recording and supine avoidance device. J Clin Sleep Med. 2011;7(4):376–83. https://doi.org/10.5664/JCSM.1194.
19. Cohen AT, Alikhan R, Arcelus JI, et al. Assessment of venous thromoboembolism risk and the benefits of thromboprophylaxis in medical patients. Thromb Haemost. 2005;94:750–9.
20. Pieracci FM, Barie PS, Pomp A. Critical care of the bariatric patient. Crit Care Med. 2006;34:1796–18.
21. Juhan-Vague MCA. Regulation of fibrinolysis in the development of atherothrombosis: role of adipose tissue. Thromb Haemost. 1999;82:832–6.
22. Batist G, Bothe A, Bistran BR, et al. Low antithrombin III in morbid obesity: return to normal with weight reduction. J Parenter Enteral Nutr. 1983;7:447–9.
23. Amin AN, Varker H, Princic N, Lin J, Thompson S, Johnston S. Duration of venous thromboembolism risk across a continuum in medically ill hospitalized patients. J Hosp Med. 2012;7:231–8.
24. Allman-Farinelli MA. Obesity and venous thrombosis: a review. Semin Thromb Hemost. 2011;37(8):903–7.
25. Carmody BJ, Sugerman HJ, Kellum JM, Jamal MK, Johnson JM, Carbonell AM, et al. Pulmonary embolism complicating bariatric surgery: detailed analysis of a single institution's 24-year experience. J Am Coll Surg. 2006;203(6):831–7.
26. Stein PD, Matta F. Pulmonary embolism and deep venous thrombosis following bariatric surgery. Obes Surg. 2013;23(5):663–8.
27. Froehling DA, Daniels PR, Mauck KF, et al. Incidence of venous thromboembolism after bariatric surgery: a population-based cohort study. Obes Surg. 2013;23(11):1874–9.
28. Lancaster RT, Hutter MM. Bands and bypasses: 30-day morbidity and mortality of bariatric surgical procedures as assessed by prospective, multi-center, risk-adjusted ACS-NSQIP data. Surg Endosc. 2008;22(12):2554–63.
29. Winegar DA, Sherif B, Pate V, Demaria EJ. Venous thromboembolism after bariatric surgery performed by Bariatric Surgery Center of Excellence Participants: analysis of the Bariatric Outcomes Longitudinal Database. Surg Obes Relat Dis. 2011;7(2):181–8.
30. Jamal MH, Corcelles R, Shimizu H, et al. Thromboembolic events in bariatric surgery: a large multi-institutional referral center experience. Surg Endosc. 2015;29(2):376–80.
31. Finks JF, English WJ, Carlin AM, et al. Predicting risk for venous thromboembolism with bariatric surgery: results from the Michigan bariatric surgery collaborative. Ann Surg. 2012;255(6):1100–4.
32. Steele KE, Schweitzer MA, Prokopowicz G, Shore AD, Eaton LC, Lidor AO, et al. The long-term risk of venous thromboembolism following bariatric surgery. Obes Surg. 2011;21:1371–6.

33. Winegar DA, Sherif B, Pate V, Demaria EJ. Venous thromboembolism after bariatric surgery performed by Bariatric Surgery Center of Excellence Participants: analysis of the Bariatric Outcomes Longitudinal Database. Surg Obes Relat Dis. 2011;7(2):181–8.
34. Jamal MH, Corcelles R, Shimizu H, et al. Thromboembolic events in bariatric surgery: a large multi-institutional referral center experience. Surg Endosc. 2015;29(2):376–80.
35. Steele KE, Schweitzer MA, Prokopowicz G, et al. The long-term risk of venous thromboembolism following bariatric surgery. Obes Surg. 2011;21(9):1371–6.
36. Abou-Nukta F, Alkhoury F, Arroyo K, et al. Clinical pulmonary embolus after gastric bypass surgery. Surg Obes Relat Dis. 2006;2(1):24–8.
37. Gonzalez R, Haines K, Nelson LG, Gallagher SF, Murr MM. Predictive factors of thromboembolic events in patients undergoing Roux-en-Y gastric bypass. Surg Obes Relat Dis. 2006;2(1):30–5.
38. Masoomi H, Buchberg B, Reavis KM, Mills SD, Stamos M, Nguyen NT. Factors predictive of venous thromboembolism in bariatric surgery. Am Surg. 2011;77(10):1403–6.
39. Sachdeva A, Dalton M, Amaragiri SV, Lees T. Elastic compression stockings for prevention of deep vein thrombosis. Cochrane Database Syst Rev. 2010;7:CD001484.
40. Urbankova J, Quiroz R, Kucher N, Goldhaber SZ. Intermittent pneumatic compression and deep vein thrombosis prevention. A meta-analysis in postoperative patients. Thromb Haemost. 2005;94(6):1181–5.
41. The CLOTS Trials Collaboration. Effectiveness of thigh-length graduated compression stockings to reduce the risk of deep vein thrombosis after stroke (CLOTS trial 1): a multicentre, randomised controlled trial. Lancet. 2009;373(9679):1958–65.
42. Cotter SA, Cantrell W, Fisher B, Shopnick R. Efficacy of venous thromboembolism prophylaxis in morbidly obese patients undergoing gastric bypass surgery. Obes Surg. 2005;15:1316–20.
43. Shepherd MF, Rosborough TK, Schwartz ML. Heparin thromboprophylaxis in gastric bypass surgery. Obes Surg. 2003;13:249–53.
44. Scholten DJ, Hoedema RM, Scholten SE. A comparison of two different prophylactic dose regimens of low molecular weight heparin in bariatric surgery. Obes Surg. 2002;12:19–24.
45. Steele KE, Canner J, Prokopowicz G, Verde F, Beselman A, Wyse R, et al. The EFFORT trial: preoperative enoxaparin versus postoperative fondaparinux for thromboprophylaxis in bariatric surgical patients: a randomized double-blind pilot trial. Surg Obes Relat Dis. 2015;11:672–83.
46. Bartlett MA, Mauck KF, Daniels PR. Prevention of venous thromboembolism in patients undergoing bariatric surgery. Vasc Health Risk Manag. 2015;11:461–77. https://doi.org/10.2147/VHRM.S73799. eCollection 2015.
47. Mechanick JI, Youdim A, Jones DB, Garvey WT, Hurley DL, McMahon MM, et al. Clinical practice guidelines for the perioperative nutritional, metabolic, and nonsurgical support of the bariatric surgery patient-2013 update: cosponsored by American association of clinical endocrinologists, the obesity society, and American society for metabolic bariatric surgery. Obesity (Silver Spring). 2013;21(Suppl 1):S1–27.
48. Aminian A, Andalib A, Khorgami Z, Cetin D, Burguera B, Bartholomew J, et al. Who should get extended thromboprophylaxis after bariatric surgery? A risk assessment tool to guide indications for post-discharge pharmacoprophylaxis. Ann Surg. 2017;265:143–50.
49. Nutescu EA, Spinler SA, Wittkowsky A, et al. Low-molecular-weight heparins in renal impairment and obesity: available evidence and clinical practice recommendations across medical and surgical settings. Ann Pharmacother. 2009;43:1064–83.
50. Li W, Gorecki P, Semaan E, Briggs W, Tortolani AJ, D'Ayala M, et al. Concurrent prophylactic placement of inferior vena cava filter in gastric bypass and adjustable banding operations in the bariatric outcomes longitudinal database. J Vasc Surg. 2012;55:1690–5.
51. Schuster R, Hagedorn JC, Curet MJ, Morton JM. Retrievable inferior vena cava filters may be safely applied in gastric bypass surgery. Surg Endosc. 2007;21:2277–9.

52. Keeling WB, Haines K, Stone PA, Armstrong PA, Murr MM, Shames ML, et al. Current indications for preoperative inferior vena cava filter insertion in patients undergoing surgery for morbid obesity. Obes Surg. 2005;15:1009–12.
53. Obeid FN, Bowling WM, Fike JS, Durant JA. Efficacy of prophylactic inferior vena cava filter placement in bariatric surgery. Surg Obes Relat Dis. 2007;3:606–8.
54. Dalal JJ, Amin P, Ansari AS, Bhave A, Bhagwat RG, Challani A, et al. Management of acute pulmonary embolism: consensus statement for Indian patients. J Assoc Physicians India. 2015 Dec;63(12):41–50.
55. Mazo V, Sabaté S, Canet J, et al. Prospective external validation of a predictive score for postoperative pulmonary complications. Anesthesiology. 2014;121:219–31.
56. Johnson RG, Arozullah AM, Neumayer L, et al. Multivariable predictors of postoperative respiratory failure after general and vascular surgery: results from the patient safety in surgery study. J Am Coll Surg. 2007;204:1188–98.
57. Kim ES, Kim YT, Kang CH, et al. Prevalence of and risk factors for postoperative pulmonary complications after lung cancer surgery in patients with early-stage COPD. Int J Chron Obstruct Pulmon Dis. 2016;11:1317–26.
58. Pouwels S1, Smeenk FW2, Manschot L3, Lascaris B3, Nienhuijs S4, Bouwman RA3, Buise MP3. Perioperative respiratory care in obese patients undergoing bariatric surgery: Implications for clinical practice. Respir Med. 2016;117:73–80. https://doi.org/10.1016/j.rmed.2016.06.004. Epub 2016 Jun 7.
59. Sonny A, Grabitz SD, Timm FP, et al. Impact of postoperative respiratory complications on discharge disposition, mortality, and re-admissions. ASA Abstr 2016. A5016. [Google Scholar]Abstract evaluating the independent impact of postoperative reintubation, pneumonia, pulmonary edema, respiratory failure, postoperative desaturation, and atelectasis on patient-centered adverse outcomes.
60. Kim M, Brady JE, Li G. Interaction effects of acute kidney injury, acute respiratory failure, and sepsis on 30-day postoperative mortality in patients undergoing high-risk intraabdominal general surgical procedures. Anesth Analg. 2015;121:1536–46.
61. Bailey JG, Davis PJB, Levy AR, et al. The impact of adverse events on healthcare costs for older adults undergoing nonelective abdominal surgery. Can J Surg. 2016;59:172–9.
62. Dimick JB, Chen SL, Taheri PA, et al. Hospital costs associated with surgical complications: a report from the private-sector National Surgical Quality Improvement Program. J Am Coll Surg. 2004;199:531–7.
63. Krodel DJ, Bittner EA, Abdulnour R, et al. Case scenario: acute postoperative negative pressure pulmonary edema. Anesthesiology. 2010;113:200–7.
64. Krodel DJ, Bittner EA, et al. Negative pressure pulmonary edema following bronchospasm. Chest. 2011;140:1351–4.
65. Piper AJ, Sullivan CE. Effects of short-term NIPPV in the treatment of patients with severe obstructive sleep apnea and hypercapnia. Chest. 1994 Feb;105(2):434–40.
66. Kheterpal S, Martin L, Shanks AM, Tremper KK. Prediction and outcomes of impossible mask ventilation: a review of 50,000 anesthetics. Anesthesiology. 2009;110:891–7.
67. Zaremba S, Mojica JE, Eikermann M. Perioperative sleep apnea: a real problem or did we invent a new disease? F1000Res. 2016;5.
68. Amato MBP, Barbas CSV, Medeiros DM, ct al. Effect of a protective-ventilation strategy on mortality in the acute respiratory distress syndrome. N Engl J Med. 1998;338:347–54.
69. [No authors listed]. Ventilation with lower tidal volumes as compared with traditional tidal volumes for acute lung injury and the acute respiratory distress syndrome. The Acute Respiratory Distress Syndrome Network. N Engl J Med. 2000;342:1301–8.
70. Ladha K, Vidal Melo MF, McLean DJ, et al. Intraoperative protective mechanical ventilation and risk of postoperative respiratory complications: hospital based registry study. BMJ. 2015;351:h3646.
71. Staehr-Rye AK, Meyhoff CS, Rasmussen LS, et al. Does high intra-operative inspiratory oxygen fraction lead to postoperative respiratory complications? ASA Abstr 2015. A2059.

[Google Scholar]Abstract reporting that high intraoperative inspiratory oxygen fraction is dose-dependently associated with major respiratory complications and 30-day mortality.
72. Fuks D, Cauchy F, Fteriche S, et al. Laparoscopy decreases pulmonary complications in patients undergoing major liver resection: a propensity score analysis. Ann Surg. 2016;263:353–61.
73. Isono S, Remmers JE, Tanaka A, et al. Anatomy of pharynx in patients with obstructive sleep apnea and in normal subjects. J Appl Physiol. 1997;82:1319–26.
74. Cartwright RD. Effect of sleep position on sleep apnea severity. Sleep. 1984;07:110–4.
75. Tagaito Y, Isono S, Tanaka A, et al. Sitting posture decreases collapsibility of the passive pharynx in anesthetized paralyzed patients with obstructive sleep apnea. Anesthesiology. 2010;113:812–8.
76. Sun Z, Sessler DI, Dalton JE, et al. Postoperative hypoxemia is common and persistent: a prospective blinded observational study. Anesth Analg. 2015;121:709–15. [PMC free article] [PubMed] [Google Scholar]This study found that hypoxemia, including prolonged hypoxemia, was relatively common in postoperative, hospitalized patients. The degree of hypoxemia is often greatly underestimated by SpO_2 recordings.
77. Lee LA, Caplan RA, Stephens LS, et al. Postoperative opioid-induced respiratory depression: a closed claims analysis. Anesthesiology. 2015;122:659–65.
78. Zaremba S, Shin CH, Hutter MM, et al. Continuous positive airway pressure mitigates opioid-induced worsening of sleep-disordered breathing early after bariatric surgery. Anesthesiology. 2016;125:92–104.
79. Taenzer AH, Pyke JB, McGrath SP, Blike GT. Impact of pulse oximetry surveillance on rescue events and intensive care unit transfers: a before-and-after concurrence study. Anesthesiology. 2010;112:282–7.
80. Clinical Issues Committee ASMBS. Perioperative management of obstructive sleep apnea. Surg Obes Relat Dis. 2012;8(3):e27–32.
81. Ray K, Bodenham A, Paramasivam E. Pulmonary atelectasis in anaesthesia and critical care. Continuing Educ Anaesthesia Crit Care Pain. 2014;14(5):236–45.
82. Pelosi P, Croci M, Ravagnan I, et al. Respiratory system mechanics in sedated, paralyzed, morbidly obese patients. J Appl Physiol. 1997;82:811–8.
83. Pelosi P, Croci M, Ravagnan I, et al. Total respiratory system, lung, and chest wall mechanics in sedated-paralyzed postoperative morbidly obese patients. Chest. 1996;109:144–51.
84. Pelosi P, Croci M, Ravagnan I, et al. The effects of body mass on lung volumes, respiratory mechanics, and gas exchange during general anesthesia. Anesth Analg. 1998;87:654–60.
85. Parikh MS, Fielding GA, Ren CJ. U.S. experience with 749 laparoscopic adjustable gastric bands: intermediate outcomes. Surg Endosc. 2005;19:1631–5. https://doi.org/10.1007/s00464-005-0302-7.
86. Avriel A, Warner E, Avinoach E, Avnon LS, Shteinberg M, Shteinberg D, et al. Major respiratory adverse events after laparoscopic gastric banding surgery for morbid obesity. Respir Med. 2012;106:1192–8. https://doi.org/10.1016/j.rmed.2012.05.002.
87. Klaus A, Weiss H. Is preoperative manometry in restrictive bariatric procedures necessary? Obes Surg. 2008;18:1039–42. https://doi.org/10.1007/s11695-007-9399-1.
88. Naef M, Mouton WG, Naef U, van der Weg B, Maddern GJ, Wagner HE. Esophageal dysmotility disorders after laparoscopic gastric banding – An underestimated complication. Ann Surg. 2011;253:285–90. https://doi.org/10.1097/SLA.0b013e318206843e.
89. Gong MN, Bajwa EK, Thompson BT, Christiani DC. Body mass index is associated with the development of acute respiratory distress syndrome. Thorax. 2010;65:44–50.
90. Anzueto A, Frutos-Vivar F, Esteban A, et al. Influence of body mass index on outcome of the mechanically ventilated patients. Thorax. 2011;66:66–73.
91. Le Moine O, Matos C, Closset J, Deviere J. Endoscopic management of pancreatic fistula after pancreatic and other abdominal surgery. Best Pract Res Clin Gastroenterol. 2004;18(5):957–75.
92. Mehran A, Ukleja A, Szomstein S, Rosenthal R. Laparoscopic partial gastrectomy for the treatment of gastropleural fistula. J Soc Laparoendosc Surgeons. 2005;9(2):213–5.

93. Campos JM, Siqueira LT, Ferraz AA, Ferraz EM. Gastrobronchial fistula after obesity surgery. J Am Coll Surg. 2007;204:711.
94. Campos JM, Siqueira LT, Meira MR, Ferraz AA, Ferraz EM, Guimaraes MJ. Gastrobronchial fistula as a rare complication of gastroplasty for obesity: a report of two cases. J Bras Pneumol. 2007;33:475–9.
95. Chin PL. Gastrobronchial fistula as a complication of laparoscopic adjustable gastric banding. Surg Obes Relat Dis. 2008;4:671–3.
96. Garrett KA, Rosati C. Gastro-broncho-pleural fistula after laparoscopic gastric band placement. Obes Surg. 2009;19:941–3.
97. Nguyen D, Dip F, Hendricks L, Lo Menzo E, Szomstein S, Rosenthal R. The surgical management of complex fistulas after sleeve gastrectomy. Obes Surg. 2016;26:245–50. https://doi.org/10.1007/s11695-015-1788-2.
98. Trelles N, Gagner M, Palermo M, Pomp A, Dakin G, Parikh M. Gastrocolic fistula after re-sleeve gastrectomy: outcomes after esophageal stent implantation. Surg Obes Relat Dis. 2010;6(3):308–12.
99. Jiramethee N, Mira-Avendano I, Phelan J. An unusual case of gastro-pleural fistula masquerading as pneumonia following bariatric surgery. Am J Respir Crit Care Med. 2017;195. View at: Google Scholar.

Management of Nutritional and Metabolic Complications of Bariatric Surgery: Hepatic Complications After Bariatric Surgery

9

Wei-Jei Lee

Liver health is a big deal. We live in an age of toxic overload, processed foods, environmental toxicity, heavy metals, poor diets and compromised digestive systems. —Anonymous

—Anonymous

9.1 Introduction

Obesity and its related diseases are among the leading causes of death globally [1]. Non-alcoholic fatty liver disease (NAFLD) is the hepatic manifestation and main complication of obesity. The spectrum of this disease is broad from steatosis and non-alcoholic steatohepatitis (NASH) through cirrhosis and liver failure. In general, more than 80% of morbidly obese patients suffer from NAFLD, with 25–55% resulting in NASH and 2–12% resulting in fibrosis and cirrhosis [2–4]. After exclusion of other forms of liver disease, the clinician needs to be able to select patients at risk of progressive disease, investigate them appropriately, and develop management strategies [5, 6].

Bariatric surgery, as the most effective therapy for patients with morbid obesity today, provides a significant improvement in pre-existing hepatic complications, including NAFLD, NASH, and fibrosis accompanied by an improvement in levels of aspartate aminotransferase (AST), alanine aminotransferase (ALT), and gamma-glutamyl transferase (GGT) [7]. However, sometimes hepatic complications might develop after bariatric surgery, leading to serious complications requiring liver transplantation or resulting in death [8–15]. The situation was notoriously known

W.-J. Lee (✉)
Department of Surgery, Min-Sheng General Hospital, Taoyuan, Taiwan, Republic of China

A. G. Bhasker et al. (eds.), *Management of Nutritional and Metabolic Complications of Bariatric Surgery*,
https://doi.org/10.1007/978-981-33-4702-1_9

after jejunoileal and jejunocolic bypass procedures that were abandoned after 1980 due to several metabolic and hepatic complications [8, 9]. The clinical outcomes of current bariatric surgical procedures have improved a great deal. However, there have still been some reports of patients post-bariatric surgeries presenting with severe hepatic complications. The reports were mainly related to Biliopancreatic Diversion with Duodenal Switch (BPD/DS), Roux-en-Y Gastric Bypass (RYGB), distal RYGB, or One Anastomosis Gastric Bypass (OAGB) [10–16].

This chapter reviews the data from the literature, with the aim of elucidating the hepatic complications of bariatric surgeries.

9.2 Incidence/Prevalence

The clinical spectrum of hepatic complications after bariatric surgery varies from elevated liver enzymes, hypoproteinemia, hyperammonemia to liver failure. The hepatic complications after bariatric surgery seem highly related to the amount of bowel not exposed to ingested food or excluded duodenum and proximal bowel, which is the biliopancreatic (BP) limb. Hepatic complications are rarely seen after restrictive surgeries, such as sleeve gastrectomy or gastric banding. The incidence of hepatic complications seems to increase along with the increase of BP limb or decrease of common channel [17–19]. One anastomosis gastric bypass (OAGB), a simplified single anastomosis gastric bypass, has a longer BP limb as compared to conventional RYGB. The weight loss was found to be better in OAGB than RYGB, but OAGB had a higher rate of abnormal hepatic enzyme and protein deficiency [20–22]. The incidence of hepatic complication according to different definitions in various bariatric procedures are listed in Table 9.1.

9.2.1 Elevated Liver Enzymes

Elevated liver enzymes were commonly found in the first 3 months after gastric bypass surgery [5, 23]. The elevation was higher after OAGB than after RYGB [17, 18, 23]. However, most of the patients had normal liver enzymes after 6 months. In a recent study, patients with NASH undergoing RYGB were more susceptible to early transit deterioration of liver function compared to SG [24]. This is why SG is now recommended for patients with liver cirrhosis [25].

9.2.2 Protein Deficiency and Hypoalbuminemia

Protein–calorie malnutrition is a possible hepatic complication after gastric bypass or other malabsorptive procedures. The incidence of hypoalbuminemia is increased along with the increase of bypass limb or decrease of common channels. The reported incidence of hypoalbuminemia varied from 1.8% to 15% after RYGB [26–30], 2.8–34% after OAGB [21, 29–31], 5–35% after SADI [32] and 15–50% after

Table 9.1 Incidence of hepatic complications after various bariatric procedures

	Hepatic enzyme elevation	Hypo-albuminemia	Hyper-ammonia	Liver failure
Gastric banding	–	0.6%	–	–
Sleeve gastrectomy	–	1.2%	–	–
RYGB (<100 cm BP)	5%	1.8–15%	0.07%	–
Distal RYGB	–		–	Case report
OAGB (150 cm BP)	–	2%	–	–
OAGB (200 cm BP)	10%	2.8%	–	Case report
OAGB (250 cm BP)	–	10.5–34%	–	Case report
SADI (200 cm CC)	–	12–35%	–	–
SADI (250 cm CC)	–	7.7–10.3%	–	–
SADI (300 cm CC)	–	5%	–	–
BPD/DS (50 cm CC)	–	15–50%	–	0.21%
Jejunal bypass (50 cm CC)	–	–	–	13%

RYGB Roux-en-Y gastric bypass, *BP* bilio-pancreatic limb, *OAGB* one anastomosis gastric bypass, *SADI* single anastomosis duodeno-ileal anastomosis, *CC* common channel, *BPD/DS* bilio-pancreatic diversion/duodenal switch

BPD/DS [28, 33] (Table 9.1). The incidence may be even higher in the Asian population where many patients are vegetarians [21, 29, 34].

9.2.3 Hyperammonemia

Hyperammonemia encephalopathy is a rare but a potentially devastating condition after bariatric surgery. A case study identified seven cases of hyperammonemic encephalopathy after bariatric surgery and five of these died [35]. Another study reviewed 20 cases of hyperammonemic syndrome after RYGB, and the outcome was fatal in half of them [36]. Hyperammonemia is usually associated with liver failure after bariatric surgery but may be found in patients without liver failure. These hyperammonemic syndromes may be associated with porto-systemic shunt, genetic defect of urea cycle, and functional inhibition of the urea cycle by nutrient deficiency or bacterial overgrowth. Late-onset Carbamoyl Phosphatase Synthase 1 (CSP1) and Ornithium Transcarbamylase (OTC) deficiency were suspected to be the cause of hyperammonemic complication. The estimated prevalence of OTC deficiency in the general population ranging between 1/14,000 and 1/70,000 [37, 38]. However, the prevalence of hyperammonemia was as high as 1:1300 to 1:1400 among RYGB patients, about 10 times higher than the normal population [39]. The reasons for this are that RYGB can reduce the nutrient intake leading to catabolism and protein breakdown. Protein breakdown will release ammonia into blood. Associated nutrient deficiencies and bacterial overgrowth may further worsen the situation.

9.2.4 Liver Insufficiency or Failure

Liver insufficiency has been described after malabsorptive bariatric procedure, mainly jejunoileal bypass, with an incidence of liver failures of up to 10% [9]. In BPD-DS, the reported incidence of hepatic complication and protein deficiency was around 2.5% and 5% [32]. Incidence of liver failure after BPD has been reported with liver transplantation in several case series [10–13]. Hepatic failure with mortality has also been reported after OAGB [15]. OAGB was found to have higher incidence of calorie–protein deficiency than RYGB due to a longer BP limb [18–24]. Hepatic complication after RYGB is very rare and usually associated with poor oral intake. Hepatic complications after RYGB were reported to be largely associated with preoperatively diagnosed cirrhosis, alcohol abuse, and intraoperative complications [26, 27]. However, distal gastric bypass was found to result in higher incidence of hepatic complications [14]. There was no report of hepatic complications after pure restrictive procedures such as SG or gastric banding. On the contrary, it has been shown that purely restrictive procedures are feasible and effective in patients with pre-existing advanced liver disease [25, 39].

9.3 Symptoms of Hepatic Complication

Symptoms of hepatic complication usually are related to hypoalbuminemia caused by protein–calorie malnutrition, characterized by edema, anemia, hair loss, and asthenia. Other associated symptoms are muscle wasting, diarrhea, atrophic gastritis, vomiting, anorexia, abdominal pain, etc. At the later stage of liver failure, patients might develop jaundice, ascites, and encephalopathy with hyperammonemia [40].

9.4 Diagnosis

Hepatic complication after bariatric surgery can be diagnosed initially with a negative impact on liver function. At a late stage, the patients can be diagnosed by low serum prealbumin or albumin, transferrin, fat-soluble vitamin, elevated serum ammonia, bilirubin, and deranged coagulation profile. Possible factors might be associated with a negative impact on liver function including preoperative diagnosed chronic liver disease, alcohol abuse, and intraoperative complications [26, 27]. Liver biopsy, usually showed severe steatohepatitis, and played a nonsignificant role in the diagnosis of hepatic complications after bariatric surgery [41].

9.5 Management

According to the high prevalence of obesity worldwide and its increasing rate, NAFLD or NASH is the most common liver injury and it is becoming the leading indication for transplantation. Therefore, it is better to perform bariatric surgeries for patients who have indications of NAFLD-NASH in order to subside it, prevent further progression to cirrhosis, and decrease the chances of needing liver transplant. However, malnutrition can be fatal after malabsorptive bariatric procedures, therefore, patients should be followed up frequently to monitor their liver enzymes and use of high-protein supplements must be encouraged and enforced.

Protein–calorie malnutrition could occur after malabsorptive bariatric procedures characterized by hypoalbuminemia, edema, anemia, and asthenia. Nutritional assistance should be started to manage the nutritional deficiency induced by bariatric surgery by itself or through bacterial overgrowth. Blind loop syndrome or small intestine bacterial overgrowth patients usually present with symptoms such as bloating, flatulence, abdominal discomfort, diarrhea, abdominal pain, weight loss, and steatorrhea. It can be recognized using the quantitative culture of the small bowel aspirate, 14C-D-xylose, hydrogen breath tests, or urinary or serum tests. Bacterial overgrowth is usually accompanied by macrocytic or microcytic anemia, lymphopenia, low serum prealbumin and transferrin, fat-soluble vitamin deficiencies, and elevated levels of serum folate and vitamin K. The management of bacterial overgrowth is based on the elimination of the underlying cause, eradication of overgrowth, and correction of nutritional deficiencies [41].

Enteral feeding is preferred to correct nutritional deficiencies after bariatric surgery. Enteral route is a more physiological and immune-enhancing route as compared to parenteral nutrition which can induce or aggravate steatosis and also lead to catheter-related complications. Pancreatic enzymes should be added to increase protein absorption. It seems reasonable to consider administering intravenous thiamine before glucose-containing solution. Other vitamins and micronutrients should also be given as needed. A nasogastric tube should be inserted to avoid aspiration in unconscious patients. Some authors advocate for gastrostomy tube insertion in the bypassed stomach to benefit from early digestion in the proximal bowel, reversal of bacterial overgrowth in the excluded digestive limb, and immune-enhancing capacity.

However, in patients who cannot benefit from enteral feeding due to low compliance or technique difficulties, TPN with vitamins and trace elements should be initiated.

If patients fail to recover with this nutritional assistance, surgery should be undertaken to shorten or eliminate the bypassed bowel [28, 30, 31, 42]. The optimal time for this intervention is unclear but quick action is needed to prevent the patient from advanced liver failure that may lead to death [43].

9.6 Take Home Message

Although bariatric surgery usually leads to amelioration of obesity-associated NAFLD or NASH, sometimes it may lead to hepatic complications. Hence, all bariatric surgeons must understand the risk factors, causes, and proper management of liver-related complications after bariatric surgery. Although, no bariatric surgeries are free of risks; however, the risk for hepatic complications seems to be higher after malabsorptive procedures. To prevent unwanted post-bariatric hepatic complications, it is crucial to individualize patient selection and management.

Key Points

1. *Weight loss after bariatric surgery frequently induces an improvement of non-alcoholic fatty liver disease, non-alcoholic steatohepatitis, and fibrosis. However, bariatric procedures have been also associated with cases of acute liver failure or of chronic liver disease evolving until cirrhosis.*
2. *The clinical manifestations of hepatic complications after bariatric surgery vary from elevated liver enzymes, hypoproteinemia, hyperammonemia to liver failure.*
3. *Possible underlying mechanisms include (1) rapid and drastic weight loss, (2) protein–calorie malnutrition, (3) gut microbiota alteration and bacterial overgrowth, and (4) pre-existing chronic hepatic diseases.*
4. *Enteral feeding is preferred to correct nutritional deficiencies after bariatric surgery.*
5. *No bariatric surgeries are free of risks; however, the risk for hepatic complications seems to be higher after malabsorptive procedures.*
6. *To prevent unwanted post-bariatric hepatic complications, it is crucial to individualize patient selection and management.*

References

1. Flegal KM, Carroll MD, Kit BK, Ogden CL. Prevalence of obesity and trends in the distribution of body mass index among US adults. 1999-2010. JAMA. 2012;307:491–7.
2. Younossi Z, et al. Global epidemiology of nonalcoholic fatty liver disease-Meta-analytic assessment of prevalence, incidence, and outcomes. Hepatology. 2016;64:73–84.
3. Farrell GC, Wong VW, Chitturi S. NAFLD in Asia-as common and important as in the West. Nat Rev Gastroenterol Hepatol. 2013;10(5):307–18.
4. Clark JM. The epidemiology of nonalcoholic fatty liver disease in adults. J Clin Gastroenterol. 2006;40(Suppl 1):S5–10.
5. Lee WJ, Wang W, Lee YC, et al. Clinical characteristics and outcome of morbidly obese bariatric patients with concurrent hepatitis B viral infection. Obes Surg. 2008;18:589–94.
6. Han ML, Lee WJ, Chen JC, et al. Clinical characteristics and outcome of morbidly obese bariatric patients with concurrent hepatitis C viral infection. Obes Surg. 2019;29:828–34.
7. Bower G, Toma T, Harling L, et al. Bariatric surgery and non-alcoholic fatty liver disease: a systematic review of liver biochemistry and histology. Obes Surg. 2015;(12):2280–9.
8. Tan CH, Nawaf AK, Ser KH, et al. Longterm effect of bariatric surgery on resolution of non-alcoholic steatohepatitis (NASH): an external validation and application of a clinical NASH score. Surg Obes Relat Dis. 2018;14(10):1600–6.
9. Requarth J, Burchard K, Colacchio T. Longterm morbidities following jejunoileal bypass: the continuing potential need for surgical reversal. Arch Surg. 1995;130:318–25.
10. Grimm I, Schindler W, Haluszka O. Steatohepatitis and fatal hepatic failure after biliopancreatic diversion. Am J Gastroenterol. 1992;87:775–9.
11. Catillo J, Fabrega E, Escalante CF, et al. Liver transplantation in a case of steatohepatitis and subacute hepatic failure after biliopancreatic diversion and morbid obesity. Obes Surg. 2001;11:640–2.
12. Baltasar A. Liver failure and transplantation after duodenal switch. Surg Obes Relat Dis. 2014;10:e93–6.

13. Cazzo E, Pareja JC, Chaim EA. Liver failure following biliopancreatic diversions: a narrative review. Sao Paulo Med J. 2017;135(1):66–70.
14. Sugerman HJ, Kellum JM, DeMaria EJ. Conversion of proximal to distal gastric bypass for failed gastric bypass for superobesity. J Gastrointest Surg. 1997;1(6):517–24. Discussion 24–6.
15. Motamedi MAK, Barzin M, Ebrahimi M, et al. Severe fatal protein malnutrition and liver failure in a morbidly obese patient after mini-gastric bypass surgery: case report. Int J Surg Case Rep. 2017;33:71–4.
16. Motamedi MAK, Rakhshani N, Khalaj A, et al. Biopsy-proven progressive fatty liver disease nine months post mini-gastric bypass surgery: a case report. Int J Surg Case Rep. 2017;39:168–71.
17. Mahawar KK, Parmar C, Graham Y, et al. Monitoring of liver function tests after Roux-en-Y gastric bypass; An examination of evidence base. Obes Surg. 2016;26(10):2516–22.
18. Mahawar KK, Parmar C, Carr WRJ, et al. Impact of biliopancreatic limb length on severe protein-calorie malnutrition requiring revisional surgery after one anastomosis (mini) gastric bypass. J Minim Access Surg. 2018;14(1):37–43.
19. Ahuja A, Tantia O, Goyal G, et al. MGB-OAGB: effect of biliopancreatic limb length on nutritional deficiency, weight loss, and comorbidity resolution. Obes Surg. 2018;28(11):3439–45.
20. Lee WJ, Ser KH, Lee YC, Tsou JJ, Chen SC, Chen JC. Laparoscopic Roux-en-Y vs. mini-gastric bypass for the treatment of morbid obesity: a 10-year experience. Obes Surg. 2012;27:623–31.
21. Jammu GS, Sharma R. A 7-year clinical audit of 1107 cases comparing sleeve gastrectomy, Roux-en-Y bypass, and mini-gastric bypass, to determine an effective and safe bariatric and metabolic procedure. Obes Surg. 2016;26(5):926–32.
22. Lee WJ, Almalki OM, Ser KH, Chen JC, Lee YC. Randomized controlled trial of one anastomosis gastric bypass versus Roux-en-Y gastric bypass for obesity: comparison of the YOMEGA and Taiwan studies. Obes Surg. 2019;29:3047–65.
23. Kruschitz R, Luger M, Kienbacher C, et al. The effect of Roux-en-Y vs. Omega-loop gastric bypass of liver, metabolic parameters, and weight loss. Obes Surg. 2016;26:2204–12.
24. Kalinowski P, Paluszkiewiez R, Ziarkiewiez-Wroblewska B, et al. Liver function in patients with non-alcoholic fatty liver disease randomized to Roux-en-Y gastric bypass versus sleeve gastrectomy: a secondary analysis of a randomized clinical trial. Ann Surg. 2017;260(5):738–45.
25. Jan A, Narwaria M, Mahawar KK. A systematic review of bariatric surgery in patients with liver cirrhosis. Obes Surg. 2015;25(8):1518–26.
26. Martin JM, Chikunguwo SM, Mosca ER, et al. Severe protein malnutrition in a morbidly obese patient after bariatric surgery. Nutrition. 2015;31:535–8.
27. Faintuch J, Matsuda M, Cruz MELF, et al. Severe protein-calories malnutrition after bariatric procedure. Obes Surg. 2004;14(1):175–8.
28. LIanos JPS, Ferrer MF, Alvarez-Sala-Walther L, et al. Protein malnutrition incidence comparison after gastric bypass versus biliopancreatic diversion. Nutr Hosp. 2015;32(1):80–6.
29. Chen JC, Shen CY, Lee WJ, Tsai PL, Lee YC. Protein deficiency after gastric bypass: the role of common limb length in revision surgery. Surg Obes Relat Dis. 2019;15(1):441–6.
30. Bhandari M, Nautiyal HK, Kosta S, Mathur W, Fobi M. Comparison of one-anastomosis gastric bypass and Roux-en-Y gastric bypass for treatment of obesity: a 5-year study. Surg Obes Relat Dis. 2019, online first.
31. Khalaj A, Motamedi MAK, Mousapour P, Valizadeh M, Barzin M. Protein–Calorie malnutrition requiring revision surgery after one-anastomosis-Mini-gastric bypass (OAGB-MGB): case series from Tehran obesity treatment study (TOTS). Obes Surg. 2019:1714–20.
32. Horsely B, Cottam D, Cottam A, et al. Bowel reconstruction to treat chronic diarrhea and hypoproteinemia following single anastomosis duodenal-ileal bypass with sleeve gastrostomy: a single-site. Obes Surg. 2019;29:2387–91.
33. Mingrone G, Panunz S, De Gaetamo A, et al. Bariatric-metabolic surgery versus conventional medical treatment in obese patients with type 2 diabetes: 5 year follow-up of an open-label, single-center, randomized controlled trials. Lancet. 2015;386:964–73.
34. Borudes S. Which is a good diet-Veg or Non-veg? Faith-based Vegetarianism for protection from obesity – a myth or actually ? Obes Surg. 2019;29(4):1276–80.

35. Estrella J, Yee G, Wilcken B, Tchan M, Talbot M. Hyperammonemic encephalopathy complicating bariatric surgery: a case study and review of the literature. Surg Obes Relat Dis. 2014;10:e35–8.
36. Fenves A, Shchelochkov OA, Mehta A. Hyperammonemic syndrome after Roux-en-Y gastric bypass. Obesity. 2015;23(4):746–9.
37. Brusilow SW, Maestri NE. Urea cycle disorders: diagnosis, pathophysiology, and therapy. Adv Pediatr. 1996;43:127–70.
38. Dionisi-Vici C, Rizzo C, Burlina AB, et al. Inborn errors of metabolism in the Italian pediatric population: a national retrospective survey. J Pediatr. 2002;140:321–7.
39. Lazzati A, Iannelli A, Schneck AS, et al. Bariatric surgery and liver transplantation: a systematic review a new frontier for bariatric surgery. Obes Surg. 2015;25(1):134–42.
40. Mocanu I, Carvalhana S, Costa P, Palma R. Liver failure after bariatric surgery – Clinical case and literature review. J Gastroenterol Metabol. 2018;1:104.
41. Keleidari B, Mahmoudieh M, Gorgi K, Sheikhbahaei E, Shahabi S. Hepatic failure after bariatric surgery: a systematic review. Hepat Mon. 2019;19(1):e86078.
42. Chen CY, Lee WJ, Lee HM, et al. Laparoscopic conversion of gastric bypass complication to sleeve gastrectomy: technique and early results. Obes Surg. 2016;26:2014–21.
43. Lammers WJ, Tilburg AJP, Apers JA, Wiebolt J. Liver failure caused by prolonged state of malnutrition following bariatric surgery. World J Hepatol. 2018;10(3):396–9.

Renal Complications After Bariatric Surgery

10

Rickesha Wilson and Ali Aminian

Superficially, it might be said that the function of the kidneys is to make urine; but in a more considered view one can say that the kidneys make the stuff of philosophy itself.

—Homer Smith

10.1 The Relationship Between Obesity, Diabetes, and Renal Disease

The pandemic crisis of obesity has worsened over the last several decades. Obesity increases the risk of diabetes and hypertension and is often part of a larger public health crisis known as the metabolic syndrome [1]. The metabolic syndrome can have a detrimental impact on an individual's renal function. The literature estimates that in 14–30% of those with chronic kidney disease (CKD), obesity plays a pathogenic role and a fifth of these patients have at least stage II obesity [2, 3]. Furthermore, epidemiological investigations have demonstrated the correlation between each component of the metabolic syndrome and increased risk of developing CKD. The overall metabolic health of an individual is more indicative of the risk of CKD development as evidence points out that metabolically healthy individuals with obesity have lower risk of CKD development than metabolically unhealthy individuals without obesity [4]. Obesity has also been found to increase the risk of nephrolithiasis and renal cell cancer [3]. Mechanisms by which obesity leads to renal dysfunction include obesity-mediated hypertension, insulin resistance, glomerular

R. Wilson · A. Aminian (✉)
Department of General Surgery, Bariatric and Metabolic Institute, Cleveland Clinic, Cleveland, OH, USA
e-mail: WILSONR13@ccf.org; AMINIAA@ccf.org

A. G. Bhasker et al. (eds.), *Management of Nutritional and Metabolic Complications of Bariatric Surgery*,
https://doi.org/10.1007/978-981-33-4702-1_10

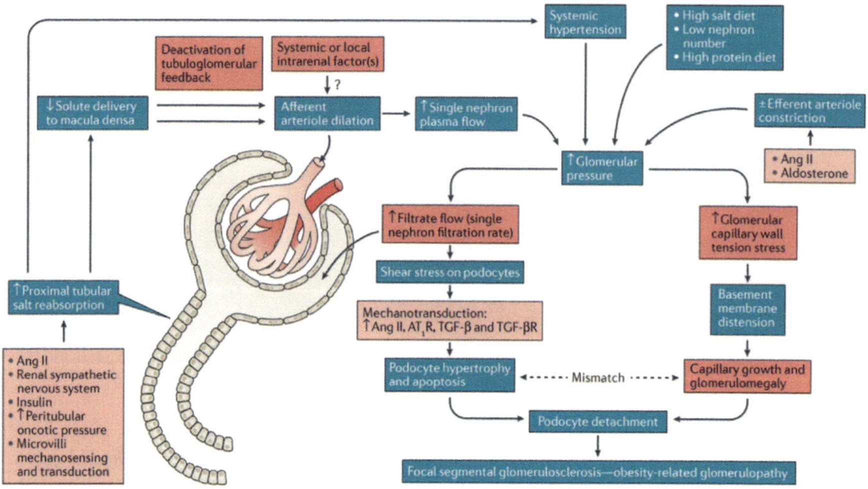

Fig. 10.1 Obesity-related glomerulopathy. Hemodynamic alterations in obesity: primary dilatation of the afferent arteriole and variable constriction of the efferent arteriole via activation of angiotensin II (Ang II) and aldosterone contribute to increases in single nephron plasma flow, glomerular intracapillary hydrostatic pressure, and filtration rate. The major driver of afferent arteriolar dilatation is unknown, but deactivation of tubuloglomerular feedback via increased proximal tubular salt reabsorption and decreased delivery to the macula densa likely has a role. A host of factors, including Ang II, the renal sympathetic nervous system, insulin, an increase in post-glomerular oncotic pressure due to increased filtration fraction, and mechanosensors of tubular flow rates, mediate the increased tubular reabsorption of sodium. The increase in filtrate flow (single nephron filtration rate) in turn promotes glomerular capillary wall stretch tension, glomerulomegaly, and maladaptive podocyte stress leading to obesity-related glomerulopathy and focal segmental glomerulosclerosis. *AT1R* type 1 angiotensin II receptor, *TGF-β*, transforming growth factor β, *TGF-βR* TGF-β receptor. Adapted with permission from *Nat Rev Nephrol* 12, 453–471 (2016)

hypertrophy, activation of the renin–angiotensin–aldosterone system, inflammation, and adipocytokine dysregulation [3].

Obesity affects the kidney through a process known as obesity-related glomerulopathy (ORG, Fig. 10.1). Obesity causes hemodynamic changes at the level of the glomerulus by reducing preglomerular vascular resistance and increasing the glomerular filtration rate (GFR). This results in glomerular hyperfiltration, known to be a major cause of ORG [5]. The resultant glomerular hypertension leads to glomerulomegaly, mild effacement of podocytes, stretching of the microvasculature in this region, and eventual microalbuminuria. The pathologic findings of ORG are focal segmental glomerulosclerosis (FSGS) lesions in the perihilar region, mesangial and tubular cell lipid deposits, and podocyte effacement from glomerular hypertrophy. In patients with obesity without diabetes, diabetic-like renal changes have been found, focal mesangial sclerosis and thickening of tubular and basement membranes [6].

Obesity-related hyperfiltration may also be impacted by increased glucose and sodium absorption in the proximal convoluted tubules via the sodium–glucose cotransporter proteins (SGLT1 and SGLT2). Obesity can cause a decreased sodium load at the distal tubule, and feedback to the macula densa promotes afferent arteriole vasodilation and subsequent glomerular hyperfiltration. Inhibitors of SGLT2 have been shown to reduce albuminuria and GFR, giving further credence to the hypothesis of a renal tubular origin of ORG [7, 8].

The most common clinical manifestation of obesity-related renal disease is proteinuria, which can be, but is usually not, detected in the nephrotic or massive range (>3.5 g/day and >20 g/day, respectively) [9, 10]. There is likely a slow progression of proteinuria over time and metabolic compensation is allowed that limits the development of nephrotic syndrome (hypoalbuminemia, edema, and hyperlipidemia). Potential mechanisms responsible for ORG-specific differences from nephrotic syndrome may be increased hepatic synthesis of albumin over time and also tubular handling of filtered proteins that may change in the setting of hyperfiltration [5]. This clinical distinction in ORG is important for clinicians to be aware of when patients with obesity are detected to have proteinuria for the most accurate diagnostic and therapeutic interventions. Furthermore, studies have shown that renal biopsies at the time of bariatric surgery reflect ORG-lesions even without clinical manifestations of proteinuria or renal derangements [11].

10.2 Early Postoperative Complications

Acute kidney injury (AKI) can complicate the postoperative course after metabolic surgery, and its incidence is approximately 1% [12]. The etiology of perioperative AKI after bariatric surgery is multifactorial in the obese population and individuals with pre-existing hypertension, diabetes, and renal disease are at increased risk of perioperative AKI [13–15]. There is a three- to sevenfold increase in postoperative AKI in patients undergoing noncardiac surgery with obesity compared to individuals without obesity [16]. Morbidity and mortality following bariatric surgery in the setting of acute renal dysfunction, especially for severe cases requiring dialysis support, is increased by 6.5-fold [17, 18].

A study published by Hanipah et al. in 2018 explored the incidence of postoperative AKI in 42 of their 4722 metabolic surgery patients along with the major causes and long-term effects on renal function. Acute kidney injury occurred due to prerenal causes in 88% of patients and renal causes in 12%. Nine patients (21%) required hemodialysis support in the postoperative period due to septic shock ($n = 7$), bleeding ($n = 1$), and worsening pre-existing CKD stage 5 ($n = 1$). Median follow-up was 28 months and 90% had a return to baseline renal function. Of the four patients who had abnormal renal function at follow-up, three had CKD stages 4 and 5 prior to surgery and required permanent dialysis, and one developed CKD stage 3 postoperatively due to short gut syndrome after multiple surgeries. This study concluded that most patients have a return to normal baseline renal function after postoperative

AKI, however, those with pre-existing renal disease are at high risk for persistent renal dysfunction [12].

Koppe et al. compared the incidence of AKI in bariatric surgery patients ($n = 2643$) compared to a matched, nonsurgical cohort ($n = 2595$) using a large, prospectively maintained database in the United Kingdom. This study found a low incidence of AKI (five events) within the first 30 days following surgery and a protective effect of bariatric surgery compared to controls beyond 30 days during the 3-year follow-up period [19].

A multicenter study based out of Australia evaluated 590 bariatric surgery patients who were admitted to the intensive care unit (ICU) postoperatively. This study found that patients who developed AKI in the ICU (17%), had increased peak plasma creatinine concentrations, hospital and ICU lengths of stay compared to those ICU patients without AKI. While most of these AKI episodes (76%) were mild, a single episode of AKI in the ICU postoperatively was associated with higher long-term mortality [13].

Appropriate management of postoperative AKI in the bariatric and metabolic surgery population involves early identification of renal dysfunction, aggressive hydration with intravenous fluids for prerenal causes such as dehydration, bleeding, and hypovolemia from sepsis. Prompt treatment for infectious etiologies and septic shock is also warranted to avoid multiorgan dysfunction and further metabolic derangements that make renal function worse. Renal causes of AKI such as rhabdomyolysis and contrast nephropathy should also be treated expectantly.

10.3 Nephrolithiasis

Obesity is a known risk factor for nephrolithiasis. Different metabolic surgery procedures are also associated with nephrolithiasis to varying degrees: purely malabsorptive procedures (22–28%), Roux-en-Y gastric bypass (RYGB) (7–13%), and lowest in restrictive procedures [SG and adjustable gastric banding (ABG)] (Fig. 10.2) [20]. Time to renal stone development after bariatric surgery ranges from 1.5 to 3.6 years [21–23]. Prior history of stones before surgery increases the risk of postoperative stone development compared to those without a history (42% vs. 14%, respectively, HR > 4.1, $p < 0.0001$) [24]. De novo stone formation after RYGB in those with no prior stone history ranges from 3 to 8% [23, 25].

Several components are at play in the pathogenesis of nephrolithiasis after metabolic surgery—namely hypovolemia, hyperoxaluria, hypocitraturia, aciduria, and supersaturation of the urine with calcium oxalate [26, 27]. Oxalate is an endogenous byproduct of amino acid metabolism and is absorbed by the stomach, small intestine, and colon. Its absorption is increased in malabsorptive states and secondary enteric hyperoxaluria (urinary excretion of >40–45 mg/day) develops due to increased absorption of oxalate from the intestine—inflammation and bile salts promote mucosal permeability. Calcium usually binds oxalate and is excreted in the stool. However, due to the presence of non-absorbed fatty acids binding calcium in enteric hyperoxaluria in malabsorptive states, more oxalate is available downstream

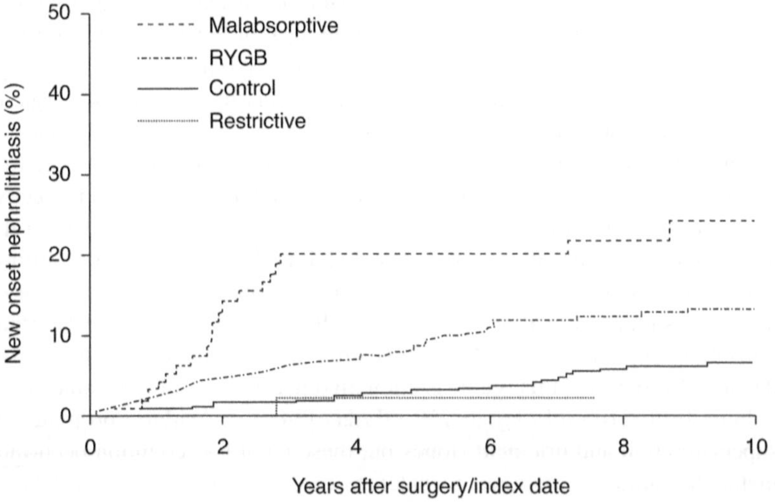

No. at risk						
Malabsorptive	101	77	58	47	36	27
RYGB	563	502	408	293	208	94
Control	729	673	572	416	282	135
Restrictive	55	54	36	18	0	0

Fig. 10.2 Risk of new-onset nephrolithiasis after bariatric surgery. The risk of incident stones was greater after RYGB or malabsorptive bariatric procedures compared with that of matched obese controls. Patients with restrictive procedures were not at increased risk. Adapted with permission from Kidney International (2015) 87, 839–845

in the colon to be passively absorbed into the bloodstream and eventually filtered and excreted by the kidneys [28, 29].

Malabsorptive procedures (RYGB, jejunoileal bypass, and biliopancreatic diversion with duodenal switch) have the highest rate of nephrolithiasis, postoperatively. In the Rochester Epidemiology Project, all patients who underwent an RYGB had higher urinary oxalate levels, and those who developed renal stones had the highest levels along with supersaturation of calcium oxalate. The number of other types of renal stones does not change significantly (hydroxyapatite, struvite, and uric acid) [24]. The makeup of the colonic flora can also have an impact on the clearance of luminal oxalate. *Oxalobacter formigenes* (*O. formigenes*) is a Gram-negative anaerobe found to be associated with lower urinary oxalate levels [30]. After malabsorptive surgery, the alteration in the gut microbial flora that reduces *O. formigenes* in addition to increased fecal fat content can promote increased oxalate absorption and lead to a higher incidence of nephrolithiasis [30, 31].

Hypocitraturia after metabolic surgery is less common than hyperoxaluria with a 24–63% incidence in the literature [20]. Citric acid is a weak acid made endogenously from the tricarboxylic acid cycle and also comes from fruits and vegetables in the diet. Its dissociated anion is citrate, which forms soluble complexes with calcium in the urine and prevents precipitation of calcium oxalate and calcium phosphate. In acidosis, the mitochondrial use of citrate increases, leading to increased renal absorption and hypocitraturia of <320 mg/day. Assuming a 2-L urinary output daily and normal urine pH and potassium levels, 640 mg/day is the urine citrate in normal, healthy individuals [32].

Obesity is associated with hypercalciuria, which also promotes stone formation. RYGB has been associated with hypocalciuria and this can exert a protective effect on stone formation by preventing supersaturation of calcium oxalate in the urine. Valezi and colleagues demonstrated in 151 RYGB patients that one-fifth of those with hypercalciuria preoperatively had none postoperatively [33]. Urinary volume decreases significantly after metabolic surgery and is a major driver of urinary crystallization. One study found the average drop in 24-h urine volume to go from 1.8 L/day to 1.4 L/day, and this is consistent with other findings of a sustained decrease in volume from 2100 mL/day to 750 mL/day [34, 35]. Aciduria promotes uric acid supersaturation and uric acid stones but these are a less common occurrence after metabolic surgery compared to calcium oxalate stones, 1.5% vs. 94%, respectively [24].

The jejunoileal bypass in the 1970s proved to be littered with complications and was eventually abandoned with a 28% risk of nephrolithiasis and a 9% risk of renal insufficiency according to a 15-year longitudinal study [36]. The now more commonly performed metabolic surgeries have a varied risk of nephrolithiasis (Fig. 10.2) [24]. Extensive gastrointestinal bypass procedures have a documented higher risk of nephrolithiasis compared to restrictive procedures. A retrospective database review of 4639 patients following RYGB compared to matched obese controls revealed a 7.65% vs. 4.63% nephrolithiasis risk (odds ratio of 1.71) and a mean time to developing renal stones of 1.5 years [37]. There is an increase in stone risk also with more distal RYGB procedures [21]. Lieske and colleagues prospectively matched 762 bariatric patients with obese controls with similar baseline nephrolithiasis incidence of 4% and 4.2%. The development of new stones tripled in the bariatric group postoperatively to 11.1% vs. 4.3% at a mean follow-up of 6 years. Baseline stone type in these two groups was largely calcium oxalate 73% vs. 65% and increased postoperatively to 94% calcium oxalate. In patients undergoing malabsorptive procedures, those at highest risk for stones are also at highest risk for CKD (hazard ratio of 1.96, $p < 0.03$), although this distinction is not detected when all bariatric procedure types are combined [24].

Restrictive procedures have demonstrated a much lower risk of nephrolithiasis compared to malabsorptive procedures, and that risk approaches that of nonsurgical matched obese controls [24, 38]. Semins and others have demonstrated that AGB patients have an even lower incidence, 1.49% vs. 5.97% that is consistent beyond 2.5 years [39]. Restrictive procedures also are associated with hypovolemia, but this effect is likely countered by the hypocalciuria and the low stone risk is maintained [20].

Mitigation and management of nephrolithiasis can be achieved to improve patient outcomes. Hyperoxaluria can be managed with a low-fat diet that would decrease the fatty acid load and promote calcium oxalate binding. A low oxalate diet and calcium supplementation would also decrease the oxalate load in the gut and decrease the incidence of hyperoxaluria. Adequate daily hydration keeps urinary volume closer to baseline levels and decreases the risk of crystallization and supersaturation of calcium oxalate in the urine [40]. Hypocitraturia can be treated with potassium citrate salts and also calcium citrate, which increases urinary citrate levels, increases hypercalciuria, and also increases the calcium load in the intestinal lumen to bind oxalate. Probiotics could potentially repopulate the gut flora with oxalate reducing species, such as *O. formigenes*.

Procedural interventions are mainly shockwave lithotripsy and ureteroscopy as reported by Matlaga and colleagues. In this study, 355 RYGB patients who developed urinary calculi in the treatment cohort were more likely to undergo shockwave lithotripsy (1.75% vs. 0.41%) or ureteroscopy (2.11% vs. 0.58%). The odds ratios for RYGB patients to develop stones and subsequently need procedures were 1.71 and 3.65, respectively [37].

Further opportunities exist for advancing our knowledge of the mechanisms for nephrolithiasis and preventing this risk in metabolic surgery patients. The SLC26 gene family encodes oxalate transport proteins in the intestines that may have altered function following RYGB. Risk stratification preoperatively of patients at highest risk for nephrolithiasis can be implemented and influence the recommended and chosen procedure type [32].

10.4 Safety of Bariatric and Metabolic Surgery in Patients with Chronic Kidney Disease

The stage of CKD does not significantly affect 30-day mortality, but there is a positive correlation between stage of renal dysfunction and postoperative complications, albeit low [41]. Thirty-day mortality for patients with ESRD range from 0.4 to 0.7% [42, 43]. The impact of varying degrees of renal dysfunction on short-term bariatric surgery outcomes was studied by Saleh and colleagues [44]. Using the American College of Surgeons National Surgical Quality Improvement Program database, over 64,000 patients were retrospectively evaluated with varying degrees of CKD based on estimated GFR (eGFR): stage I (61.7%), stage 2 (32%), stage 3 (5.3%), and stages 4 and 5 (1%). There was an increasing trend in overall and major complications with increasing renal insufficiency, however, there was no statistical significance. There was only a significant difference in the RYGB group who had stage I vs III renal disease for overall complications and stage I vs IV for major complications ($p < .001$).

Cohen and others conducted one of the largest retrospective cohort studies [45] using the Metabolic and Bariatric Surgery Accreditation and Quality Improvement Program to determine the effect of CKD and ESRD on short-term postoperative outcomes in bariatric surgery. Using matching techniques to account for differences in patient characteristics, they evaluated 323,034 bariatric surgery patients without CKD, 1694 with CKD, and 925 with ESRD. There was an increase in 30-day reoperation rate with an odds ratio of 2.25 and 3.1 for CKD and ESRD, respectively, and an increased mortality rate with an odds ratio of 11.59 for ESRD patients. Also, men with CKD had higher readmission rates compared to men without CKD, while women in both groups had similar rates in this category. Overall adverse outcomes were considered low at less than 15% and bariatric surgery was still deemed safe for patients with CKD and ESRD. The mortality rates for those with renal disease were comparable to those in the literature without bariatric surgery. This study was reflective of the current trends in bariatric surgery with approaches being minimally invasive and the majority of patients in each group undergoing SG. It was limited by the lack of delineation in renal dysfunction between patient groups and the limited data from the database not capturing specific parameters such as creatinine levels and proteinuria [45].

A longitudinal population-based study of Medicare beneficiaries who underwent bariatric surgery from 2006 to 2016 compared the postoperative outcomes of those with and without ESRD [46]. Over the course of the study period, there was a 9-fold increase in patient volume and an 1.5-fold increase in ESRD prevalence. Readmission rates and length of stay were higher for those with ESRD than those without. During this time there was also a surge in the number of SG procedures from less than 1% to 84%. This study captures the current trends in procedure type across the country and captures a large proportion of the ESRD community that is served by Medicare.

Metabolic and bariatric surgery is safe in select patients with CKD and should not be perceived as a contraindication for surgery. There is a slightly higher risk for early postoperative complications in patients with CKD but long-term evidence shows a benefit in overall renal function.

10.5 Considerations in Transplant Candidates/Recipients

Obesity increases the risk of CKD and eventually contributes to development of ESRD [47]. As defined by the United States Renal Data System (USRDS), ESRD patients are formally registered to receive hemodialysis or transplantation as a form of renal replacement therapy [48]. The incidence of ESRD at the end of 2016 according to the USRDS was 1887 per million individuals and the two primary causes were diabetes and hypertension. Obesity is the most preventable risk factor in ESRD and 60% of affected individuals are either overweight or obese [49, 50]. Renal transplantation for ESRD patients have clear benefits, however, many patients with class III or higher obesity are not able to be listed for transplantation due to the associated relative and absolute contraindications at some institutions (BMI greater than 35 and 40, respectively) [51, 52].

Bariatric surgery serves as an effective bridge to transplantation for ESRD patients who are unable to be listed due to class III or higher obesity, and this is a more reliable weight loss strategy than nonoperative management [53]. A registry-based study from a single center in Florida by Modanlou et al. reported that 72 obese patients (BMI 38 ± 12) who underwent bariatric surgery had an average time to activation on the transplant list of 16 ± 13 months ($n = 72$) and an actual time to transplantation from bariatric surgery of 17 ± 11 months ($n = 29$) [53]. Al-Bhari et al. at a single center in Florida retrospectively reviewed the outcomes of 16 patients on hemodialysis who underwent bariatric surgery from 1998 to 2016. Median follow-up was 2.8 years (range 1–10), preoperative BMI was 48 ± 8 kg/m^2 and postoperative BMI was 31 ± 7 kg/m^2 with an average percent excess body weight loss of 62 ± 24%. At the time of publication, four patients (25%) had undergone renal transplantation at 4.3 ± 1.4 years post-bariatric surgery, five patients were currently listed, five patients were still not listed due to persistent comorbid conditions, and two patients died due to comorbidities. Waiting times for transplantation in the bariatric surgery population continue to be due to a shortage of organs and regional factors such as pretransplantation work up [54].

Transplant recipients who are obese have a higher risk of posttransplant diabetes, surgical site complications, delayed graft function, and higher mortality due to obesity-related comorbidities [55, 56]. Remission or mitigation of obesity-related comorbidities through metabolic surgery can improve outcomes for renal transplant recipients.

10.6 Risk Reduction After Metabolic Surgery

Improving the major risk factors of CKD through metabolic surgery can significantly address the global health and economic strains that ESRD carries. Long-term evidence demonstrates that metabolic surgery significantly reduces the overall risk of renal dysfunction in patients with significant metabolic risk factors.

The investigators of the STAMPEDE trial published their long-term 5-year results after randomizing patients with T2D to receive either medical therapy or RYGB or SG. The primary endpoint of glycated hemoglobin less than 6% without diabetes medications was met by 5% of participants in the medical cohort versus 29% in the surgical cohort [57]. In addition to improved glycemic control, patients who underwent metabolic surgery had a significant decrease in the use of medications for diabetes, hypertension, and dyslipidemia. These long-term results suggest that the overall metabolic improvement with surgery compared to medical therapy alone leads to reduced risk of eventual renal dysfunction that the metabolic syndrome causes.

In the prospective, matched Swedish Obese Subjects study, patients with obesity and diabetes who underwent bariatric surgery compared to usual care experienced higher rates of diabetes remission, which subsequently correlated to reduced incidence of microvascular complications after 15 years. When analyzing these outcomes based on glycemic status, surgery was found to have the greatest risk reduction among participants with prediabetes compared to usual care. In those with prediabetes who underwent surgery, the risk of renal microvascular complications was reduced even among those who develop diabetes during follow-up [58].

Aminian and colleagues evaluated 131 patients with diabetes and the impact of RYGB on the long-term risk reduction of various end-organ complications using various risk prediction models. Median follow-up was 6 years after RYGB, and excess weight loss was 60.7 ± 25.1% with a diabetes remission rate of 61%.

Significant percentages of patients had other metabolic syndrome components to fall within appropriate range at follow-up according to the American Diabetes Association criteria: glycated hemoglobin (85%), LDL (73%), and blood pressure (63%). The predicted relative risk reduction for cardiovascular disease (CHD, Stroke, and PVD) was 27% and for moderate–severe chronic kidney disease was 45% [59, 60].

Other studies have also documented strong evidence for the remission of metabolic syndrome components. Adams and colleagues report a 62% diabetes remission after RYGB at 6 year follow-up [61]. The Swedish Obese Subjects study after 10-year follow-up found improved recovery for diabetes, hypertriglyceridemia, low HDL, hypertension, and hyperuricemia with metabolic surgery [62]. Brethauer et al. who investigated 217 patients with diabetes after metabolic surgery also found a diabetes remission rate of 50%, improvement in 34%, and no change in 16%. The usual normo-albuminuria to albuminuria transition rate of 2–4% per year reported in the literature, was less than 1% per year after metabolic surgery in this small study. Regression of established diabetic nephropathy was seen in approximately half of patients [63, 64].

Reducing the incidence of microvascular complications from diabetes are critical outcomes to measure the efficacy of metabolic surgery compared to medical therapy. A large multicenter-matched cohort study retrospectively evaluated adults with T2D and severe obesity. There were 4024 patients who had bariatric surgery compared to 11,059 nonsurgical controls. The surgical cohort demonstrated a lower incidence of composite microvascular disease as well as nephropathy at 1, 3, 5, and 7 years after the index date. Specifically, at 5 years, incident composite microvascular disease and nephropathy was 59% lower with surgical treatment [65].

Similarly, another large, retrospective, matched-cohort study from the Cleveland Clinic Health System compared metabolic surgery and usual care for patients with T2D and obesity. The primary outcome was incidence of extended major adverse cardiovascular events (MACE): all-cause mortality, coronary artery events, cerebrovascular events, heart failure, nephropathy, and atrial fibrillation. Patients who underwent metabolic surgery had a 40% reduction in MACE (hazard ratio, HR, of 0.61) and a 60% reduction in risk of nephropathy (HR 0.40) in 8 years (Fig. 10.3) [66].

Studies have also shown that metabolic surgery reduces the risk of CKD, stage 3 or higher, from progressing to kidney failure. Funes et al. reported a risk reduction of 70% at 2 years and 60% at 5 years [67]. These studies demonstrate the profound impact that metabolic surgery has on obesity-related renal dysfunction when compared to medical therapy. Substantial and sustained weight loss accounts for much of the metabolic, hemodynamic, and neurohormonal changes that occur after metabolic surgery. However, there is growing evidence that some of these significant changes are weight independent [68–70]. The risk reduction that metabolic surgery affords to individuals with obesity and metabolic risk factors makes this treatment a powerful tool going forward to treat and prevent chronic diseases that affect the kidneys and other organ systems.

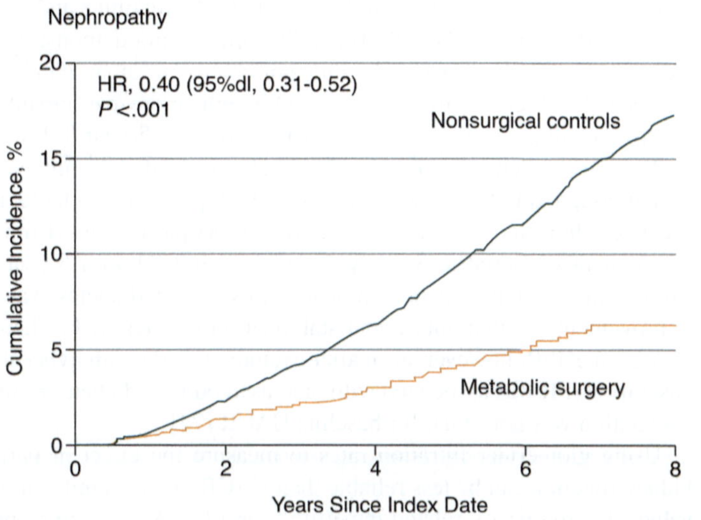

No. at risk					
Nonsurgical controls	9190	7056	4515	2262	893
Metabolic surgery	1937	1216	838	506	293

Fig. 10.3 Kaplan-Meier curve of the cumulative incidence of nephropathy at 8 years. Adapted with permission from *JAMA*. 2019;322(13):1271–1282

10.7 Improvement of Kidney Function After Metabolic Surgery

There is a close relationship between obesity and albuminuria, a marker of kidney damage defined as a urinary albumin-to-creatine ratio (UACR) of greater than 30 mg/g. Albuminuria is also a known risk factor for renal and cardiovascular disease but is linked to obesity independent of other comorbidities [64, 71].

A systematic review and meta-analysis by Upala and colleagues evaluated 15 observational studies assessing the effect of bariatric surgery on patients with diabetic nephropathy. The results from this meta-analysis revealed a significant reduction in UACR (−6.6 mg/g of creatinine) and a reduction in albuminuria (−55.76 mg in 24 h) after bariatric surgery with short-term follow-up [72].

Young and colleagues retrospectively evaluated the long-term changes of UACR in 101 patients with preoperative diabetes and albuminuria. The median UACR decreased from 80 mg/g prior to surgery to 30 mg/g at last follow-up (61 months). Along with significant weight reduction and glycemic control, albuminuria resolved in 77% of these patients and improved in 51% [73].

The STAMPEDE trial reported its 5-year renal outcomes. There was a significant decrease in UACR only in the sleeve gastrectomy group compared to medical therapy. There was a significant decrease in both creatinine and GFR from baseline among participants in the RYGB and SG cohorts, not demonstrated in the medical therapy cohort. There was no significant change in albuminuria status at 5 years between the three treatment groups, although, more participants in the surgical groups had albuminuria at baseline that resolved by 5-year follow-up [57].

To assess whether remission of diabetes is related to improvement in eGFR, proteinuria, and risk for CKD, Friedman et al. performed a large, multicenter, prospective cohort study of over 700 bariatric surgery participants (from the Longitudinal Assessment of Bariatric Surgery-2 study) with T2D with 5-year follow-up. This study found that partial or complete remission of diabetes was associated with improvement in albuminuria and stabilization of CKD risk. There was negligible change in eGFR, however, even after excluding those with hyperfiltration. A higher baseline eGFR was associated with increased odds of diabetes remission, while this association was not found for baseline UACR [74].

Using glomerular filtration rates to measure the effect of bariatric surgery on kidney function can be less reliable than UACR due to significant variation in GFR values due to obesity-related hyperfiltration [75]. A large, retrospective, matched-cohort study from Kaiser Permanente Southern California's patient registry evaluated patients with CKD, stages 3 and 4, before and after bariatric surgery ($n = 714$) and compared them to a group of nonsurgical controls ($n = 714$). The primary endpoint was change in eGFR over a median 3-year follow-up period. There was a significant increase in eGFR in surgery patients compared to controls (9.84 mL/min/1.73 m^2 greater) and also in those undergoing RYGB compared to SG (6.60 mL/min/1.73 m^2 greater) [76].

MicroRNAs (miR) are endogenous RNAs that regulate gene expression through silencing the translation of mRNAs. They have emerged as a viable biomarker in several disease states due to their stability in biofluids and simple detectability through PCR and other platforms. At the urinary level, miRNAs have been detected in immunoglobulin A nephropathy and bladder cancer. A longitudinal, prospective study of 24 bariatric surgery patients (compared to obese and healthy controls) revealed that miR 192, mi200a, and mi200b were upregulated in urine following bariatric surgery with a profile reflecting controls with obesity preoperatively to healthy controls over 100 days postoperatively. Obesity and diabetes share a similar mechanism in the development of CKD through epithelial-to-mesenchymal transition (EMT). MicroRNAs 192 and those in the 200 family inhibit EMT by down-regulating ZEB1 and ZEB2 and consequently decreasing collagen deposition in the extracellular matrix [77]. Continuing research into reliable markers to measure kidney function will further establish metabolic surgery's impact on renal function.

10.8 Conclusions

There is mounting evidence that metabolic and bariatric surgery has a beneficial impact on renal function for at-risk patients with obesity and metabolic disease. Risk of postoperative complications such as acute kidney injury and nephrolithiasis may be higher in those with baseline renal dysfunction, however, metabolic surgery remains a safe option for this population. Furthermore, long-term evidence is favorable for metabolic surgery reducing the risk of microvascular complications from obesity and diabetes. Select patients awaiting transplantation may also benefit from metabolic surgery to reduce waiting times and reduce the relative contraindications related to obesity. Several markers are available to assess and follow renal function in and beyond the perioperative period to monitor at-risk patients and their response to surgery. The high-risk patients with pre-existing advanced CKD, multiple comorbidities, and advanced age are at risk for developing renal dysfunction and must be monitored closely.

Key Points

1. *Mechanisms by which obesity leads to renal dysfunction include obesity-mediated hypertension, insulin resistance, glomerular hypertrophy, activation of the renin–angiotensin–aldosterone system, inflammation, and adipocytokine dysregulation.*
2. *Obesity affects the kidney through a process known as obesity-related glomerulopathy.*
3. *The most common clinical manifestation of obesity-related renal disease is proteinuria.*
4. *Appropriate management of postoperative AKI in the bariatric and metabolic surgery population involves early identification of renal dysfunction, aggressive hydration with intravenous fluids for prerenal causes such as dehydration, bleeding, and hypovolemia from sepsis.*
5. *De novo kidney stone formation after RYGB in those with no prior stone history ranges from 3 to 8%.*
6. *Metabolic and bariatric surgery is safe in select patients with CKD and should not be perceived as a contraindication for surgery.*
7. *There is a slightly higher risk for early postoperative complications in patients with CKD but long-term evidence shows a benefit in overall renal function.*
8. *Bariatric surgery serves as an effective bridge to transplantation for ESRD patients who are unable to be listed due to class III or higher obesity, and this is a more reliable weight loss strategy than nonoperative management.*
9. *Remission or mitigation of obesity-related comorbidities through metabolic surgery can improve outcomes for renal transplant recipients.*
10. *Metabolic surgery reduces the risk of CKD, stage 3 or higher, from progressing to kidney failure.*

References

1. Nor Hanipah Z, Punchai S, Augustin T, Brethauer SA, Schauer PR, Aminian A. Impact of early postbariatric surgery acute kidney injury on long-term renal function. Obes Surg. 2018;28:3580–5.
2. Wang Y, Chen X, Song Y, Caballero B, Cheskin LJ. Association between obesity and kidney disease: a systematic review and meta-analysis. Kidney Int. 2008;73:19–33.
3. Chang AR, Grams ME, Navaneethan SD. Bariatric surgery and kidney-related outcomes. Kidney Int Rep. 2017;2:261–70.

4. Hashimoto Y, Tanaka M, Okada H, et al. Article metabolically healthy obesity and risk of incident CKD. Clin J Am Soc Nephrol. 2015;10:578–83.
5. Praga M, Morales E. The fatty kidney: obesity and renal disease. Nephron. 2017;136:273–6.
6. D'agati VD, Kaskel FJ, Falk RJ. Medical progress focal segmental glomerulosclerosis. N Engl J Med. 2011;365:2398–411.
7. Zinman B, Wanner C, Lachin JM, et al. Empagliflozin, cardiovascular outcomes, and mortality in type 2 diabetes. N Engl J Med. 2015;373:2117–28.
8. Novikov A, Vallon V, Diego S. SGLT2 inhibition in the diabetic kidney-an update HHS Public Access. Curr Opin Nephrol Hypertens. 2016;25:50–8.
9. Praga M, Herna Â, Ndez E, Morales E, Pe A, Campos Â, Âa M, Valero A, Martõ Ânez MA, Leo M. Clinical features and long-term outcome of obesity-associated focal segmental glomerulosclerosis. Nephrol Dial Transplant. 2001;1790:98.
10. Kambham N, Markowitz GS, Valeri AM, Lin J, D'agati VD. Obesity-related glomerulopathy: an emerging epidemic. Kidney Int. 2001;59:1498–509.
11. Serra A, Romero R, Lopez D, Navarro M, Esteve A, Perez N, Alastrue A, Ariza A. Renal injury in the extremely obese patients with normal renal function. Kidney Int. 2008;73:947–55.
12. Hanipah ZN, Punchai S, Augustin T, Brethauer SA, Schauer PR, Aminian A. Impact of early postbariatric surgery acute kidney injury on long-term renal function. Obes Surg. 2018;28:3580–5.
13. Morgan DJR, Ho KM. Acute kidney injury in bariatric surgery patients requiring intensive care admission: a state-wide, multicenter, cohort study. Surg Obes Relat Dis. 2015;11:1300–6.
14. Currie A, Chetwood A, Ahmed AR, Currie A, Chetwood A, Ahmed AR. Bariatric surgery and renal function. Obes Surg. 2011;21:528–39.
15. Sharma SK, McCauley J, Cottam D, et al. Acute changes in renal function after laparoscopic gastric surgery for morbid obesity. Surg Obes Relat Dis. 2006;2:389–92.
16. Glance LG, Wissler R, Mukamel DB, Li Y, Ann Diachun CB, Salloum R, Fleming FJ, Dick AW. PERIOPERATIVE MEDICINE perioperative outcomes among patients with the modified metabolic syndrome who are undergoing noncardiac surgery. Anesthesiology. 2010;113:859.
17. Thakar CV, Worley S, Arrigain S, Yared JP, Paganini EP. Influence of renal dysfunction on mortality after cardiac surgery: modifying effect of preoperative renal function. Kidney Int. 2005;67:1112–9.
18. Uchino S, Kellum J, Bellomo R, et al. Acute renal failure in critically ill patients. JAMA. 2005;294:813–8.
19. Koppe U, Nitsch D, Mansfield KE, Mathur R, Bhaskaran K, Batterham RL, Smeeth L, Douglas IJ. Long-term effects of bariatric surgery on acute kidney injury: a propensity-matched cohort in the UK Clinical Practice Research Datalink. BMJ Open. 2018;8:1–8.
20. Hasan Bhatti U, Duffy AJ, Eric Roberts K, Hafeez Shariff A. Nephrolithiasis after bariatric surgery: a review of pathophysiologic mechanisms and procedural risk. Int J Surg. 2016;36:618–23.
21. Sinha MK, Collazo-Clavell ML, Rule A, Milliner DS, Nelson W, Sarr MG, Kumar R, Lieske JC. Hyperoxaluric nephrolithiasis is a complication of Roux-en-Y gastric bypass surgery. Kidney Int. 2007;72:100–7.
22. Asplin JR, Coe FL. Hyperoxaluria in kidney stone formers treated with modern bariatric surgery. J Urol. 2007;177:565–9.
23. Durrani O, Morrisroe S, Jackman S, Averch T. Analysis of stone disease in morbidly obese patients undergoing gastric bypass surgery. J Endourol. 2006;20:749–52.
24. Lieske JC, Mehta RA, Milliner DS, Rule AD, Bergstralh EJ, Sarr MG. Kidney stones are common after bariatric surgery. Kidney Int. 2015;87:839–45.
25. Encinosa WE, Bernard DM, Chen C-C, Steiner CA. Healthcare utilization and outcomes after bariatric surgery. Med Care. 2006;44:706–12.
26. Kok DJ, Papapoulos SE, Bijvoet OLM. Crystal agglomeration is a major element in calcium oxalate urinary stone formation. Kidney Int. 1990;37:51–6.
27. Kok DJ, Papapoulos SE, Bijvoet OLM. Excessive crystal agglomeration with low citrate excretion in recurrent stone-formers. Lancet. 1986;327:1056–8.

28. Nazzal L, Puri S, Goldfarb DS. Enteric hyperoxaluria: an important cause of end-stage kidney disease. Nephrol Dial Transplant. 2016;31:375–82.
29. Dobbins JW, Binder HJ. Importance of the colon in enteric hyperoxaluria. N Engl J Med. 1977;296:298–301.
30. Kaufman DW, Kelly JP, Curhan GC, Anderson TE, Dretler SP, Preminger GM, Cave DR. Oxalobacter formigenes may reduce the risk of calcium oxalate kidney stones. J Am Soc Nephrol. 2008;19:1197–203.
31. Kumar R, Lieske JC, Collazo-Clavell ML, Sarr MG, Olson ER, Vrtiska TJ, Bergstralh EJ, Li X. Fat malabsorption and increased intestinal oxalate absorption are common after Roux-en-Y gastric bypass surgery. Surgery. 2011;149:654–61.
32. Canales BK, Hatch M. Kidney stone incidence and metabolic urinary changes after modern bariatric surgery: review of clinical studies, experimental models, and prevention strategies. Surg Obes Relat Dis. 2014;10:734–42.
33. Carlos Valezi A, Emilio Fuganti P, Mali Junior J, Daher Delfino V. Urinary evaluation after RYGBP: a lithogenic profile with early postoperative increase in the incidence of urolithiasis. Obes Surg. 2013:1575–80.
34. Park AM, Storm DW, Fulmer BR, Still CD, Wood GC, Hartle JE. A prospective study of risk factors for nephrolithiasis after Roux-en-Y gastric bypass surgery. J Urol. 2009;182:2334–9.
35. Agrawal V, Liu XJ, Campfield T, Romanelli J, Enrique Silva J, Braden GL. Calcium oxalate supersaturation increases early after Roux-en-Y gastric bypass. Surg Obes Relat Dis. 2014;10:88–94.
36. Requarth JA, Burchard KW, Colacchio TA, Stukel TA, Mott LA, Greenberg ER, Weismann RE. Long-term morbidity following jejunoileal bypass. Arch Surg. 1995;130:318.
37. Matlaga BR, Shore AD, Magnuson T, Clark JM, Johns R, Makary MA. Effect of gastric bypass surgery on kidney stone disease. J Urol. 2009;181:2573–7.
38. Chen T, Godebu E, Horgan S, Mirheydar HS, Sur RL. The effect of restrictive bariatric surgery on urolithiasis. J Endourol. 2013;27:242–4.
39. Semins MJ, Matlaga BR, Shore AD, Steele K, Magnuson T, Johns R, Makary MA. The effect of gastric banding on kidney stone disease. Urology. 2009:746–9.
40. Noun R, Skaff J, Riachi E, Daher R, Abi Antoun N, Nasr M. One thousand consecutive mini-gastric bypass: short-and long-term outcome. Obes Surg. 2012:697–703.
41. Turgeon NA, Perez S, Mondestin M, Scott Davis S, Lin E, Tata S, Kirk AD, Larsen CP, Pearson TC, Sweeney JF. CLINICAL EPIDEMIOLOGY The impact of renal function on outcomes of bariatric surgery. J Am Soc Nephrol. 2012;23:885–94.
42. Mozer AB, Pender Iv JR, Chapman WHH, Sippey ME, Pories WJ, Spaniolas K. Bariatric surgery in patients with dialysis-dependent renal failure. Obes Surg. 2015:2088–92.
43. Andalib A, Aminian A, Khorgami Z, Navaneethan SD, Schauer PR, Brethauer SA. Safety analysis of primary bariatric surgery in patients on chronic dialysis. Surg Endosc. 2016;30:2583–91.
44. Saleh F, Kim SJ, Okrainec A, Jackson TD. Bariatric surgery in patients with reduced kidney function: an analysis of short-term outcomes. Surg Obes Relat Dis. 2015;11:828–35.
45. Cohen JB, Tewksbury CM, Torres Landa S, Williams NN, Dumon KR. National postoperative bariatric surgery outcomes in patients with chronic kidney disease and end-stage kidney disease. Obes Surg. 2019:975–82.
46. Sheetz KH, Woodside KJ, Shahinian VB, Dimick JB, Montgomery JR, Waits SA. Trends in bariatric surgery procedures among patients with ESKD in the United States. Clin J Am Soc Nephrol CJN.01480219. 2019.
47. Cacciola RAS, Pujar K, Ilham MA, Puliatti C, Asderakis A, Chavez R. Effect of degree of obesity on renal transplant outcome. Transpl Proc. 2008;40:3408–12.
48. McCullough KP, Morgenstern H, Saran R, Herman WH, Robinson BM. Projecting ESRD incidence and prevalence in the United States through 2030. J Am Soc Nephrol. 2019;30:127–35.
49. Kramer H, Luke A. Obesity and kidney disease: a big dilemma. Curr Opin Nephrol Hypertens. 2007;16:237–41.

50. Friedman AN, Miskulin DC, Rosenberg IH, Levey AS. Demographics and trends in overweight and obesity in patients at time of kidney transplantation. Am J Kidney Dis. 2003;41:480–7.
51. Segev DL, Simpkins CE, Thompson RE, Locke JE, Warren DS, Montgomery RA, Segev D. Obesity impacts access to kidney transplantation. Clin Epidemiol J Am Soc Nephrol. 2008;19:349–55.
52. Glanton CW, Kao T-C, Cruess D, Agodoa LYC, Abbott KC. CLINICAL NEPHROLOGY-EPIDEMIOLOGY-CLINICAL TRIALS Impact of renal transplantation on survival in end-stage renal disease patients with elevated body mass index. Kidney Int. 2003;63:647–53.
53. Modanlou KA, Muthyala U, Xiao H, Schnitzler MA, Salvalaggio PR, Brennan DC, Abbott KC, Graff RJ, Lentine KL. Bariatric surgery among kidney transplant candidates and recipients: analysis of the United States renal data system and literature review. Transplantation. 2009;87:1167–73.
54. Al-Bahri S, Fakhry TK, Gonzalvo JP, Murr MM. Bariatric surgery as a bridge to renal transplantation in patients with end-stage renal disease. Obes Surg. 2017;27:2951–5.
55. Gore JL, Pham PT, Danovitch GM, Wilkinson AH, Rosenthal JT, Lipshutz GS, Singer JS. Obesity and outcome following renal transplantation. Am J Transplant. 2006;6:357–63.
56. Udgiri NR, Kashyap R, Minz M. The impact of body mass index on renal transplant outcomes: a significant independent risk factor for graft failure and patient death. Transplantation. 2003;75:249.
57. Schauer PR, Bhatt DL, Kirwan JP, et al. Bariatric surgery versus intensive medical therapy for diabetes — 5-year outcomes. N Engl J Med. 2017;376:641–51.
58. Carlsson LM, Sjöholm K, Karlsson C, et al. Long-term incidence of microvascular disease after bariatric surgery or usual care in patients with obesity stratified by baseline glucose status. Lancet Diabetes Endocrinol. 2017;5:271–9.
59. Aminian A, Daigle CR, Romero-Talamás H, Kashyap SR, Kirwan JP, Brethauer SA, Schauer PR. Risk prediction of complications of metabolic syndrome before and 6 years after gastric bypass. Surg Obes Relat Dis. 2014;10:576–82.
60. Hippisley-Cox J, Coupland C. Predicting the risk of chronic kidney disease in men and women in England and Wales: prospective derivation and external validation of the QKidney®Scores. BMC Fam Pract. 2010;11:49.
61. Adams TD, Davidson LE, Litwin SE, et al. After 6 years. JAMA. 2012;308:1122–31.
62. Sjöström L, Lindroos AK, Peltonen M, et al. Lifestyle, diabetes, and cardiovascular risk factors 10 years after bariatric surgery. N Engl J Med. 2004;351:2683–93.
63. Stacy Brethauer MA, Aminian A, Romero-Talamás H, et al. Can diabetes be surgically cured?: Long-term metabolic effects of bariatric surgery in obese patients with type 2 diabetes. Ann Surg. 2013;258:628–37.
64. Heneghan HM, Cetin D, Navaneethan SD, Orzech N, Brethauer SA, Schauer PR. Effects of bariatric surgery on diabetic nephropathy after 5 years of follow-up. Surg Obes Relat Dis. 2013;9:7–14.
65. O'Brien R, Johnson E, Haneuse S, et al. Microvascular outcomes in patients with diabetes after bariatric surgery versus usual care. Ann Intern Med. 2018;169:300–10.
66. Aminian A, Zajichek A, Arterburn DE, Wolski KE, Brethauer SA, Schauer PR, Kattan MW, Nissen SE. Association of metabolic surgery with major adverse cardiovascular outcomes in patients with type 2 diabetes and obesity. JAMA. 2019;322:1271–82.
67. Funes DR, Blanco DG, Gómez CO, Frieder JS, Menzo EL, Szomstein S, White KP, Rosenthal RJ. Metabolic surgery reduces the risk of progression from chronic kidney disease to kidney failure. Ann Surg. 2019;270:511–8.
68. Douros JD, Tong J, D'Alessio DA. The effects of bariatric surgery on islet function, insulin secretion, and glucose control. Endocr Rev. 2019;40:1394–423.
69. Batterham RL, Cummings DE. Mechanisms of diabetes improvement following bariatric/metabolic surgery. Diabetes Care. 2016;39:893–901.
70. Chondronikola M, Harris LLS, Klein S. Bariatric surgery and type 2 diabetes: are there weight loss-independent therapeutic effects of upper gastrointestinal bypass? J Intern Med. 2016;280:476–86.

71. Rossi MCE, Nicolucci A, Pellegrini F, et al. Obesity and changes in urine albumin/creatinine ratio in patients with type 2 diabetes: the DEMAND study. Nutr Metab Cardiovasc Dis. 2010;20:110–6.
72. Upala S, Wijarnpreecha K, Congrete S, Rattanawong P, Sanguankeo A. Bariatric surgery reduces urinary albumin excretion in diabetic nephropathy: a systematic review and meta-analysis. Surg Obes Relat Dis. 2016;12:1037–44.
73. Young L, Hanipah ZN, Brethauer SA, Schauer PR, Aminian A. Long-term impact of bariatric surgery in diabetic nephropathy. Surg Endosc. 2019;33:1654–60.
74. Friedman AN, Wang J, Wahed AS, Docherty NG, Fennern E, Pomp A, Purnell JQ, le Roux CW, Wolfe B. The association between kidney disease and diabetes remission in bariatric surgery patients with type 2 diabetes. Am J Kidney Dis. 2019;74:761–70.
75. Abouchacra S, Chaaban A, Gebran N, Hussein Q, Ahmed M, Bernieh B, Torab F, Kayyal Y, Omary HA, Nagelkerke N. GFR estimation in the morbidly obese pre- and postbariatric surgery: one size does not fit all. Int Urol Nephrol. 2013;45:157–62.
76. Imam TH, Fischer H, Jing B, Burchette R, Henry S, Derose SF, Coleman KJ. Estimated GFR before and after bariatric surgery in CKD. Am J Kidney Dis. 2017;69:380–8.
77. Micic DD, Ramos-Molina B, Stocker CJ, et al. Bariatric surgery modulates urinary levels of microRNAs involved in the regulation of renal function. Front Endocrinol 2019;10:319. www.frontiersin.org.

Endocrine and Metabolic Complications After Bariatric Surgery

11

J. Michael Gonzalez-Campoy, Catherine B. Proebstle, Andrea Pierson, Bronwyn Knaebe, and Bruce W. Richardson

Hormones are powerful things, we are helpless in their wake

—Meg Cabot

Abbreviations

1,25(OH)2D	1,25Dihydroxy-vitamin D
25(OH)D	25-Hydroxy-vitamin D
ASBMS	American Society for Bariatric and Metabolic Surgery
BMI	Body mass index
BPD-DS	Biliopancreatic diversion with duodenal switch
EWL	Excess weight loss
GIP	Gastric inhibitory polypeptide
GLP-1	Glucagon-like peptide-1
LAGB	Laparoscopic adjustable gastric banding
mg	Milligrams
mg/dL	Milligrams per deciliter
ng/mL	Nanograms per milliliter
NIPHS	Noninsulinoma pancreatogenous hypoglycemia syndrome
PCOS	Polycystic ovarian syndrome
PTH	Parathyroid hormone
RYGB	Roux-en-Y gastric bypass
SAGB	Single anastomosis gastric bypass

J. M. Gonzalez-Campoy (✉) · C. B. Proebstle · A. Pierson · B. Knaebe · B. W. Richardson
Minnesota Center for Obesity, Metabolism and Endocrinology, Eagan, MN, USA
e-mail: drmike@mncome.com; Catherine@mncome.com; Andrea@mncome.com; Bronwyn@mncome.com

A. G. Bhasker et al. (eds.), *Management of Nutritional and Metabolic Complications of Bariatric Surgery*,
https://doi.org/10.1007/978-981-33-4702-1_11

SG	Sleeve gastrectomy
SHPT	Secondary hyperparathyroidism
T2DM	Type 2 diabetes mellitus
TSH	Thyroid stimulating hormone
VBG	Vertical banded gastroplasty
VIP	Vasoactive intestinal peptide

11.1 Introduction

Adipose tissue is not simply a site for energy storage. It is an active endocrine organ and a major regulator of metabolism. Adipocytes are endocrine cells. They release hormones, including leptin and adiponectin, which have effects on major organs that participate in the regulation of metabolism. Further, adipocytes have receptors for many hormones, including epinephrine and insulin, which allows for extensive cross-communication with other organs and subsequent effect on metabolic homeostasis [1].

In the right environment, susceptible individuals accumulate fat mass (***adiposity***). The outdated concept of overweight and obesity as defined by thresholds of body mass index has given way to a more contemporary view. With adiposity there are changes to function and structure of adipocytes and adipose tissue (including vasculature, nerves, and connective matrix). Adipocytes, like any other cells in the body, may become diseased. Adipose tissue as a whole may become diseased too. Analogous to ophthalmopathy, cardiomyopathy, nephropathy, neuropathy, and encephalopathy, there is also ***adiposopathy***. Adiposopathy includes changes in adipocyte cytology and function, and changes in adipose tissue anatomy, distribution, and function, which then contribute to metabolic derangements (Table 11.1). Adiposopathy, or "sick fat," is an endocrine disease, and is the primary treatment target to correct the metabolic and endocrine derangements of overweight or obesity

Table 11.1 Anatomical and functional changes of adipose tissue in adiposopathy

Anatomical changes	Functional changes
Adipocyte hypertrophy Growth of adipose tissue beyond its vascular supply Increased number of adipose tissue immune cells • Macrophage ring structures surrounding dying adipocytes Ectopic fat deposition (in other body tissues) Heterogeneous adipose tissue distribution • Visceral adiposity linked to metabolic diseases	Impaired adipogenesis and adipocyte hypertrophy Adipocyte lipolysis in excess of lipogenesis • Increased free fatty acids Pathogenic adipose tissue endocrine responses • Hypoadiponectinemia • Hyperleptinemia Pathogenic adipose tissue immune responses • High levels of inflammatory markers Pathogenic crosstalk between fat and other organs

[2–5]. Bariatric endocrinology is the sub-sub-specialty of endocrinology that deals with adiposopathy as an endocrine disease [6].

Adiposopathy helps to explain why not all patients with adiposity develop metabolic and endocrine complications. Those individuals whose adipose tissue remains functionally intact with a gain in fat mass do not develop metabolic or endocrine complications. Conversely, individuals with adiposopathy are unable to compensate and have progression of disease. Cardiovascular events (i.e., myocardial infarction and cerebrovascular accident), and damage to other organs (i.e., hepatic cirrhosis from non-alcoholic steatohepatitis) are the ultimate complications of this disease process over time. It is optimal to intervene as early as possible in the natural history of adiposopathy (Fig. 11.1). Adiposopathy also explains why some individuals develop metabolic and endocrine derangements at varying degrees of adiposity.

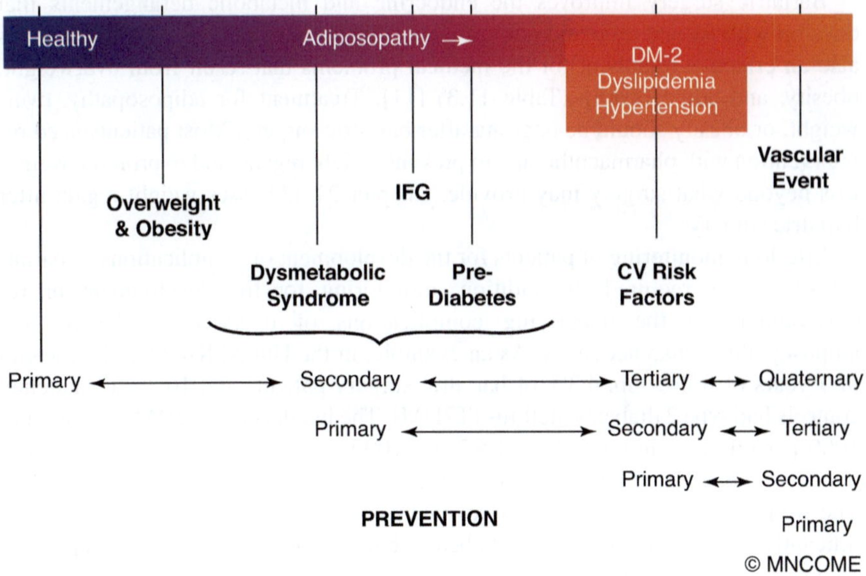

Fig. 11.1 Prevention of cardiovascular disease. The accumulation of fat mass leads to changes in adipose tissue function and the development of an inflammatory milieu. The top bar indicates the progression from healthy adipose tissue to progressively worsening adiposopathy. Adiposopathy is etiological in the progression of the disease processes that eventually lead to organ damage. A vascular event implies long-standing disease. Treating a patient after a vascular event makes this a primary intervention and represents a lack of prevention. Interventions to modify known cardiovascular risk factors as a primary intervention make treatment of vascular events secondary intervention. Interventions to modify the risk factors of the known cardiovascular risk factors make treatment of a vascular event a tertiary intervention. Early intervention to preserve a healthy lifestyle and prevent the development of overweight, obesity, and adiposopathy makes treatment of a vascular event a quaternary intervention. Early intervention prevents, or at least significantly delays a vascular event. The corollary to this is that primary prevention of vascular events starts with the implementation of a healthy lifestyle early in life. Abbreviations: *DM-2* type 2 diabetes mellitus, *IFG* impaired fasting glucose, *MNCOME* Minnesota Center for Obesity, Metabolism and Endocrinology, PA. © Copyright Minnesota Center for Obesity, Metabolism and Endocrinology, PA (MNCOME)

The best approach to the management of overweight, obesity, and adiposopathy is to regard them as any other chronic disease. Chronic diseases may be treated, managed, and controlled. They may go into remission. Chronic diseases, however, are not curable. Each patient needs to understand that weight management, and monitoring for complications of the disease continuum, are both for life. Treatment should be individualized and designed to address the duration and severity of disease [6–8].

Most patients accomplish effective weight loss with medical treatment. Bariatric surgery should be reserved for patients whose disease is refractory to medical management, and the burden of disease warrants a more aggressive approach [9]. Referral to bariatric surgery must underscore that this is not a cure for overweight, obesity or adiposopathy. Patients need to understand that the benefit of bariatric surgery carries implicit risks.

Bariatric surgery improves the endocrine and metabolic derangements that develop with weight gain and adiposopathy (Table 11.2) [10]. Bariatric surgery is also an effective treatment for the medical problems that result from overweight, obesity, and adiposopathy (Table 11.3) [11]. Treatment for adiposopathy, overweight, or obesity should be ongoing after bariatric surgery. Most patients need re-intervention with pharmacotherapy to prevent weight regain, and to promote weight loss beyond what surgery may provide. Chapter 21 addresses weight regain after bariatric surgery.

Life-long monitoring of patients for the development of complications of bariatric surgery is required. In addition, monitoring for the development or re-development of the underlying complications of overweight, obesity, and adiposopathy is also necessary. As an example, in the United Kingdom by the end of 7 years of follow-up, 4.3% of bariatric surgery patients and 16.2% of matched controls had type 2 diabetes mellitus (T2DM). The incidence of T2DM was 28.2 per 1000 person-years in controls and 5.7 per 1000 person-years in bariatric surgery patients. The adjusted hazard ratio was 0.20 (95% CI 0.13–0.30, $p < 0.0001$) [12]. The weight loss and metabolic improvements achieved with bariatric surgery significantly decreased the risk of diabetes, but did not eliminate it. Chapter 22 addresses this subject further.

This chapter will address endocrine and metabolic complications of bariatric surgery. This chapter will not address endocrinology and metabolism subjects dealt with in other chapters of this textbook. (Nutritional deficiencies are covered in Chap. 23, and reproductive complications are covered in Chap. 15).

11.2 Incidence of Endocrine and Metabolic Complications of Bariatric Surgery

The incidence of endocrine and metabolic complications following bariatric surgery varies widely. The type of bariatric surgery procedure, and the time elapsed after the procedure, each determine the incidence of endocrine and metabolic complications. Malabsorptive procedures are more likely to cause endocrine problems than

Table 11.2 Changes in metabolic parameters with the bariatric procedures most commonly done

	Procedure			
	Malabsorptive	Restrictive		Mixed
	Bilio-pancreatic diversion duodenal switch	Adjustable gastric banding	Vertical sleeve gastrectomy	Roux en-Y gastric bypass
Excess weight loss	82%	44%	66%	50%
Mean weight loss	30–40%	15–30%	20–30%	25–35%
BMI change	−18	−7.1	−10.9	−16.7
Diabetes remission	98%	59%	81%	78%
Dyslipidemia remission	99%	36%	67%	61%
Hypertension remission	83%	56%	78%	66%
Energy expenditure	n/a	↓	↓	↑
Ghrelin	↓↓	↓→↑	↓↓	↓→↑
Glucagon like peptide-1	↑	→↓	↑	↑
Peptide YY	↑	↑	↑	↑
Oxyntomodulin	↑	→	↑	↑
GIP	↓	→	→↑	↓→↑
Cholecystokinin	n/a	n/a	→	→
Pancreatic polypeptide	↓	→	→	→
Amylin	n/a	→	→	↓
Glucagon secretion	↑	n/a	n/a	↓→↑
Postpandial insulin secretion	↑	→↓	↑	→↓
Hepatic insulin sensitivity	↑	↑	↑	↑
Muscle insulin sensitivity	↑	↑	↑	↑
Plasma glucose	↓	↓	↓	↓
Hemoglobin A1c	↓3.8%	↓1.8%	↓2.9	↓2.9%
Glucose effect	Weight-independent	Weight-dependent	Weight-independent	Weight-independent
Triglycerides	↓	↓	↓	↓
LDL-C	↓	↓↑	↓	↓
HDL-C	→	→	↑	↑
Visceral fat mass (Waist circumference)	↓	↓	↓	↓
Resistin	n/a	↑	↓	→
Leptin	↓	↓	↓	↓
Adiponectin	↑	↑	→	↑
Leptin to adiponectin ratio	↓	↓	↓	↓
Thyroid hormone requirements	↓	↓	↓	↓
Testosterone levels in men	↑	↑	↑	↑
Estrogen to testosterone ratio in women	↑	↑	↑	↑

Multiple arrows denote equivocal data

BMI body mass index, *GIP* glucose-dependent insulinotropic polypeptide, *HDL-C* high density lipoprotein cholesterol, *LDL-C* low density lipoprotein cholesterol, *n/a* no data available

Table 11.3 Outcomes of bariatric surgery on metabolic, endocrine, and atherosclerotic diseases

Obesity-related endocrine disease	Outcome after bariatric surgery
Cardiovascular disease	82% risk reduction
Diabetes mellitus, type 2	82–98% resolved
Dyslipidemia	63% resolved
Dysmetabolic syndrome	80% resolved
Gout	72–77% resolved
Hirsutism in women	75–79% resolution
Hypertension	52–92% resolved
Mortality from diabetes mellitus, type 2	92% reduction
Mortality from heart disease	56% reduction
Non-alcoholic fatty liver disease	37% resolution
Polycystic ovarian syndrome	100% resolution of menstrual irregularity

restrictive procedures. It is not possible to predict which individual patient may develop endocrine problems after a bariatric procedure. Therefore, regardless of the published incidence data, reviewed below, each patient needs a pre-operative assessment of glycemia, calcium and bone metabolism, thyroid function, and the gonadal axis. Each patient also needs education, best delivered by a team of healthcare professionals, so there is a clear understanding of the benefits and risks of bariatric surgery, including endocrine and metabolic complications. After bariatric surgery, education and monitoring are necessary on an ongoing basis [13].

Nutritional and vitamin deficiencies in patients after malabsorptive surgeries develop from lack of adherence to meal planning and nutritional supplementation recommendations over time [9]. Nutritional deficiencies are the subject of Chap. 5.

11.2.1 Incidence of Derangements of Calcium Metabolism

Vitamin D deficiency is prevalent throughout the world [14]. In Boston, Massachusetts, USA, serum 25-hydroxyvitamin D (25(OH)D) plasma concentrations of 30 nanograms per milliliter (ng/mL) or less, are found in 64% of healthy adults. One-third of adults have 25(OH)D levels of 20 ng/mL or less [15]. Decreased intestinal calcium absorption due to vitamin D deficiency causes a drop in the plasma calcium concentration. The parathyroid hormone (PTH) plasma concentration goes up secondary to the drop in plasma calcium. Eucalcemia is maintained by the multiple actions of elevated PTH, which makes secondary hyperparathyroidism common and actual hypocalcemia less common.

Derangements of calcium metabolism are prevalent in patients who have had bariatric surgery. In 80 patients who had surgery in France, 10 years after biliopancreatic diversion with duodenal switch (BPD-DS) 78% of the patients maintain a BMI < 35. At the same 10-year mark, vitamin D levels are normal in 35.4% of patients, the rest having low levels. The low level of vitamin D coupled with a short gut and hindered calcium absorption causes secondary hyperparathyroidism (SHPT) in 62% of patients [16]. A study of 1436 Canadian patients had similar results, where 68.6% of patients had SHPT 5 years after BPD-DS [17]. The prevalence of SHPT was higher than the prevalence of low vitamin D, which reached a plateau at 15.5% 36 months after surgery. This is a strong indicator that the decreased length for absorption of the gut plays a major role in the development of SHPT, regardless of vitamin D status. The prevalence of hypocalcemia was 26.9% 2 years after surgery [17].

Data on 1470 patients who had bariatric surgery in Taiwan shows that the overall prevalence of SHPT is 21.0% before bariatric surgery [18]. Multivariate analysis shows that vitamin D level is the only independent predictor of SHPT before surgery. The prevalence of SHPT increases after bariatric surgery.

- 1 year after surgery the prevalence of SHPT is:
  - 35.4% overall
  - 50.6% for One anastomosis gastric bypass (OAGB)
  - 33.2% for Roux-en-Y gastric bypass (RYGB)
  - 25.8% for laparoscopic adjustable gastric banding (LAGB)
  - 17.8% for sleeve gastrectomy (SG)
- 5 years after surgery the prevalence of SHPT is:
  - 63.3% overall
  - 73.6% for SAGB
  - 56.6% for RYGB
  - 38.5% for LAGB
  - 41.7% for SG

Serum PTH at 1 year after surgery correlated with decreased BMI and weight loss. Multivariate analysis showed that age, sex, calcium level, and bypass procedure were independent predictors of SHPT after surgery [18].

11.2.2 Incidence of Bone Density Loss and Fracture Risk

Weight loss causes bone mineral density loss [19–21]. Following bariatric surgery, this bone mineral density loss places patients at higher risk for fractures [22]. In Olmsted County, Minnesota, USA, with a median follow-up of 7.7 years, 79 subjects from a cohort of 258 patients who had bariatric surgery between 1985 and 2004, had 132 fractures. This represented a 2.3-fold increase in fracture risk [23]. In Quebec, Canada, 12,676 patients who had bariatric surgery between 2001 and 2014 had a higher risk of fracture compared to control patients with obesity after a mean of 4.4 years of follow-up. Fracture risk was highest after BPD-DS [24].

Taken together, the prevalence of hypovitaminosis D, hypocalcemia, SHPT, bone mineral density loss, and increased fracture risk warrant an aggressive approach to the preservation of calcium homeostasis and bone integrity in patients with obesity who have bariatric surgery.

11.2.3 Incidence of Hypoglycemia

On the other hand, the incidence of hypoglycemia is much lower. In a Swedish nationwide cohort of 5040 patients who had gastric bypass surgery between 1986 and 2006, the incidence of hypoglycemia was as low as 0.2%. The rate of hospitalization for hypoglycemia and other related diagnoses, including confusion, syncope, epilepsy, and seizures was two- to sevenfold higher in gastric bypass patients, compared to matched controls. There was no hypoglycemia after vertical banded gastroplasty (VBG) or LAGB. The absolute risk of hypoglycemia in this study underestimates the incidence of hypoglycemia because it excluded outpatient episodes from the analysis [25].

In a study at Catholic University in Rome, 120 patients were randomized 1:1 to RYGB or SG and followed for a year. Of these, 117 patients (93%) completed the 12-month follow-up. Reactive hypoglycemia was detected in 14% of SG patients and 29% of RYGB patients ($p = 0.079$) [26]. Daily hypoglycemic episodes during continuous glucose monitoring did not differ between groups ($p = 0.75$). Four of 59 RYGB subjects (6.8%) had 1–3 hospitalizations for symptomatic hypoglycemia. There were no hospitalizations for hypoglycemia in patients who had an SG [26].

The incidence of hypoglycemia at the Geisinger Health Systems was studied in a cohort of 1206 patients without preoperative diagnoses of T2DM or hypoglycemia [27]. One-hundred fifty eight patients had a diagnosis of hypoglycemia, a glucose less than 60 milligrams per deciliter (mg/dL), or documentation of the use of medications to treat hypoglycemia (13%). Only 8 of the 158 patients had severe hypoglycemia, defined as a glucose of <40 mg/dL, need for emergency room care, or hospitalization. This is the only study to date that documented that hypoglycemia risk over 5 years after surgery is higher in patients whose preoperative hemoglobin A1c was under 5.5%, body mass index (BMI) was under 39 kilograms per meter^2 (kg/m^2), and percent of excess weight loss (EWL) was 75% or more [27].

11.2.4 Incidence of Derangements of the Thyroid Axis

Weight loss after bariatric surgery causes a fall in the thyroid-stimulating hormone (TSH) level, which reflects a decreased need for thyroid hormone [28–33]. Patients with hypothyroidism requiring treatment with thyroid hormone need a reduction of the thyroid dose after bariatric surgery.

11.2.5 Incidence of Changes in the Gonadal Axis

Overweight, obesity, and adiposopathy impair fertility in both men and women [34, 35]. Bariatric surgery improves fertility and increases the likelihood of an unintended pregnancy [36–38]. In 2016, the Centers for Disease Control included bariatric surgery within the past 2 years as a risk for adverse health events in pregnancy [39]. There is no data on the prevalence of undesired pregnancy after bariatric surgery.

Table 11.4 Endocrine complications of malabsorptive weight loss surgeries (Roux-en-Y, sleeve gastrectomy, biliopancreatic diversion, and biliopancreatic diversion with duodenal switch)

Endocrine complication	Highest prevalence	Testing needed	Monitoring frequency
Vitamin D deficiency	64%	25-Hydroxyvitamin D	Baseline, every 2 months until stable, and then annually
Hypocalcemia	27%	Total plasma calcium Total protein Phosphorus 24-h urinary calcium	Baseline, every 2 months until stable, and then annually
Secondary hyperparathyroidism	74% at 5 years	Parathyroid hormone	Baseline, every 2 months until stable, and then annually
Metabolic bone disease	30%	DEXA scan	Baseline, yearly until stable, then every 2 years
Reactive hypoglycemia	29%	Mixed meal glucose tolerance test Glucose (fingerstick) CGMS if available	As needed
Severe hypoglycemia with neuroglycopenia	7%	Glucose and c-peptide during episode	As needed
Increased fertility (may lead to undesired pregnancy)	Not reported	Log of menses (women) Total testosterone (men)	Baseline and annually
Decreased thyroid hormone requirements in patients with corrected hypothyroidism	100%	Free T3, Free T4, TSH	Baseline, every 6 weeks until stable, and then annually

Abbreviations: *DEXA* dual energy X-ray absorptiometry, *CGMS* continuous glucose monitoring system, *T3* triiodothyronine, *T4* tetraiodothyronine, *TSH* thyroid stimulating hormone

11.3 Adverse Endocrine and Metabolic Sequelae After Bariatric Surgery

Table 11.4 lists the major endocrine and metabolic complications of bariatric surgery. Disorders of glycemia and calcium metabolism are more likely after malabsorptive procedures. All bariatric procedures lead to increased fertility and decreased thyroid hormone requirements.

11.4 Pathophysiology of the Enlisted Adverse Sequelae

11.4.1 Pathophysiology of Calcium and Bone Metabolism

Calcium intake is frequently inadequate to meet calcium needs after bariatric surgery [40].

Bariatric procedures that decrease the receptive capacity of the stomach will result in decreased exposure of ingested calcium salts to the acid of the stomach. This is especially so following RYGB, where most of the stomach is removed from the alimentary canal. The acidity of the stomach contributes to the solubilization of calcium salts, and bypassing the stomach contributes to calcium malabsorption [41–43].

Bariatric procedures that result in a shortened alimentary canal limit the absorptive capacity of the gut for calcium. In addition to a decreased absorptive surface, there is also a shortened time for absorption to happen. Competition for absorption with other cations further decreases calcium absorption. Coupled with the prevalent hypovitaminosis D, calcium absorption from the intestine decreases [44–46]. Figure 11.2 illustrates the major mechanisms involved in the decreased intestinal calcium absorption following malabsorptive bariatric surgeries.

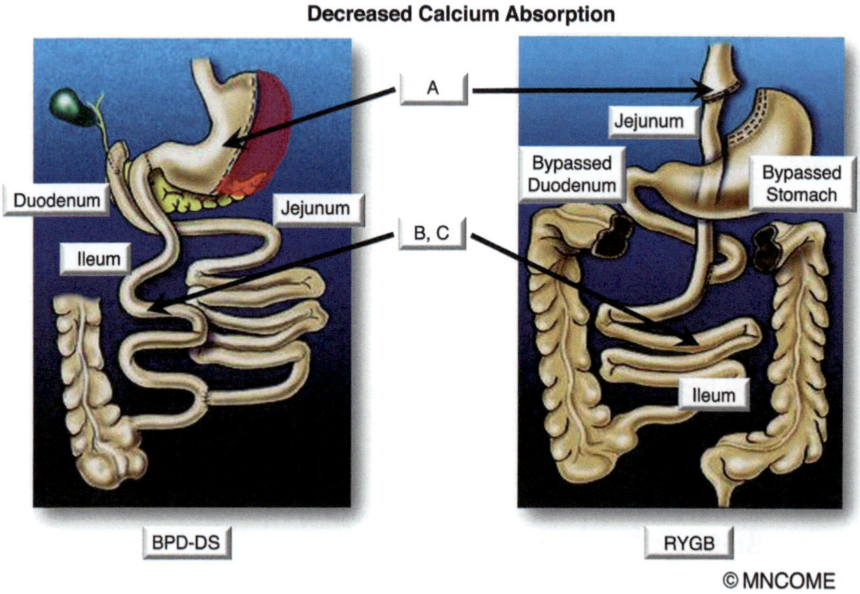

Fig. 11.2 Decreased calcium absorption after malabsorptive procedures. Following bariatric surgery calcium absorption is impaired. The red area in the left panel represents the partial gastrectomy that is part of the BPD-DS procedure. The major mechanisms involved are (**a**) decreased gastric acid exposure limiting solubilization of calcium salts; (**b**) decreased length of small intestine for absorption of calcium (including competing cation absorption), also leading to a decreased time for calcium absorption; and (**c**) decreased activity of 1, 25-dihydroxy-vitamin D. Additionally, most patients have inadequate calcium intake over time. Abbreviations: *BPD-DS* biliopancreatic diversion with duodenal switch, *RYGB* Roux-en-Y gastric bypass, *MNCOME* Minnesota Center for Obesity, Metabolism and Endocrinology, PA. © Copyright Minnesota Center for Obesity, Metabolism and Endocrinology, PA (MNCOME)

Hypocalcemia due to decreased intestinal calcium absorption stimulates the secretion of PTH from the parathyroid glands, resulting in SHPT [17, 18, 47, 48]. SHPT returns the plasma calcium concentration to normal. The effects of SHPT include increased calcium reabsorption from the renal tubules, with an associated phosphaturic effect. In addition to returning calcium to the circulation directly, the lower plasma phosphate decreases the formation of calcium phosphate, increasing the plasma calcium indirectly. SHPT also leads to increased activity of the renal hydroxylase that converts 25(OH)D to 1,25 dihydroxy-vitamin D (1,25$(OH)_2$D). Through the activation of vitamin D, SHPT indirectly increases intestinal calcium absorption [49].

SHPT causes increased bone resorption, which frees calcium from bone stores. Over time, continuous bone resorption accelerates bone mineral density loss and increases fracture risk [21, 49–51]. The development of primary hypogonadism, leading to the menopause, worsens the bone mineral density loss in women after bariatric surgery [52]. The use of contraception that suppresses gonadal function leading to estrogen deficiency (i.e., progesterone only products), should be avoided in premenopausal women after bariatric surgery.

Figure 11.3 Summarizes the pathophysiology of calcium metabolism after bariatric surgery.

11.4.2 Pathophysiology of Glucose Metabolism

Immediately after RYGB, before a patient with T2DM experiences weight loss, first-phase insulin secretion, and hepatic insulin sensitivity increase [53]. Blood glucose levels drop within 48 h after SG and RYGB [54]. Patients with insulin-requiring T2DM prior to surgery have an 87% reduction in their total daily insulin requirements by postoperative day 2 [55]. These dramatic changes in glycemia, irrespective of fat mass, are due to multiple effects of bariatric surgery (Table 11.2). Patients have an increased risk of hypoglycemia after malabsorptive bariatric surgeries.

The dumping syndrome, which affects more than 15% of patients after bariatric surgery, includes the following symptoms:

- Abdominal cramping and diarrhea
- Nausea and vomiting
- Flushing
- Hypotension
- Tachycardia
- Lightheadedness (and syncope)

The dumping syndrome occurs following the ingestion of simple carbohydrates without the anatomy to slow absorption (i.e., bypassing the pyloric sphincter) [56, 57]. Sugar in the small intestine causes an osmotic overload and fluid shifts into the

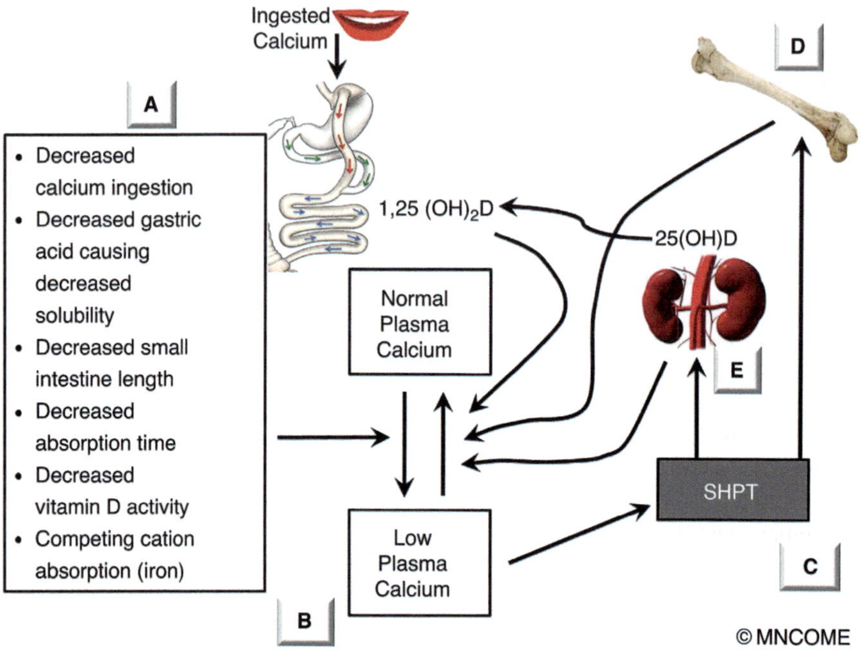

Fig. 11.3 Pathophysiology of derangements of calcium metabolism. Following bariatric surgery, there are significant changes to calcium homeostasis. (**a**) Intestinal absorption of calcium is decreased. (**b**) This causes a fall in the plasma calcium. (**c**) Hypocalcemia stimulates the secretion of parathyroid hormone, which will return calcium levels to normal. (**d**) SHPT increases bone resorption, freeing calcium into the circulation. Over time this causes bone mineral density loss (osteomalacia). (**e**) In the kidneys parathyroid hormone increases calcium reabsorption and promotes phosphaturia. This adds to the plasma calcium directly, and indirectly by lowering the mass effect of phosphate on calcium. Parathyroid hormone increases the activity of the renal hydroxylase that converts 25(OH)D to the activated 1,25(OH)2D. Activated vitamin D increases intestinal calcium absorption, which adds to the plasma calcium. Abbreviations: *1,25 (OH)2D* 1,25 Dihydroxy-vitamin D, *25(OH)D* 25-hydroxy-vitamin D, *SPTH* secondary hyperparathyroidism, *MNCOME* Minnesota Center for Obesity, Metabolism and Endocrinology, PA. © Copyright Minnesota Center for Obesity, Metabolism and Endocrinology, PA (MNCOME)

intestinal lumen leading to watery diarrhea. The small intestine releases vasoactive intestinal peptide (VIP), gastric inhibitory polypeptide (GIP), and glucagon-like peptide-1 (GLP-1) in response to the presence of nutrients in the gut. These enteric hormones vasodilate the splanchnic vessels drawing volume away from the peripheral circulation. A decrease in peripheral circulating volume is the cause of the tachycardia and eventual hypotension [56, 58]. This "early dumping syndrome" is common after RYGB and generally occurs within minutes to 1 h after the ingestion of calorie-dense foods, especially refined sugars and fats [59].

Postprandial or reactive hypoglycemia is part of the dumping syndrome. [56–58, 60, 61] The small intestine releases GIP and GLP-1. As elevated glucose levels reach the pancreatic islets, they stimulate the beta cells to release insulin. GLP-1 boosts the release of insulin. Both insulin and GLP-1 inhibit glucagon release from the alpha cells, which are downstream in the islet circulation. The result is an exaggerated insulin release in excess of need. Insulin levels remain high even as glucose levels go down past normal. This hyperinsulinemic hypoglycemia is clinically manifested about 1–3 h after meal ingestion and usually develops months to years after surgery [26, 62–64]. The American Society for Bariatric and Metabolic Surgery (ASBMS) issued a position statement on this subject in 2017. In contrast to the "early dumping syndrome," hyperinsulinemic hypoglycemia is what historically was termed "late dumping syndrome."

Severe hypoglycemia after bariatric surgery is uncommon. In this situation, patients develop neuroglycopenia, which can cause cognitive impairment, loss of consciousness, or seizures 1–3 h after ingesting simple carbohydrate [65–67]. Neuroglycopenia is not present when fasting, and this is a distinction from patients with insulinoma where fasting hypoglycemia is common [68]. Neuroglycopenia may occur in association with physical activity and is associated with hypoglycemia unawareness due to loss of adrenergic and cholinergic symptoms [59].

Noninsulinoma pancreatogenous hypoglycemia syndrome (NIPHS) includes neuroglycopenic symptoms and mimics the clinical presentation of insulinoma. However, neuroglycopenia develops 2–4 h after ingestion of meals, and imaging studies of the pancreas are negative for a pancreatic mass. Histologically, the pancreas in these patients shows islet hypertrophy and nesidioblastosis [68, 69].

11.4.3 Pathophysiology of the Thyroid Axis

A healthy hypothalamic–pituitary–thyroid axis adjusts thyroid hormone production to meet needs. Patients with a normal thyroid axis prior to surgery are ensured a continued euthyroid state.

Autoimmune thyroiditis is common and therefore it is the most common thyroid problem in patients who undergo bariatric surgery. For most patients their disease is evolving. The stage of thyroid gland destruction determines the need to replace thyroid hormone at the time of bariatric surgery. One-fifth of patients undergoing bariatric surgery already require thyroid hormone replacement [28]. The scant literature on thyroid function after bariatric surgery is consistent in documenting a drop in TSH [32, 70]. The pathophysiology behind this observation is not yet defined.

11.4.4 Pathophysiology of Gonadal Axis

A discussion of the pathophysiological changes of the gonadal axis with obesity or with bariatric surgery is beyond the scope of this chapter, and is complex [34, 35]. Men with hypogonadotropic hypogonadism due to obesity will return their gonadal axis to normal after bariatric surgery. Women with polycystic ovarian syndrome (PCOS; which is largely due to adiposopathy and insulin resistance affecting ovarian function), or with hypogonadotropic hypogonadism due to obesity, will return to normal after bariatric surgery. For both men and women, there is increased fertility after surgery.

11.5 Diagnosis

In 2008, we authored the first guideline for the perioperative nutritional, metabolic, and nonsurgical support of the bariatric patient [71]. This was a joint effort of the American Association of Clinical Endocrinologists and the American Society for Metabolic and Bariatric Surgery. The newest revision of the guideline is now available and is a valuable reference to have along with this textbook.

11.5.1 Diagnosis of Derangements of Calcium and Bone Metabolism

All patients should have baseline measurements of total calcium, total protein, 25(OH)D, phosphorus, and PTH prior to any malabsorptive procedure (Table 11.4) [9]. We recommend close monitoring of 25(OH)D, total calcium (with concomitant total protein), phosphorus, and PTH every 2 months until PTH levels are normalized on two consecutive draws. Patients should then be encouraged to maintain their calcium and vitamin D intake, and repeat measurements may then be made annually.

A baseline measurement of bone mineral density with dual-energy X-ray absorptiometry (DEXA) should be done prior to any malabsorptive procedure. Any subsequent DEXA scans should be done on the same densitometer, by the same technician if possible, to allow for direct comparisons to baseline [72, 73]. A repeat DEXA scan 1 year after surgery establishes which patients have had rapid bone loss, and would require close observation over time [72, 73].

11.5.2 Diagnosis of Derangements of Glucose Metabolism

All patients undergoing bariatric surgery should have baseline hemoglobin A1c, fasting glucose, and fasting insulin or c-peptide levels documented. Glycemic measures should be part of the ongoing management of all patients because some will develop or redevelop hyperglycemic derangements [12]. Patients with symptoms of hypoglycemia should be tested for this (Table 11.4).

Any patient who had a malabsorptive procedure, who now has symptoms consistent with reactive hypoglycemia, but not neuroglycopenia, should be provided with a glucose meter. Self-monitoring of capillary glucose by fingerstick sampling and food logging provides documentation of the temporal relationship of meals to symptoms, and the level of glycemia with symptoms. For most patients with postprandial hyperinsulinemic hypoglycemia medical nutrition therapy (MNT) will correct the symptoms [59, 65, 74].

Patients who have persistent symptoms despite nutritional intervention should undergo a mixed meal glucose tolerance test. Testing should be done in a facility with expertise, where personnel are prepared to assist any patient who develops severe hypoglycemia during the test period. Although the mixed meal contains protein, carbohydrate, and fat, the carbohydrate content is not standardized. Most mixed meal tests will include 40–75 g of carbohydrate [75, 76].

The conventional oral glucose tolerance test, where a patient ingests 75 g of soluble glucose and plasma glucose is measured at intervals up to 4 h post ingestion, is not recommended in patients who had malabsorptive bariatric surgery. The glucose load may precipitate the dumping syndrome during testing and is otherwise not well tolerated [75].

Where insulinoma or NIPHS is suspected, patients should be admitted to the hospital for observation and testing. Whipple's triad is:

1. The presence of neuroglycopenia
2. A concomitant low plasma glucose (less than 50 mg/dL)
3. Resolution of the symptoms with glucose treatment [77–79]

Patients who meet the criteria for Whipple's triad are considered to have verified hypoglycemia, and an etiology for it should be defined. NIPHS is a diagnosis of exclusion (factitious or iatrogenic causes, dumping syndrome, and insulinoma are excluded). Plasma glucose is required to avoid the pitfalls of capillary testing. A c-peptide level should always be drawn with the plasma glucose [80, 81].

Imaging of the pancreas is needed to exclude an insulinoma. This includes an ultrasound of the pancreas (transabdominal, endoscopic, and/or intraoperative), and computerized tomography with thin slices through the pancreas. Negative imaging excludes insulinoma. Selective calcium stimulation of the arterial supply of the pancreas helps define a gradient of insulin release, and can guide a partial pancreatectomy to ameliorate symptoms in NIPHS [82].

11.5.3 Diagnosis of Derangements of the Thyroid Axis

All patients undergoing bariatric surgery should have baseline thyroid function tests documented, including free T3, free T4, and thyroid-stimulating hormone (TSH). In patients with a family history of thyroid disease, or with a goiter on physical examination, we recommend documentation of thyroid peroxidase and thyroglobulin antibodies. Pre-existing thyroid abnormalities of structure or function should lead to closer follow-up of the thyroid status of these patients after surgery (Table 11.4) [83].

11.5.4 Diagnosis of Derangements of the Gonadal Axis

All patients undergoing bariatric surgery should have a thorough sexual history documented. If there is sexual dysfunction a baseline set of gonadal hormones should be done.

11.6 Management

A multidisciplinary team approach results in the best care of patients with adiposopathy, overweight, or obesity [6, 8, 84–86]. This holds true for patients whose disease warrants bariatric surgery [11, 13]. The team approach to patient care ensures that patients receive the knowledge they need to make decisions about their health, and that options are discussed at a level that is educationally, linguistically, and culturally appropriate for each patient. MNT is essential to good outcomes in bariatric surgery patients. The team should include registered dieticians, nurse educators/coaches, psychologists, and physicians or physician extenders [6]. A major goal is to maintain patient engagement, to avoid sequelae of bariatric surgery, or complications that develop over time, that may go undiagnosed and untreated.

11.6.1 Management of Derangements of Calcium and Bone Metabolism

The prevalence of SHPT makes it necessary to monitor and adequately supplement vitamin D and calcium in all patients who have had bariatric surgery, especially malabsorptive procedures [16, 18]. Calcium citrate supplementation allows for better absorption of calcium than calcium carbonate in the absence of gastric acid [87]. The total daily elemental calcium dose from all sources for patients who had BPD-DS is 1800–2400 mg. For all other patients, the total daily elemental calcium dose from all sources is 1500 mg [9, 72]. Calcium supplementation in multiple daily doses that add up to the needed total daily elemental calcium dose is necessary. Large oral doses at once overcome the absorptive capacity of the gut for calcium and result in the passage of the ingested calcium without absorption. The goal of treatment is to optimize intestinal calcium absorption to avoid the development of SHPT [87, 88].

Oral bisphosphonates are contraindicated in patients who had a malabsorptive procedure with a stomach resection because they require the acidity of the stomach for absorption. They are contraindicated in patients who had a restrictive procedure because the tablets may cause ulcerations. Intravenous bisphosphonate therapy should be considered for patients with documented bone mineral density loss [72, 83]. Other treatments for low bone mineral density may be considered as needed (i.e., denosumab). Consideration should be given to the use of estrogen replacement in women who transition to a postmenopausal state (primary hypogonadism) as a means to preserve bone mineral density.

11.6.2 Management of Derangements of Glucose Metabolism

MNT for patients after bariatric surgery is best provided by registered dieticians with expertise in overweight, obesity, adiposopathy, and the metabolic and endocrine complications of the various bariatric procedures. MNT should include recommendations for meals with low-carbohydrate, low-glycemic index, adequate protein, and heart-healthy fats. Patients should restrict alcohol and caffeine intake. Most patients with post-bariatric surgery hypoglycemia will respond to MNT [59, 83, 89].

Continuous glucose monitoring is now an important tool in the management of patients with hypoglycemia after bariatric surgery. Self-awareness of the glucose level in response to meals helps most patients modify their meal plan to prevent hypoglycemia [90–92].

Pharmacological interventions that help treat hypoglycemia from NIPHS after bariatric surgery include [93, 94]:

- Decreased glucose absorption from the intestine by blockade of intestinal disaccharidases.
  - acarbose, 50–100 mg three times a day, with each meal, [94, 95]
- Inhibition of insulin release from the beta cells in the pancreas
  - diazoxide, 50 mg two times a day, [96]
  - octreotide, 100 mcg two times a day, subcutaneously, [97–99]
  - calcium channel blockers (i.e., verapamil, 80 mg two times a day; nifedipine, 120 mg/day), [95, 100]
- Modulation of insulin release by the beta cells in the pancreas
  - GLP-1 receptor agonists, (i.e., liraglutide, 1.2–1.8 mg a day, subcutaneously) [101].

Gastric feeding through a gastric tube placed into the gastric remnant reverses the hypoglycemia in NIPHS, and has been advanced as a treatment option. This also serves to document that nutrient delivery alterations are the major cause of NIPHS, and not a change in pancreatic islet mass [102].

Reversal of the bariatric procedure should be done for any patient who continues to have neuroglycopenia that cannot be managed medically. This is mostly applicable to patients who had RYGB. Since reversal of RYGB effectively cures hypoglycemia, this also favors a non-pancreatic cause of severe hypoglycemia [103, 104]. Therefore, partial or total pancreatectomy should be reserved for rare recalcitrant cases [59, 68, 81, 83].

11.6.3 Management of Derangements of the Thyroid Axis

Thyroid function should be followed closely in all patients with pre-existing thyroid disease. Levothyroxine dosing needs adjustments to normalize TSH values, and to keep the TSH at the low end of its reference range. It is expected that weight loss will decrease thyroid needs, and the dose of levothyroxine will need to be adjusted down. However, many patients will have progression of their autoimmune thyroiditis over time, with loss of endogenous thyroid hormone production. The levothyroxine dose will need to be increased in these patients. Decreased absorption of levothyroxine in malabsorptive procedures is possible. Liquid forms of levothyroxine may improve absorption after malabsorptive procedures, and benefit patients with swallowing difficulties after bariatric surgery [83]. Softgel levothyroxine may also be considered for these patients [83].

11.6.4 Management of Derangements of the Gonadal Axis

Women with overweight or obesity, of reproductive age with intact anatomy, should be advised that their fertility status will improve with weight loss and correction of adiposopathy. Bariatric surgery could lead to an unintended pregnancy, and counseling to prevent this is necessary [83]. Women with PCOS reach bariatric surgery with years of irregular or absent menses. They will resume normal menses after bariatric surgery, and should be prepared to deal with them.

Men with pre-existing hypogonadotropic hypogonadism have a rise in the circulating testosterone with weight loss and reversal of adiposopathy. This translates into increased libido and improved erectile function after bariatric surgery. Men should be counseled about these changes, and be forewarned about possible unintended pregnancy.

Key Points

- *Bariatric endocrinology deals with derangements of structure and function of the adipocyte as an endocrine cell, and adipose tissue as an endocrine organ. In addition to adiposity, overweight and obesity lead to adiposopathy. Adiposopathy then contributes to derangements of metabolism that are the complications of this disease.*
- *Weight loss, in addition to reducing adiposity, treats adiposopathy. This is true both with medical and surgical weight loss.*
- *Bariatric surgery is an effective treatment of overweight, obesity, and adiposopathy in patients whose disease is refractory to medical management.*
- *Bariatric procedures carry a significant risk of metabolic and endocrine complications, which falls under the scope of practice or bariatric endocrinology. SHPT and NIPHS are two situations where a bariatric endocrinology team should be included in the care of patients.*
- *All patients with overweight, obesity, and adiposopathy benefit from a team approach to medical care that includes ongoing medical nutrition therapy, coaching to achieve effective behavior modification for a healthier lifestyle, and pharmacotherapy to treat complications of surgery but also to allow for ongoing weight loss beyond what surgery can accomplish.*

References

1. Gonzalez-Campoy J. Hormonal regulation of energy balance and energy stores. In: Gonzalez-Campoy JM, et al., editors. Bariatric endocrinology. Switzerland: Springer International; 2018. p. 37–58.
2. Bays HE, Gonzalez-Campoy JM. Adiposopathy. In: Friedberg E, et al., editors. New-opathies. Singapore: World Scientific; 2012. p. 105–68.

3. Bays HE, Gonzalez-Campoy JM, Henry RR, et al. Is adiposopathy (sick fat) an endocrine disease? Int J Clin Pract. 2008;62(10):1474–83. Epub 2008/08/07.
4. Christofides E, Gonzalez-Campoy J. Adiposopathy. In: Friedberg E, et al., editors. Bariatric endocrinology. Switzerland: Springer International; 2018. p. 99–120.
5. Gonzalez-Campoy J. Bariatric endocrinology, adiposopathy, and disorders of regional fat distribution. AACE Clin Case Rep. 2017;3(4):e387–e90.
6. Gonzalez-Campoy JM, Richardson B, Richardson C, et al. Bariatric endocrinology: principles of medical practice. Int J Endocrinol. 2014;2014:917813. Epub 2014/06/06.
7. Gonzalez-Campoy JM. The birth of bariatric endocrinology and the coming of age of obesity medicine. US Endocrinol [Internet]. 2016;12(1):10-1. https://doi.org/10.17925/USE.2016.12.01.10.
8. Gonzalez-Campoy J. Bariatric endocrinology. In: Gonzalez-Campoy JM, et al., editors. Bariatric Endocrinology. Switzerland: Springer International; 2018. p. 1–18.
9. Mechanick JI, Apovian C, Brethauer S, et al. Clinical Practice Guidelines for the Perioperative Nutrition, Metabolic, and Nonsurgical Support of Patients Undergoing Bariatric Procedures – 2019 Update: cosponsored by American Association of Clinical Endocrinologists/American College of Endocrinology, the Obesity Society, American Society for Metabolic & Bariatric Surgery, Obesity Medicine Association, and American Society of Anesthesiologists. Endocr Pract. 2019. Epub 2019/11/05.
10. Bays HE, Laferrere B, Dixon J, et al. Adiposopathy and bariatric surgery: is 'sick fat' a surgical disease? Int J Clin Pract. 2009;63(9):1285–300. Epub 2009/08/21.
11. Gonzalez-Campoy J. Bariatric procedures. In: Gonzalez-Campoy JM, et al., editors. Bariatric endocrinology. Switzerland: Springer International; 2018. p. 413–42.
12. Booth H, Khan O, Prevost T, et al. Incidence of type 2 diabetes after bariatric surgery: population-based matched cohort study. Lancet Diabetes Endocrinol. 2014;2(12):963–8. Epub 2014/12/04.
13. McMahon MM, Sarr MG, Clark MM, et al. Clinical management after bariatric surgery: value of a multidisciplinary approach. Mayo Clin Proc. 2006;81(10 Suppl):S34–45. Epub 2006/10/14.
14. Roth DE, Abrams SA, Aloia J, et al. Global prevalence and disease burden of vitamin D deficiency: a roadmap for action in low- and middle-income countries. Ann N Y Acad Sci. 2018;1430(1):44–79. Epub 2018/09/19.
15. Mitchell DM, Henao MP, Finkelstein JS, et al. Prevalence and predictors of vitamin D deficiency in healthy adults. Endocr Pract. 2012;18(6):914–23. Epub 2012/09/18.
16. Topart P, Becouarn G, Delarue J. Weight loss and nutritional outcomes 10 years after biliopancreatic diversion with duodenal switch. Obes Surg. 2017;27(7):1645–50. Epub 2017/01/05.
17. Tardio V, Blais JP, Julien AS, et al. Serum parathyroid hormone and 25-hydroxyvitamin D concentrations before and after biliopancreatic diversion. Obes Surg. 2018. Epub 2018/01/13.
18. Wei JH, Lee WJ, Chong K, et al. High incidence of secondary hyperparathyroidism in bariatric patients: comparing different procedures. Obes Surg. 2018;28(3):798–804. Epub 2017/09/19.
19. Coates PS, Fernstrom JD, Fernstrom MH, et al. Gastric bypass surgery for morbid obesity leads to an increase in bone turnover and a decrease in bone mass. J Clin Endocrinol Metab. 2004;89(3):1061–5. Epub 2004/03/06.
20. Collazo-Clavell ML, Jimenez A, Hodgson SF, et al. Osteomalacia after Roux-en-Y gastric bypass. Endocr Pract. 2004;10(3):195–8. Epub 2004/08/18.
21. Williams SE. Metabolic bone disease in the bariatric surgery patient. J Obes. 2011;2011:634614. Epub 2011/01/29.
22. Saad R, Habli D, El Sabbagh R, et al. Bone health following bariatric surgery: an update. J Clin Densitometry. 2019. Epub 2019/09/15.
23. Nakamura KM, Haglind EG, Clowes JA, et al. Fracture risk following bariatric surgery: a population-based study. Osteoporos Int. 2014;25(1):151–8. Epub 2013/08/06.
24. Rousseau C, Jean S, Gamache P, et al. Change in fracture risk and fracture pattern after bariatric surgery: nested case-control study. BMJ. 2016;354:i3794. Epub 2016/11/05.
25. Marsk R, Jonas E, Rasmussen F, et al. Nationwide cohort study of post-gastric bypass hypoglycaemia including 5,040 patients undergoing surgery for obesity in 1986-2006 in Sweden. Diabetologia. 2010;53(11):2307–11. Epub 2010/05/25.

26. Capristo E, Panunzi S, De Gaetano A, et al. Incidence of hypoglycemia after gastric bypass versus sleeve gastrectomy: a randomized trial. J Clin Endocrinol Metab. 2018; Epub 2018/03/29.
27. Lee CJ, Wood GC, Lazo M, et al. Risk of post-gastric bypass surgery hypoglycemia in non-diabetic individuals: a single center experience. Obesity (Silver Spring). 2016;24(6):1342–8. Epub 2016/05/27.
28. Zendel A, Abu-Ghanem Y, Dux J, et al. The impact of bariatric surgery on thyroid function and medication use in patients with hypothyroidism. Obes Surg. 2017;27(8):2000–4. Epub 2017/03/04.
29. Julia H, Benaiges D, Molla P, et al. Changes in thyroid replacement therapy after bariatric surgery: differences between laparoscopic Roux-en-Y gastric bypass and laparoscopic sleeve gastrectomy. Obes Surg. 2019;29(8):2593–9. Epub 2019/04/27.
30. Juiz-Valina P, Outeirino-Blanco E, Pertega S, et al. Effect of weight loss after bariatric surgery on thyroid-stimulating hormone levels in euthyroid patients with morbid obesity. Nutrients. 2019;11(5). Epub 2019/05/30.
31. Gokosmanoglu F, Aksoy E, Onmez A, et al. Thyroid homeostasis after bariatric surgery in obese cases. Obes Surg. 2019. Epub 2019/10/17.
32. Neves JS, Castro Oliveira S, Souteiro P, et al. Effect of weight loss after bariatric surgery on thyroid-stimulating hormone levels in patients with morbid obesity and normal thyroid function. Obes Surg. 2018;28(1):97–103. Epub 2017/07/21.
33. Zhang H, Liu W, Han X, et al. Effect of laparoscopic Roux-en-Y gastric bypass surgery on thyroid hormone levels in chinese patients, could it be a risk for thyroid nodules? Obes Surg. 2017;27(10):2619–27. Epub 2017/05/05.
34. Gonzalez-Campoy J. Gonadal dysfunction in males with overweight, obesity and adiposopathy. In: Gonzalez-Campoy JM, et al., editors. Bariatric endocrinology. Switzerland: Springer International; 2018. p. 271–82.
35. Gonzalez-Campoy J. Gonadal dysfunction and infertility in women with obesity. In: Gonzalez-Campoy JM, et al., editors. Bariatric endocrinology. Switzerland: Springer International; 2018. p. 283–92.
36. Kominiarek MA, Jungheim ES, Hoeger KM, et al. American Society for Metabolic and Bariatric Surgery position statement on the impact of obesity and obesity treatment on fertility and fertility therapy endorsed by the American College of Obstetricians and Gynecologists and the Obesity Society. Surg Obes Relat Dis. 2017;13(5):750–7. Epub 2017/04/19.
37. Moran LJ, Norman RJ. The effect of bariatric surgery on female reproductive function. J Clin Endocrinol Metab. 2012;97(12):4352–4. Epub 2012/12/12.
38. Legro RS, Dodson WC, Gnatuk CL, et al. Effects of gastric bypass surgery on female reproductive function. J Clin Endocrinol Metab. 2012;97(12):4540–8. Epub 2012/10/16.
39. Curtis KM, Tepper NK, Jatlaoui TC, et al. U.S. medical eligibility criteria for contraceptive use, 2016. MMWR Recomm Rep/Centers for Disease Control. 2016;65(3):1–103. Epub 2016/07/29.
40. Duran de Campos C, Dalcanale L, Pajecki D, et al. Calcium intake and metabolic bone disease after eight years of Roux-en-Y gastric bypass. Obes Surg. 2008;18(4):386–90. Epub 2008/02/01.
41. Tondapu P, Provost D, Adams-Huet B, et al. Comparison of the absorption of calcium carbonate and calcium citrate after Roux-en-Y gastric bypass. Obes Surg. 2009;19(9):1256–61. Epub 2009/05/14.
42. Sakhaee K, Pak C. Superior calcium bioavailability of effervescent potassium calcium citrate over tablet formulation of calcium citrate after Roux-en-Y gastric bypass. Surg Obes Relat Dis. 2013;9(5):743–8. Epub 2012/01/10.
43. Kopic S, Geibel JP. Gastric acid, calcium absorption, and their impact on bone health. Physiol Rev. 2013;93(1):189–268. Epub 2013/01/11.
44. Schafer AL. Vitamin D and intestinal calcium transport after bariatric surgery. J Steroid Biochem Mol Biol. 2017;173:202–10. Epub 2016/12/29.
45. Karefylakis C, Naslund I, Edholm D, et al. Vitamin D status 10 years after primary gastric bypass: gravely high prevalence of hypovitaminosis D and raised PTH levels. Obes Surg. 2014;24(3):343–8. Epub 2013/10/29.

46. Hewitt S, Sovik TT, Aasheim ET, et al. Secondary hyperparathyroidism, vitamin D sufficiency, and serum calcium 5 years after gastric bypass and duodenal switch. Obes Surg. 2013;23(3):384–90. Epub 2012/09/28.
47. Switzer NJ, Marcil G, Prasad S, et al. Long-term hypovitaminosis D and secondary hyperparathyroidism outcomes of the Roux-en-Y gastric bypass: a systematic review. Obes Rev. 2017;18(5):560–6. Epub 2017/03/09.
48. Sethi M, Chau E, Youn A, et al. Long-term outcomes after biliopancreatic diversion with and without duodenal switch: 2-, 5-, and 10-year data. Surg Obes Relat Dis. 2016;12(9):1697–705. Epub 2016/07/19.
49. Corbeels K, Verlinden L, Lannoo M, et al. Thin bones: vitamin D and calcium handling after bariatric surgery. Bone Rep. 2018;8:57–63. Epub 2018/06/30.
50. Ivaska KK, Huovinen V, Soinio M, et al. Changes in bone metabolism after bariatric surgery by gastric bypass or sleeve gastrectomy. Bone. 2017;95:47–54. Epub 2016/11/08.
51. Uebelhart B. Effects of bariatric surgery on bone. Joint Bone Spine. 2016;83(3):271–5. Epub 2016/03/20.
52. Luhrs AR, Davalos G, Lerebours R, et al. Determining changes in bone metabolism after bariatric surgery in postmenopausal women. Surg Endosc. 2019. Epub 2019/06/19..
53. Martinussen C, Bojsen-Moller KN, Dirksen C, et al. Immediate enhancement of first-phase insulin secretion and unchanged glucose effectiveness in patients with type 2 diabetes after Roux-en-Y gastric bypass. Am J Physiol Endocrinol Metab. 2015;308(6):E535–44. Epub 2015/01/30.
54. de Oliveira LF, Tisott CG, Silvano DM, et al. Glycemic behavior in 48 hours postoperative period of patients with type 2 diabetes mellitus and non diabetic submitted to bariatric surgery. Arquivos brasileiros de cirurgia digestiva: ABCD/Brazil Archiv Digest Surg. 2015;28 Suppl 1:26–30. Epub 2015/11/06.
55. Diemer DM, Terry KL, Matthews M, et al. Postoperative insulin requirements in bariatric surgery. Endocr Pract. 2017;23(12):1369–74. Epub 2017/10/12.
56. van Beek AP, Emous M, Laville M, et al. Dumping syndrome after esophageal, gastric or bariatric surgery: pathophysiology, diagnosis, and management. Obes Rev. 2017;18(1):68–85. Epub 2016/10/18.
57. Mesureur L, Arvanitakis M. Metabolic and nutritional complications of bariatric surgery: a review. Acta Gastro-Enterologica Belgica. 2017;80(4):515–25. Epub 2018/03/22.
58. Chaves YD, Destefani AC. Pathophysiology, diagnosis and treatmentof dumping syndrome and its relation to bariatric surgery. Arquivos brasileiros de cirurgia digestiva: ABCD/Brazil Archiv Digest Surg. 2016;29(Suppl 1):116–9. Epub 2016/09/30.
59. Eisenberg D, Azagury DE, Ghiassi S, et al. ASMBS position statement on postprandial hyperinsulinemic hypoglycemia after bariatric surgery. Surg Obes Relat Dis. 2017;13(3):371–8. Epub 2017/01/24.
60. Ramadan M, Loureiro M, Laughlan K, et al. Risk of dumping syndrome after sleeve gastrectomy and Roux-en-Y gastric bypass: early results of a multicentre prospective study. Gastroenterol Res Pract. 2016;2016:2570237. Epub 2016/06/01.
61. Berg P, McCallum R. Dumping syndrome: a review of the current concepts of pathophysiology, diagnosis, and treatment. Dig Dis Sci. 2016;61(1):11–8. Epub 2015/09/24.
62. Roslin MS, Oren JH, Polan BN, et al. Abnormal glucose tolerance testing after gastric bypass. Surg Obes Relat Dis. 2013;9(1):26–31. Epub 2012/03/09.
63. Roslin M, Damani T, Oren J, et al. Abnormal glucose tolerance testing following gastric bypass demonstrates reactive hypoglycemia. Surg Endosc. 2011;25(6):1926–32. Epub 2010/12/25.
64. Kim SH, Liu TC, Abbasi F, et al. Plasma glucose and insulin regulation is abnormal following gastric bypass surgery with or without neuroglycopenia. Obes Surg. 2009;19(11):1550–6. Epub 2009/06/27.
65. Honka H, Salehi M. Postprandial hypoglycemia after gastric bypass surgery: from pathogenesis to diagnosis and treatment. Curr Opin Clin Nutr Metab Care. 2019;22(4):295–302. Epub 2019/05/15.
66. Salehi M, Vella A, McLaughlin T, et al. Hypoglycemia after gastric bypass surgery: current concepts and controversies. J Clin Endocrinol Metab. 2018;103(8):2815–26. Epub 2018/08/14.

67. Yaqub A, Smith EP, Salehi M. Hyperinsulinemic hypoglycemia after gastric bypass surgery: what's up and what's down? Int J Obes (Lond). 2017. Epub 2017/11/01.
68. Vella A, Service FJ. Incretin hypersecretion in post-gastric bypass hypoglycemia–primary problem or red herring? J Clin Endocrinol Metab. 2007;92(12):4563–5. Epub 2007/12/07.
69. Service FJ, Natt N, Thompson GB, et al. Noninsulinoma pancreatogenous hypoglycemia: a novel syndrome of hyperinsulinemic hypoglycemia in adults independent of mutations in Kir6.2 and SUR1 genes. J Clin Endocrinol Metab. 1999;84(5):1582–9. Epub 1999/05/14.
70. Guan B, Chen Y, Yang J, et al. Effect of bariatric surgery on thyroid function in obese patients: a systematic review and meta-analysis. Obes Surg. 2017;27(12):3292–305. Epub 2017/10/19.
71. Mechanick JI, Kushner RF, Sugerman HJ, et al. American Association of Clinical Endocrinologists, The Obesity Society, and American Society for Metabolic & Bariatric Surgery Medical guidelines for clinical practice for the perioperative nutritional, metabolic, and nonsurgical support of the bariatric surgery patient. Endocr Pract. 2008;14(Suppl 1):1–83. Epub 2008/09/06.
72. Gagnon C, Schafer AL. Bone health after bariatric surgery. JBMR Plus. 2018;2(3):121–33. Epub 2018/10/05.
73. Kendler DL, Compston J, Carey JJ, et al. Repeating measurement of bone mineral density when monitoring with dual-energy X-ray absorptiometry: 2019 ISCD Official Position. J Clin Densitometry. 2019;22(4):489–500. Epub 2019/08/06.
74. Ohrstrom CC, Worm D, Hansen DL. Postprandial hyperinsulinemic hypoglycemia after Roux-en-Y gastric bypass: an update. Surg Obes Relat Dis. 2017;13(2):345–51. Epub 2016/11/21.
75. Patti ME, Li P, Goldfine AB. Insulin response to oral stimuli and glucose effectiveness increased in neuroglycopenia following gastric bypass. Obesity (Silver Spring). 2015;23(4):798–807. Epub 2015/03/11.
76. Patti ME, Goldfine AB. Hypoglycaemia following gastric bypass surgery–diabetes remission in the extreme? Diabetologia. 2010;53(11):2276–9. Epub 2010/08/24.
77. Himpens JM, Vilallonga R, Cadiere GB, et al. Metabolic consequences of the incorporation of a Roux limb in an omega loop (mini) gastric bypass: evaluation by a glucose tolerance test at mid-term follow-up. Surg Endosc. 2016;30(7):2935–45. Epub 2015/10/22.
78. Z'Graggen K, Guweidhi A, Steffen R, et al. Severe recurrent hypoglycemia after gastric bypass surgery. Obes Surg. 2008;18(8):981–8. Epub 2008/04/29.
79. Abellan P, Camara R, Merino-Torres JF, et al. Severe hypoglycemia after gastric bypass surgery for morbid obesity. Diabetes Res Clin Pract. 2008;79(1):e7–9. Epub 2007/09/07.
80. Cryer PE, Axelrod L, Grossman AB, et al. Evaluation and management of adult hypoglycemic disorders: an Endocrine Society Clinical Practice Guideline. J Clin Endocrinol Metab. 2009;94(3):709–28. Epub 2008/12/18.
81. Service GJ, Thompson GB, Service FJ, et al. Hyperinsulinemic hypoglycemia with nesidioblastosis after gastric-bypass surgery. N Engl J Med. 2005;353(3):249–54. Epub 2005/07/22.
82. Thompson SM, Vella A, Thompson GB, et al. Selective arterial calcium stimulation with hepatic venous sampling differentiates insulinoma from nesidioblastosis. J Clin Endocrinol Metab. 2015;100(11):4189–97. Epub 2015/08/28.
83. Mechanick JI, Apovian C, Brethauer S, et al. Clinical Practice Guidelines for the perioperative nutrition, metabolic, and nonsurgical support of patients undergoing bariatric procedures – 2019 update: cosponsored by American Association of Clinical Endocrinologists/American College of Endocrinology, the Obesity Society, American Society for Metabolic & Bariatric Surgery, Obesity Medicine Association, and American Society of Anesthesiologists – Executive Summary. Endocr Pract. 2019;25(12):1346–59. Epub 2019/11/05.
84. Atlantis E, Langford K, Piya M, et al. Physical capacity outcomes in patients with severe obesity after 12 months of physician-led multidisciplinary team care: a case series from a public hospital clinical obesity service. Clin Obes. 2019;9(6):e12337. Epub 2019/09/03.
85. Foster D, Sanchez-Collins S, Cheskin LJ. Multidisciplinary team-based obesity treatment in patients with diabetes: current practices and the state of the science. Diabetes Spectrum. 2017;30(4):244–9. Epub 2017/11/21.
86. Shealy K, Wagner S, Clements J, et al. Team-based approach to obesity management. J South Carolina Med Assoc. 2014;110(3):98–100. Epub 2014/09/01.

87. Baretta GA, Cambi MP, Rodrigues AL, et al. Secondary hyperparathyroidism after bariatric surgery: treatment is with calcium carbonate or calcium citrate? Arquivos brasileiros de cirurgia digestiva: ABCD/Brazil Archiv Digest Surg. 2015;28 Suppl 1:43–5. Epub 2015/11/06.
88. Alexandrou A, Tsoka E, Armeni E, et al. Determinants of secondary hyperparathyroidism in bariatric patients after Roux-en-Y gastric bypass or sleeve gastrectomy: a pilot study. Int J Endocrinol. 2015;2015:984935. Epub 2015/05/08.
89. Suhl E, Anderson-Haynes SE, Mulla C, et al. Medical nutrition therapy for post-bariatric hypoglycemia: practical insights. Surg Obes Relat Dis. 2017;13(5):888–96. Epub 2017/04/11.
90. Wysocki M, Szopa M, Stefura T, et al. Continuous glucose monitoring in bariatric patients undergoing laparoscopic sleeve gastrectomy and laparoscopic Roux-En-Y gastric bypass. Obes Surg. 2019;29(4):1317–26. Epub 2019/02/10.
91. Novodvorsky P, Walkinshaw E, Rahman W, et al. Experience with FreeStyle Libre Flash glucose monitoring system in management of refractory dumping syndrome in pregnancy shortly after bariatric surgery. Endocrinol Diabetes Metab Case Rep. 2017;2017. Epub 2018/01/06.
92. Nielsen JB, Abild CB, Pedersen AM, et al. Continuous glucose monitoring after gastric bypass to evaluate the glucose variability after a low-carbohydrate diet and to determine hypoglycemia. Obes Surg. 2016;26(9):2111–8. Epub 2016/01/13.
93. Mordes JP, Alonso LC. Evaluation, medical therapy, and course of adult persistent hyperinsulinemic hypoglycemia after Roux-en-Y gastric bypass surgery: a case series. Endocr Pract. 2015;21(3):237–46. Epub 2014/08/08.
94. Valderas JP, Ahuad J, Rubio L, et al. Acarbose improves hypoglycaemia following gastric bypass surgery without increasing glucagon-like peptide 1 levels. Obes Surg. 2012;22(4):582–6. Epub 2011/12/14.
95. Moreira RO, Moreira RB, Machado NA, et al. Post-prandial hypoglycemia after bariatric surgery: pharmacological treatment with verapamil and acarbose. Obes Surg. 2008;18(12):1618–21. Epub 2008/06/21.
96. Gonzalez-Gonzalez A, Delgado M, Fraga-Fuentes MD. Use of diazoxide in management of severe postprandial hypoglycemia in patient after Roux-en-Y gastric bypass. Surg Obes Relat Dis. 2013;9(1):e18–9. Epub 2011/07/05.
97. Vilarrasa N, Goday A, Rubio MA, et al. Hyperinsulinemic hypoglycemia after bariatric surgery: diagnosis and management experience from a Spanish Multicenter Registry. Obes Facts. 2016;9(1):41–51. Epub 2016/02/24.
98. Myint KS, Greenfield JR, Farooqi IS, et al. Prolonged successful therapy for hyperinsulinaemic hypoglycaemia after gastric bypass: the pathophysiological role of GLP1 and its response to a somatostatin analogue. Eur J Endocrinol. 2012;166(5):951–5. Epub 2012/03/13.
99. Ritz P, Vaurs C, Bertrand M, et al. Usefulness of acarbose and dietary modifications to limit glycemic variability following Roux-en-Y gastric bypass as assessed by continuous glucose monitoring. Diabetes Technol Ther. 2012;14(8):736–40. Epub 2012/08/03.
100. Koklu E, Ozkan KU, Sayar H, et al. Treatment of hyperinsulinemic hypoglycemia because of diffuse nesidioblastosis with nifedipine after surgical therapies in a newborn. J Pediatr Endocrinol Metab. 2013;26(11–12):1153–6. Epub 2013/06/12.
101. Abrahamsson N, Engstrom BE, Sundbom M, et al. GLP1 analogs as treatment of postprandial hypoglycemia following gastric bypass surgery: a potential new indication? Eur J Endocrinol. 2013;169(6):885–9. Epub 2013/10/03.
102. Davis DB, Khoraki J, Ziemelis M, et al. Roux en Y gastric bypass hypoglycemia resolves with gastric feeding or reversal: confirming a non-pancreatic etiology. Molec Metab. 2018;9:15–27. Epub 2018/02/17.
103. Shoar S, Nguyen T, Ona MA, et al. Roux-en-Y gastric bypass reversal: a systematic review. Surg Obes Relat Dis. 2016;12(7):1366–72. Epub 2016/10/26.
104. Rao BB, Click B, Eid G, et al. Management of refractory noninsulinoma pancreatogenous hypoglycemia syndrome with gastric bypass reversal: a case report and review of the literature. Case Rep Endocrinol. 2015;2015:384526. Epub 2015/11/03.

Cardiovascular Complications After Bariatric and Metabolic Surgery

12

Md Tanveer Adil, Alan Askari, and Kamal Mahawar

The central problem in heart failure is not that patients are short of breath or that they retain fluid: the problem is that they die. Heart failure is a mortal illness, more serious than most malignancies.

—Arnold M. Katz, MD

Abbreviations

AF	Atrial Fibrillation
ASMBS	American Society for Metabolic and Bariatric Surgery
BMS	Bariatric and Metabolic Surgery
DVT	Deep Vein Thrombosis
HF	Heart Failure
IVC	Inferior Vena Cava
LMWH	Low Molecular Weight Heparin
MI	Myocardial Infarction

M. T. Adil (✉)
Consultant Surgeon, Department of Upper GI and Bariatric Surgery, Luton and Dunstable University Hospital, Luton, UK
e-mail: mdtanveer.adil@ldh.nhs.uk

A. Askari
Specialty Trainee, East of England Surgical Rotation, Watford General Hospital, Watford, UK
e-mail: alan.askari@nhs.net

K. Mahawar
Consultant Surgeon, Department of General Surgery, Sunderland Royal Hospital, Sunderland, UK
e-mail: Kamal.mahawar@chsft.nhs.uk

A. G. Bhasker et al. (eds.), *Management of Nutritional and Metabolic Complications of Bariatric Surgery*,
https://doi.org/10.1007/978-981-33-4702-1_12

PE	Pulmonary Embolism
USA	United States of America
VTE	Venous Thromboembolism

12.1 Introduction

Bariatric and Metabolic Surgery (BMS) is major abdominal surgery and is associated with a definite risk of post-operative cardiovascular events [1, 2]. Though BMS leads to an improvement in physical function, cardiovascular fitness, and reduced incidence of cardiac disease/events in the long term [2, 3], it is associated with a definite risk of cardiovascular events in the immediate post-operative period. In this regard, cardiovascular complications after BMS are no different from the complications following any major abdominal surgery and include Venous Thromboembolism (VTE), Myocardial Infarction (MI), arrhythmias, and Heart Failure (HF), but the demographic profile of patients undergoing BMS puts them at a substantially higher risk of developing these complications.

Although, majority of BMS procedures are currently performed laparoscopically with a relatively short anaesthetic time, surgery can still place considerable demand on the physiological reserves of these patients, especially if the patient develops major post-operative complications that can happen in approximately 3.0–5.0% of patients. The preoperative cardiac assessment should, therefore, attempt to determine if the patient has enough cardiac reserve for not just the procedure but also any major complications that might follow.

It is important to recognize that patients who undergo BMS are at a higher risk of cardiovascular events compared to the normal population. They are at moderate or high risk for developing VTE as per the American Society of Metabolic and Bariatric Surgeons (ASMBS) [1]. Besides, they suffer from many other associated co-morbidities such as type 2 diabetes, hypertension, and obstructive sleep apnoea. These conditions further increase the risk of post-operative cardiovascular complications.

12.2 Incidence/Prevalence

The reported incidence of cardiac complications like arrhythmia, MI, and HF and vascular complications such as DVT and PE varies in literature ranging from 0.1 to 12% [4–8]. Of the potential cardiac complications, Atrial Fibrillation (AF) appears to be the most common [4].

VTE is one of the most disastrous complications after BMS, affecting 0.3–1.3% of patients undergoing BMS within 30 days [5, 6]. In a large nationwide cohort of 110,000 BMS patients in France, patients with previous history of VTE, post-operative complications, heart failure, or open surgery appeared to be at the highest risk of post-operative VTE. Furthermore, the study demonstrated that there was an ongoing risk of VTE beyond the initial 30 days, with rates of embolism rising from 0.3% at 30 days to 0.5% at 90 days [5]. Another study encompassing over 73,000 patients from the United States of America (USA) confirmed that the overall VTE rate is low (0.4%) and open surgery is associated with nearly a three-fold increase in VTE rates compared to laparoscopic bariatric surgery [7]. A meta-analysis including over 107,000 patients across 71 studies put the thromboembolic risk at 1.2%. The same study put the risk of myocardial infarction at 0.4% [8].

In one study from the USA encompassing over 108,000 patients who underwent BMS, 116 patients (0.1%) had a cardiac event in the immediate post-operative period [9]. Overall, the incidence of serious cardiac complications appears to be low after BMS.

Though stroke has been reported following BMS, it appears to be rare [10]. Unfortunately, there is no high-quality data, reporting the incidence of stroke after BMS. The risk of stroke in patients undergoing major abdominal surgery has been estimated to be in the range of 0.2–0.6% [11], but in the experience of authors, it is much lower after BMS probably because a majority of patients undergoing BMS are relatively younger.

Table 12.1 summarizes the risk of various cardiovascular complications after BMS.

12.2.1 Mortality Risk After Cardiovascular Complication

Although cardiovascular complications are relatively uncommon in the immediate post-operative period, they can be life-threatening. Mortality from VTE (largely from PE) has been reported to be around 0.18% following BMS. This figure is substantially lower with gastric banding (0.09%) compared with sleeve gastrectomy (0.25%) [8]. The same meta-analysis reported a pooled mortality rate of 0.37% following myocardial infarction [8]. Another study reported the incidence of

Table 12.1 Risk of various cardiovascular complications after bariatric surgery

Venous Thromboembolism	**Incidence**
Deep vein thrombosis	0.3–3.0%
Pulmonary embolism	0.3–2.0%
Cardiac complications	
Myocardial infarction	0.1–0.4%
Atrial fibrillation/ arrhythmias	2.0–12%
Heart failure	<1%
Stroke	0.2–0.6%

cardiovascular complication to be low, but associated with a significant risk of mortality [12].

12.3 Pathophysiology

12.3.1 Arrhythmia

Up to 2% of obese patients will have AF before surgery and around 2–8% may go on to develop new-onset AF in the immediate post-operative period [13]. Older age group and male gender appear to be significant risk factors for new-onset AF after bariatric surgery and BMI appears to be less significant [13]. It is not entirely clear as to why bariatric patients are susceptible to new-onset AF. It could be because factors predisposing to AF are common in a significant proportion of patients undergoing BMS. For example, BMS, like any major gastrointestinal surgery can cause fluid shifts and changes in electrolyte composition. This coupled with an increased sympathetic tone, poor baseline nutrition (with or without anaemia), direct fatty infiltration of the of cardiac myocytes, cardiac hypertrophy, intraoperative hypotension, and catecholamine release as part of the stress response to surgery may all play a role [14]. Furthermore, a significant proportion of patients undergoing BMS also suffer from hypertension which itself increases the chance of developing AF by 70–80% [15].

12.3.2 Venous Thromboembolism

Obesity is an independent risk factor for VTE. Patients with advanced obesity such as those with BMI of >50 kg/m^2 and those with larger waist circumferences are at particularly high risk due to a combination of reduced mobility and increased intra-abdominal pressure resulting in reduced venous return and venous stasis. Furthermore, hypoventilation due to large truncal size and reduced venous return in the chest can also contribute to clot formation in the lungs. These factors combined with the effects of laparoscopic surgery can lead to reduced venous return and peripheral venous stasis in the lower extremities and predispose to peripheral venous thrombosis.

Furthermore, obesity also leads to hypercoagulable state and is associated with a higher level of pro-thrombotic agents such as fibrinogen, von Willebrand's factor, and factor VII [16]. Chronic intra-vascular inflammation secondary to obesity and impaired fibrinolysis could also play a role. Increased adipose tissue is believed to lead to a systemic inflammatory state driven by adipocyte secreted inflammatory mediators, in particular, cytokines [17].

Obesity is also associated with a significantly higher proportion of visceral fat which has a higher concentration of macrophages as part of the inflammatory response caused by adipose tissue hypoxia. This higher concentration of macrophages results in the activation of pro-thrombotic processes via the release of inflammatory mediators such as anti-TNF, clotting factors, and interleukins. On top of this, there is the added inflammatory effect of the surgery itself.

12.3.3 Cardiac Complications

MI and HF are the other significant cardiac complications after bariatric surgery. The pathophysiology of myocardial ischaemia in post-operative patients is no different from that with the rest of the population. An autopsy study of 67 patients who died as a result of myocardial infarction found that the mechanism of infarction was identical in those who had undergone recent surgery (of various types) in comparison to those who had not had surgery recently. The most common mechanism of MI is one of coronary atheromatous plaque rupture, embolus, occlusion of the vessel followed by myocardial ischaemia, and finally muscle death.

Though BMS has been found to improve HF by approximately one half compared to lifestyle modification in a study from two large Swedish registries [18], patients undergoing BMS with pre-existing HF are at risk of decompensation intra-operatively and post-operatively. New-onset HF is rare after BMS. Systolic dysfunction may occur as a result of a myocardial ischaemic event, sepsis, or inappropriate fluid therapy, while diastolic dysfunction can be precipitated in

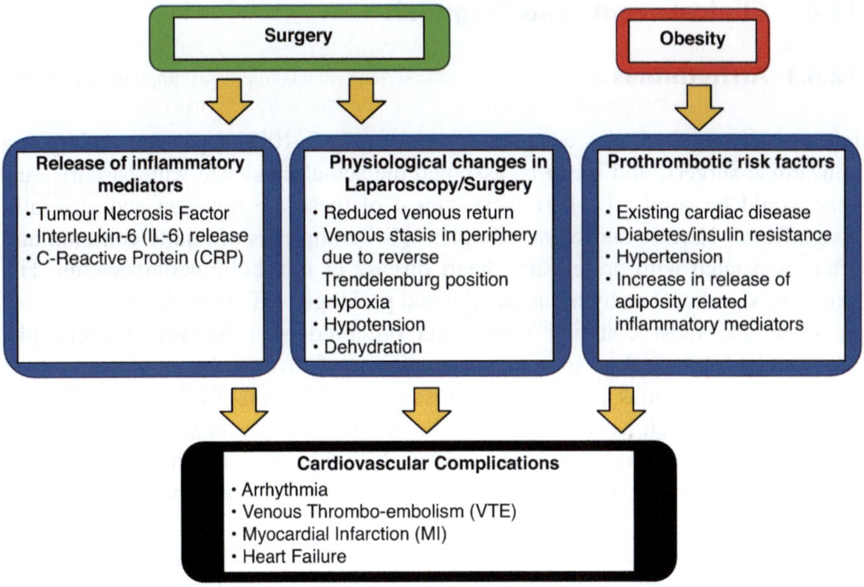

Fig. 12.1 Pathophysiology of cardiovascular complications after bariatric surgery

patients with pre-existing hypertensive left ventricular hypertrophy or cardiomyopathy.

The pathophysiology of cardiac complications after bariatric surgery is illustrated in Fig. 12.1.

12.3.4 Cardiovascular Effect of BMS

A large review evaluating the effect of bariatric surgery on cardiac function showed significant improvement in atherogenesis, cardiac electro conduction, systolic function, diastolic function, and symptoms of heart failure after surgery [19]. Even though BMS has a small risk of various cardiovascular complications, in the long term it is associated with a significant improvement in cardiovascular health [20, 21]. A study of the effect of bariatric surgery on cardiac structure and function showed significant improvements in the left ventricular mass index, left ventricular end-diastolic volume, left atrial diameter, and left ventricular ejection fraction [22]. The mechanism underlying this benefit is likely remodelling of the cardiac myocytes and epicardial adipose tissue [20, 21]. Another large prospective nationwide Swedish study showed that BMS leads to a significant reduction in total and fatal cardiovascular events like MI and stroke compared to non-surgical controls [23].

12.4 Clinical events and Diagnosis

12.4.1 Arrhythmias

Intraoperative arrhythmias occur in approximately 3–10% of patients undergoing noncardiac surgery, and it can be assumed the actual incidence with bariatric surgery would be similar [24]. However, most of these are transient and clinically insignificant. Narrow and broad complex QRS complexes are quite common and often associated with pre-existing heart disease or metabolic derangements. The two most significant arrhythmias are AF and prolonged QT interval.

AF is the most common arrhythmia observed after bariatric surgery [4]. Uncontrolled AF can lead to more serious forms of rhythm abnormalities such as ventricular arrhythmias and can predispose to embolization of clots from the heart to other organs such as the lungs and the brain. Obesity and obesity-related co-morbidities such as diabetes, hypertension, dyslipidaemia, and electrolyte abnormalities are known risk factors for repolarization disturbances, and prolonged QT interval [25].

A new-onset cardiac arrhythmia, especially AF, after BMS should lead one to suspect an intra-abdominal complication. Along with sinus tachycardia, AF in a previously healthy patient is often an early sign of staple line leak after sleeve gastrectomy (SG), or anastomotic dehiscence and bowel obstruction after gastric bypass. Therefore, any abdominal discomfort in association with AF after BMS should prompt urgent imaging/ laparoscopy as appropriate. Most patients with AF in the absence of intra-abdominal complications would remain asymptomatic. However, those with pre-existing diastolic dysfunction or hypertension can deteriorate rapidly and become haemodynamically unstable.

12.4.2 Venous Thromboembolism

Venous thromboembolism (VTE) after bariatric surgery is estimated to occur in approximately 0.3% patients within 7 days, 1.9% within 30 days, 2.1% within 90 days, and 2.1% within 180 days of bariatric surgery [26]. Risk factors identified for VTE after bariatric surgery are male gender, older age, higher BMI, longer operating time, type of procedure (higher following gastric bypass and duodenal switch compared to the gastric band), pre-existing chronic heart failure, renal disease, lung disease and alcohol abuse. A study of 27,818 patients undergoing BMS identified 93 patients (0.33%) with VTE, including 51 patients (0.18%) with pulmonary embolism (PE) [27]. Risk factors for VTE in this study were male gender (odds ratio (OR) 2.08), operating time more than 3 hours (OR 1.86), BMI category (per 10 units) (OR 1.37), and procedure type (reference adjustable gastric band): duodenal switch (OR 9.45), laparoscopic gastric bypass (OR 3.97), open gastric bypass (OR 6.48), and sleeve gastrectomy (OR 3.50) [27]. Another study identified alcohol abuse (OR 8.7), renal failure (OR 2.3), congestive heart failure (OR 2.0), and chronic lung disease (OR 1.4) as additional risk factors [27].

The diagnosis of VTE requires a high index of clinical suspicion. The two-level Wells score (Tables 12.2 and 12.3) serves as a useful guide to establish the risk of VTE and is recommended by National Institute for Health and Care Excellence (NICE) [28, 30, 31].

Table 12.2 Two-level DVT Wells score [28, 29]

Clinical feature	Points
Active cancer (treatment ongoing, within 6 months, or palliative)	1
Paralysis, paresis, or recent plaster immobilization of the lower extremities	1
Recently bedridden for 3 days or more or major surgery within 12 weeks requiring general or regional anaesthesia	1
Localized tenderness along the distribution of the deep venous system	1
Entire leg swollen	1
Calf swelling at least 3 cm larger than asymptomatic side	1
Pitting edema confined to the symptomatic leg	1
Collateral superficial veins (non-varicose)	1
Previously documented DVT	1
An alternative diagnosis is at least as likely as DVT	−2
DVT *likely*	2 points or more
DVT *unlikely*	1 point or less

Table 12.3 Two-level PE Wells score [28, 29]

Clinical feature	Points
Clinical signs and symptoms of DVT (minimum of leg swelling and pain with palpation of the deep veins)	3
An alternative diagnosis is less likely than PE	3
Heart rate > 100 beats per minute	1.5
Immobilization for more than 3 days or surgery in the previous 4 weeks	1.5
Previous DVT/PE	1.5
Hemoptysis	1
Malignancy (on treatment, treated in the last 6 months, or palliative)	1
PE *likely*	More than 4 points
PE *unlikely*	4 points or less

Unilateral calf or thigh pain, leg swelling, and redness are the usual clinical features of deep venous thrombosis (DVT). The usual symptoms and signs of PE are chest pain, dyspnoea, palpitations, cough, and in severe cases it may be associated with syncope and haemodynamic collapse. D-dimer, although typically elevated in acute VTE, may be unreliable early after BMS due to low specificity. However, it does have a role in the diagnosis of late VTE after BMS and carries a sensitivity of 95% and specificity of 50% in the diagnosis of DVT and PE [29].

Compression duplex ultrasound is the imaging modality of choice for the diagnosis of DVT and has largely superseded other modalities such as doppler and invasive techniques like contrast venography. For PE, the imaging modality of choice is the computed tomographic pulmonary angiogram (CTPA) due to its high sensitivity, non-invasive nature, easy availability, and simpler reporting system. CTPA has largely replaced other modalities such as invasive pulmonary angiography, ventilation-perfusion scan, chest X-ray, thoracic ultrasonography, and magnetic resonance angiography in clinical practice. According to a study comparing CTPA with ventilation-perfusion radionuclide lung scan, CTPA offered superior sensitivity (94.1% versus 80.8%), specificity (93.6% versus 73.8%), positive predictive value (95.5% versus 82%) and negative predictive value (96.2% versus 75.9%) than ventilation-perfusion scan [32]. In patients with allergy to contrast or with renal impairment, ventilation-perfusion SPECT or planar scans can be considered as an alternative.

12.4.3 Myocardial Ischaemia and Infarction

MI can be defined as myocardial injury with clinical evidence of myocardial ischaemia, rise and/or fall of cardiac troponin value with at least one value above the 99th percentile and at least one of the following—symptoms of myocardial ischaemia, new ischaemic ECG changes, development of pathological Q waves, imaging evidence of new loss of viable myocardium, new regional wall motion abnormality in a pattern consistent with ischaemic aetiology, or identification of coronary thrombus by angiography or autopsy [33]. Perioperative MI can be difficult to diagnose.

Two distinct mechanisms of perioperative MI are identified—(1) acute coronary syndrome (Type 1 MI), and (2) imbalance in the myocardial oxygen supply-demand (Type 2 MI) [34]. Type 1 MI is often predisposed by tachycardia and hypertension, both of which are fairly common in perioperative bariatric settings due to catecholamine and cortisol surge during surgery along with increased endogenous procoagulants, decreased anticoagulants, and decreased fibrinolysis that predominates in the perioperative setting. Type 2 MI is precipitated by tachycardia, hypotension, hypertension, anaemia, hypoxia, and hypercarbia. It presents as silent ischaemia with ST-depression more common than ST-elevation. According to studies, ST-elevation occurs in <2% of post-operative cardiac events and is a rare accompaniment of perioperative MI [33, 35]. In a bariatric setting, however, the incidence of STEMI (ST Elevation Myocardial infarction) is expected to be higher due to obesity and co-existent co-morbidities such as diabetes, dyslipidaemia, and hypertension. The rise in cardiac troponin levels has been found to occur after prolonged, transient ST-depression with peak troponin levels corroborating with the duration of ST-depression [36].

Chest pain, as a classical symptom of MI, is unreliable in the perioperative setting due to the presence of confounding variables, such as the use of analgesics. A pooled data analysis found chest pain to occur in only 14% of patients with perioperative MI [37]. Common clinical findings suggestive of perioperative MI are persistent hypotension, nausea, and diaphoresis. Diagnosis is aided by post-operative ECG changes such as ST-depression (non-ST elevation myocardial infarction or NSTEMI), or ST-elevation (ST-elevation myocardial infarction or STEMI), left bundle branch block, and pathological Q waves. Biomarker assay with cardiac troponin as a standard fourth-generation assay is usually sufficient to establish the diagnosis of perioperative MI. Fifth-generation highly sensitive assays for cardiac troponin can be used to detect more subtle elevations suggestive of MI. According to the VISION study, cardiac troponin measurement of at least 20 ng/L in men and 14 ng/L in women was significantly associated with 30-day mortality [38]. Transoesophageal echocardiography shows segmental wall motion abnormalities highly sensitive and specific for myocardial ischaemia and is integral to the monitoring of perioperative MI. Once a diagnosis of perioperative MI is established, all patients should probably undergo coronary angiography and be looked after under an expert cardiologist. Coronary angiography can differentiate Type 1 MI from Type 2 MI in the setting of NSTEMI. Type 1 NSTEMI and STEMI would require invasive intervention that can be guided only by coronary angiography.

12.4.4 Heart Failure

HF, as a complication after bariatric surgery, almost universally occurs in patients with a pre-existing cardiac disease such as coronary artery disease, pre-existing HF, valvular heart disease, hypertension, tachyarrhythmias, and anaemia. It is precipitated by intraoperative stress, inappropriate fluid management, or myocardial ischaemia. It can be defined as a clinical syndrome characterized by typical symptoms, such as breathlessness, swelling, and fatigue, and signs such as peripheral oedema, pulmonary crepitations, elevated jugular venous pressure, and cardiogenic shock in advanced cases. The diagnosis is supported by chest X-ray, electrocardiogram, echocardiography, and biomarkers. Signs of HF on chest X-ray are Kerley B lines, pleural effusion, and cardiomegaly while findings on electrocardiogram include abnormal Q wave, ST-depression, abnormal T wave, atrial fibrillation or flutter, left bundle branch block, and left ventricular hypertrophy. In patients clinically suspected of having an HF during or after bariatric surgery, echocardiography is the gold standard investigation for confirmation of the diagnosis [39]. Intraoperative and post-operative transoesophageal or post-operative transthoracic echocardiography provides rapid evaluation of regional and global right and left ventricular function, preload estimation, presence of cardiac thrombi, and valvular dysfunction. The European Society of Cardiology defines HF based on ejection fraction (EF) into (a) HF with preserved EF (EF $\geq$ 50%), (b) HF with midrange EF (EF 40%–49%), and (c) HF with reduced EF (EF < 40%) [40]. Patients suspected of HF with preserved and midrange EF should have B-type natriuretic peptide (BNP) levels >35 pg/mL or N-terminal pro-BNP (NT-pro-BNP) levels >125 pg/mL, along with at least one additional criterion such as diastolic dysfunction or structural cardiac disease like left ventricular hypertrophy or left atrial enlargement [39]. These biomarkers have the potential to strengthen the diagnosis of acute HF in a bariatric setting in conjunction with clinical findings and echocardiography, but may not be routinely available in all centres. According to a recent meta-analysis, post-operative rise in BNP and NT-pro-BNP levels after noncardiac surgery were found to be independently associated with increased risk of HF, MI, and mortality at 30 days and 180 days after surgery [40].

12.4.5 Chronic Cardiovascular Complications

Chronic cardiovascular complications after BMS have been reported, although these appear to be rare. Cardiomyopathy and subsequent heart failure have been shown to occur due to selenium deficiency after gastric bypass [41]. Selenium deficiency, although seemingly minor, can result in life-threatening heart failure after BMS [42]. Zinc deficiency after BMS has also been reported to cause significant cardiac dysfunction [43]. In the vast majority of cases, these deficiencies are due to poor adherence on the part of patients to recommended micronutrient supplements. The clinical signs and symptoms are often classical of cardiac dysfunction, i.e. dyspnoea, lethargy, and leg oedema. Cardiomyopathy and consequent decline in cardiac function in this setting is often reversible and occurs due to a reduction in antioxidant reserve within the cells of cardiac musculature. Since both zinc and selenium are required by the myocardium for antioxidant activity, symptoms have been reported to resolve or at least improve once the micronutrient deficiency is resolved. Another reported cause of heart failure after BMS is Takotsubo syndrome (stress-induced cardiomyopathy). This phenomenon is more acute and usually due to cardiac stress resulting in catecholamine release, tachycardia and ultimately left ventricular failure [44], In a few other cases, BMS did not directly contribute to cardiovascular complications but has exacerbated pre-existing cardiac conditions. These are largely confined to case reports in the literature. One such report highlighted that vomiting after laparoscopic gastric band worsened hypertrophic obstructive cardiomyopathy (HOCM) through triggering of the Valsalva manoeuvre resulting in occlusion of the outlet of the left ventricle, ultimately causing syncope [45]. Some of the cardiovascular complications may be due to mechanical/technical causes of BMS. Two unusual reports exist in the literature, highlighting that misplaced bands can potentially lead to cardiovascular complications, particularly if the band is inadvertently placed around the aorta [46] or if the marginal ulcer following a gastric bypass penetrates surrounding structures leading to an aorto-enteric fistula [47].

12.5 Management

12.5.1 Arrhythmias

Intraoperatively detected significant arrhythmias need close co-operation between the surgeon and anaesthetist for optimal management. The anaesthetist may want an immediate deflation of the pneumoperitoneum and change in the positioning of the patient to supine. It is of paramount importance to ensure adequate oxygenation and ventilation to maintain optimum PaO2, PaCO2, acid-base, electrolyte, and temperature of the patient. Alteration in the depth of anaesthesia may be required. Anti-arrhythmic drugs, anti-ischaemic drugs, pacing, or DC cardioversion may be necessary for unstable patients.

Post-operative atrial fibrillation in the first week may be reflective of an intraoperative complication like anastomotic or staple line leaks, bowel obstruction, and acute gastric dilatation, and should be viewed with suspicion. Post-operative cardiac arrhythmias are best managed in consultation with a cardiologist.

The management of post-operative atrial fibrillation is illustrated in Fig. 12.2.

12.5.2 Venous thromboembolism

VTE after BMS should be managed in consultation with an Internist or a Haematologist. Systemic anticoagulation is the therapy of choice in the treatment of VTE in the acute, short-term, and long-term setting after bariatric surgery. Catheter-directed thrombolysis is reserved for acute limb-threatening thrombosis of the ilio-femoral vein, provided the symptoms are present for less than 14 days, and the patient has a low risk of bleeding with good functional status [30]. Systemic thrombolysis is reserved for life-threatening massive PEs with haemodynamic instability but carries a high risk of bleeding complications. Mechanical thrombectomy is

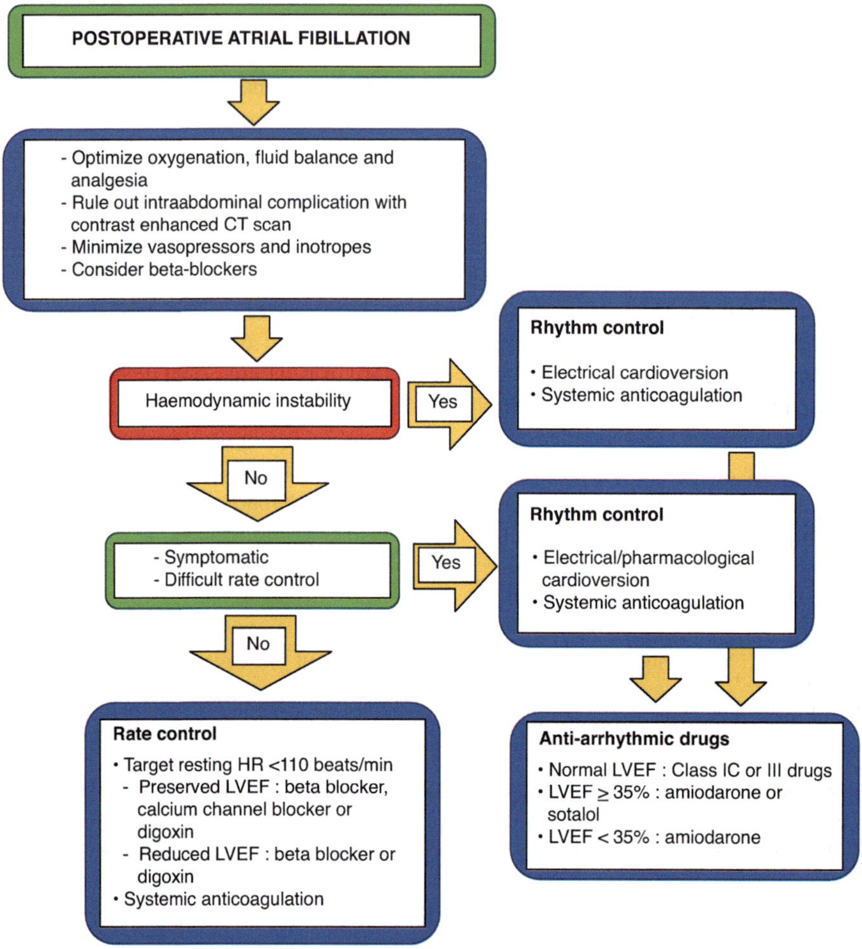

Fig. 12.2 Treatment of post-operative atrial fibrillation after bariatric surgery

rarely used in conjunction with thrombolysis. The duration of anticoagulation in the acute phase of VTE is between 7 and 10 days of parenteral therapy with unfractionated, or preferably, low molecular weight heparin (LMWH), followed by a vitamin K antagonist like warfarin which is continued for short or long term depending on the risks. For calf DVTs, the duration of treatment is usually 6 weeks. A longer duration of at least 3 months is advocated for proximal DVTs. Patients with a significantly high risk of recurrent VTE like those suffering from pro-thrombotic conditions such as Factor V Leiden mutation, prosthetic cardiac valves, or recurrent history of PEs are often kept on lifelong anticoagulation. In patients of DVT with a contraindication to anticoagulation, but at a high risk of PE, inferior vena cava (IVC) filter placement can be considered.

Table 12.4 Treatment options for acute venous thromboembolism

– ***Unfractionated heparin:*** 80 U/kg intravenous bolus followed by 18 U/kg/h adjusted to activated partial thromboplastin time (aPTT) ratio
– ***Low molecular weight heparins:***
Tinzaparin 175 U/kg s/c every 24 h
(Renal dose: Same as no evidence of accumulation in the IRIS study [42])
Alteparin 200 U/kg s/c every 24 h
(Renal dose: No official recommendation to use with caution, consider anti-Xa monitoring)
Enoxaparin 1.5 mg/kg s/c every 24 h
(Renal dose: 1 mg/kg s/c every 24 h for CrCl <30 mL/min)
– ***Pentasaccharide***
Fondaparinux 5-10 mg s/c every 24 h (7.5 mg for 50–100 kg body weight; 10 mg for >100 kg body weight)
(Renal dose: Avoid in patients with CrCl <30 mL/min; caution in patients with CrCl 30–50 mL/min)
– ***Direct oral anticoagulants***
Apixaban (oral direct factor Xa inhibitor)—10 mg BD for 7 days, followed by 5 mg BD
Dabigatran (oral direct thrombin inhibitor)—150 mg BD after 5–10 days of parenteral anticoagulation
Edoxaban (oral direct factor Xa inhibitor)—60 mg OD
Rivaroxaban (oral direct factor Xa inhibitor)—15 mg BD for 3 weeks followed by 20 mg OD.
– ***Inferior vena cava filter***

The various anticoagulant agents used for the treatment of VTE are enumerated in Table 12.4.

Prevention of VTE in bariatric surgery has been extensively studied as it is one of the most common causes of mortality after laparoscopic bariatric surgery [48]. Strategies employed to reduce VTE after bariatric surgery include early ambulation, lower extremity compression with elastic stockings, intermittent pneumatic compression or sequential compression device, and pharmacological prophylaxis, most commonly with Low Molecular Weight Heparin. There is emerging evidence towards extended prophylaxis after bariatric surgery in terms of lowering the incidence of VTE [5, 49] and many surgeons now recommend post-discharge VTE prophylaxis for 14–28 days.

12.5.3 Myocardial Infarction

MI after BMS involves multidisciplinary management involving the anaesthetist, cardiologist, and critical care team. The goal of the management of perioperative MI is to optimize the myocardial oxygen supply-demand balance whilst maintaining the haemodynamic stability of the patient. If detected intraoperatively, surgery is paused till the situation is stabilized and the surgeon should consider abandoning the procedure if possible. The physiological goals to be achieved include normalization of heart rate, blood pressure, oxygen saturations with the minimum possible FiO2, and avoidance of fluid overload. If detected post-operatively, management

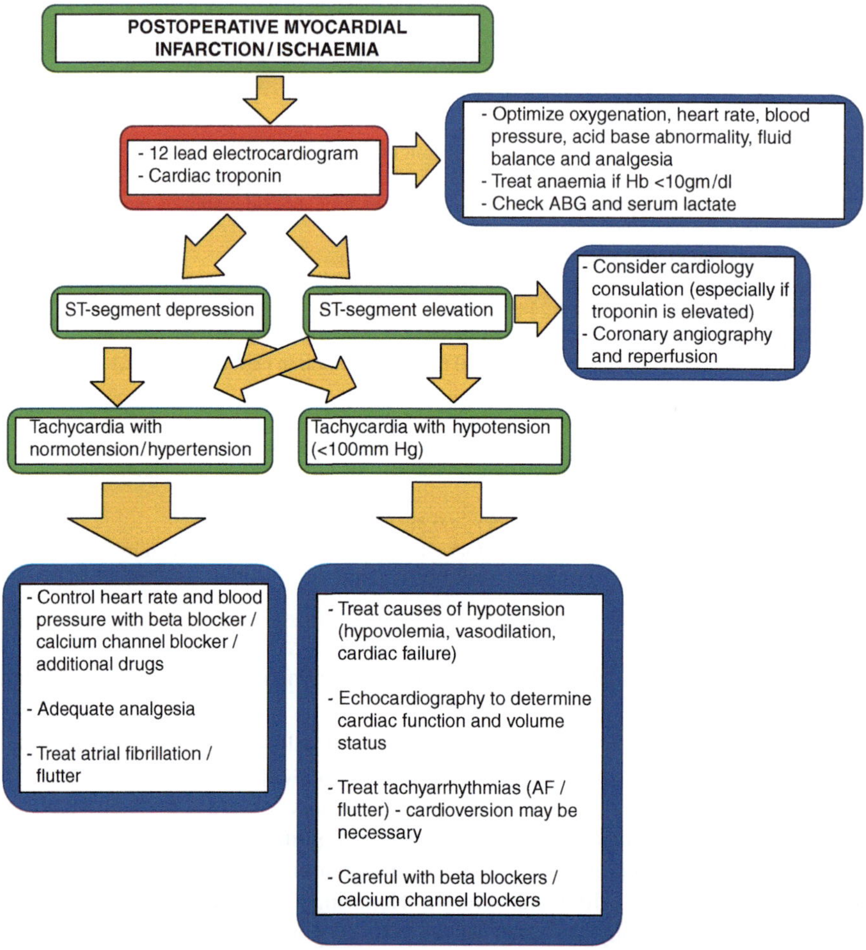

Fig. 12.3 Treatment of post-operative myocardial infarction/ischaemia after bariatric surgery

principles remain the same along with adequate analgesia. Management principles of post-operative MI after bariatric surgery are illustrated in Fig. 12.3.

12.5.4 Heart Failure

The aim of intraoperative and post-operative management of acute HF in BMS involves a rapid diagnosis of HF, including that of the cause. Treatment is aimed to prevent further organ dysfunction and myocardial damage. This is best accomplished with inputs from an experienced cardiologist and critical care team.

The diagnosis of the cause of HF allows definitive treatment through the use of specific therapy. HF secondary to fluid overload requires fluid restriction and diuretics while that due to MI may prompt angiography and reperfusion with angioplasty or stenting. The goals of treatment of acute HF in the bariatric setting would include [50]:

1. Diagnosis of the cause of HF and treatment of the cause.
2. Maximize oxygenation/ventilation, correction of heart rate, and blood pressure.
3. Correction of acid-base and electrolyte abnormalities.
4. Adequate analgesia in the post-operative setting.
5. Optimization of preload, afterload, heart rate, rhythm, and contractility.
   (a) Preload—Diuretics if volume status is high, fluids if volume status is low.
   (b) Afterload—Nitroglycerine and sodium nitroprusside if high, norepinephrine if afterload is low.
   (c) Stable heart rate and rhythm—digoxin to stabilize the heart.
   (d) Contractility—Inotropes if contractility is reduced.
6. If medical management fails—use of mechanical assistance such as intra-aortic balloon pump, percutaneous cardiopulmonary bypass system, and mechanical assist devices.
7. Ultrafiltration in diuretic-refractory HF.
8. Ventricular pacing in left ventricular dysfunction and atrioventricular block.

12.6 Prevention of Cardiovascular Complications After BMS

Surgeons practicing BMS are increasingly becoming aware of patients suffering from obesity whose risks of surgery outweigh the benefits. Patients with pre-existing ischaemic heart disease or other significant cardiovascular diseases might fall into this category. These patients should be discussed in a multidisciplinary team and surgery should only be offered to a well-counselled patient after careful consideration of all the risks and benefits in conjunction with an anaesthetist and/or a cardiologist. The Revised Cardiac Risk Index lists six known risk factors for the development of cardiovascular complications after surgery [51]. These are—(1) high-risk surgery (and bariatric surgery happens to be one), (2) history of coronary heart disease, (3) history of HF, (4) history of cerebrovascular disease, (5) preoperative treatment with insulin, and (6) preoperative serum creatinine levels >2.0 mg/dL [51]. Patients with no risk factors can safely be cleared for bariatric surgery, however, those with ≥3 risk factors or with confirmed coronary artery disease may require further non-invasive testing and cardiac optimization, and should be referred to a cardiologist for optimization before BMS is offered [52].

The addition of pharmacological prophylaxis for an extended duration beyond hospital stay is advocated by most BMS guidelines and LMWH appears to be the agent of choice compared to unfractionated heparin and direct oral anticoagulants due to low risk of bleeding and easy monitoring [5, 49, 53]. The utility of IVC filter in high-risk patients of BMS for VTE appears conflicting with some authors reporting a reduction in PE [54, 55] while others reporting an increased incidence of VTE due to IVC filter [7] and complication due to insertion of the device [56].

Though BMS has been successfully performed in patients with heart failure, the data is confined to case series and observational studies with the potential for significant type II error in published data [56]. There are no randomized trials, evaluating the safety of bariatric surgery in patients of significant heart failure. Surgery should only be offered to these patients in highly specialized centres with significant expertise in BMS as well as management of cardiac diseases after careful discussion of risks versus benefits with the patient.

Other preoperative optimization strategies that may reduce the risk of perioperative cardiovascular complications after bariatric surgery include preoperative weight loss, especially in technically difficult patients, and choosing a simpler procedure that can be performed quickly without the need for prolonged anaesthesia like sleeve gastrectomy or one anastomosis gastric bypass over a roux-en-y gastric bypass or duodenal switch [57, 58]. Cardiovascular risk optimization also includes control of other co-morbidities like diabetes, obstructive sleep apnoea, anaemia, and hypertension before BMS.

Key Points

- Patients at higher risk of cardiovascular risk factors such as those with advanced age, limited exercise tolerance, and pre-existing cardiopulmonary disorders should undergo a careful risk versus benefit analysis for BMS in a multidisciplinary setting before surgery is offered.
- High-risk patients can benefit from several optimization strategies such as correction of anaemia, improved control of diabetes and blood pressure, significant preoperative weight loss, and selection of a BMS procedure that takes less time to perform with shorter anaesthetic time.
- Patients undergoing BMS are at high risk for VTE and generally benefit from extended duration mechanical and pharmacological thromboprophylaxis. IVC filters are probably best avoided.
- Cardiac arrhythmias occurring after BMS must alert the surgeon to a potential anastomotic or staple line leak or bowel obstruction.
- Surgery should only be offered to such high-risk patients in high-volume centres with significant expertise in both BMS and cardiology after consultation with cardiologists and anaesthetists.
- Patients with pre-existing heart failure should only be offered BMS in dedicated specialist centres following a careful discussion with the patient regarding potential risks and benefits.
- Arrhythmias and cardiomyopathy leading to heart failure after the initial postoperative period are often due to micronutrient deficiency and reflects the importance of adequate micronutrient monitoring and supplementation.

Declarations

Consent to Publish

We declare that the "consent to publish" form has been submitted along with the chapter.

Availability of Data and Materials

All data generated or analyzed are included in this chapter and has been appropriately referenced.

Competing Interests
The authors declare that they have no competing interests in relation to this chapter.
Funding
We declare that we were not funded materially or financially by any organization, government, or university.

References

1. Jamal MH, Corcelles R, Shimizu H, Kroh M, Safdie FM, Rosenthal R, et al. Thromboembolic events in bariatric surgery: a large multi-institutional referral center experience. Surg Endosc [Internet]. 2015 Feb;29:376–80.
2. Romeo S, Maglio C, Burza MA, Pirazzi C, Sjöholm K, Jacobson P, et al. Cardiovascular events after bariatric surgery in obese subjects with type 2 diabetes. Diabetes Care [Internet]. 2012 Dec;35:2613–7.
3. Adil MT, Jain V, Rashid F, Al-Taan O, Whitelaw D, Jambulingam P. Meta-analysis of the effect of bariatric surgery on physical function. The British Journal of Surgery [Internet]. 2018;105:1107–18.
4. Jamaly S, Carlsson L, Peltonen M, Jacobson P, Sjöström L, Karason K. Bariatric surgery and the risk of new-onset atrial fibrillation in Swedish obese subjects. J Am Coll Cardiol [Internet]. 2016 Dec 13;68:2497–504.
5. Thereaux J, Lesuffleur T, Czernichow S, Basdevant A, Msika S, Nocca D, et al. To what extent does Posthospital discharge chemoprophylaxis prevent venous thromboembolism after bariatric surgery? Results from a Nationwide cohort of more than 110,000 patients. Ann Surg [Internet]. 2018;267:727–33.
6. Stein PD, Matta F. Pulmonary embolism and deep venous thrombosis following bariatric surgery. Obes Surg [Internet]. 2013 May;23:663–8.
7. Winegar DA, Sherif B, Pate V, DeMaria EJ. Venous thromboembolism after bariatric surgery performed by bariatric surgery Center of Excellence Participants: analysis of the bariatric outcomes longitudinal database. Surgery for Obesity and Related Diseases: Official Journal of the American Society for Bariatric Surgery [Internet]. 2011;7:181–8.
8. Chang S-H, Freeman NLB, Lee JA, Stoll CRT, Calhoun AJ, Eagon JC, et al. Early major complications after bariatric surgery in the USA, 2003–2014: a systematic review and meta-analysis. Obesity Reviews: an Official Journal of the International Association for the Study of Obesity [Internet]. 2018;19:529–37.
9. Khorgami Z, Jackson TN, Aminian A, Sahawneh JM, Sclabas GM, Chow GS. Early cardiac complications after bariatric surgery: does the type of procedure matter? *Surgery for Obesity and Related Diseases: Official Journal of the American Society for Bariatric Surgery* [Internet]. 2019 Mar 23; Available from: http://www.ncbi.nlm.nih.gov/pubmed/31151890
10. Choi JY, Scarborough TK. Stroke and seizure following a recent laparoscopic Roux-en-Y gastric bypass. Obesity Surg [Internet]. 2004;14:857–60.
11. Bateman BT, Schumacher HC, Wang S, Shaefi S, Berman MF. Perioperative acute ischemic stroke in noncardiac and nonvascular surgery: incidence, risk factors, and outcomes. Anesthesiology [Internet]. 2009 Feb;110:231–8.
12. Afolabi BA, Novaro GM, Szomstein S, Rosenthal RJ, Asher CR. Cardiovascular complications of obesity surgery in patients with increased preoperative cardiac risk. Surgery for Obesity and Related Diseases: Official Journal of the American Society for Bariatric Surgery [Internet]. 2009;5:653–6.
13. Shoemaker MB, Gidfar S, Pipilas DC, Tamboli RA, Savio Galimberti E, Williams DB, et al. Prevalence and predictors of atrial fibrillation among patients undergoing bariatric surgery. Obes Surg [Internet]. 2014 Apr;24:611–6.

14. Abed HS, Wittert GA, Leong DP, Shirazi MG, Bahrami B, Middeldorp ME, et al. Effect of weight reduction and cardiometabolic risk factor management on symptom burden and severity in patients with atrial fibrillation: a randomized clinical trial. JAMA [Internet]. 2013 Nov 20;310:2050–60.
15. Kannel WB, Wolf PA, Benjamin EJ, Levy D. Prevalence, incidence, prognosis, and predisposing conditions for atrial fibrillation: population-based estimates. The American Journal of Cardiology [Internet]. 1998 Oct 16;82:2N–9N.
16. De Pergola G, Pannacciulli N. Coagulation and fibrinolysis abnormalities in obesity. J Endocrinol Investig [Internet]. 2002 Nov;25:899–904.
17. Tchernof A, Després J-P. Pathophysiology of human visceral obesity: an update. Physiol Rev [Internet]. 2013 Jan;93:359–404.
18. Sundström J, Bruze G, Ottosson J, Marcus C, Näslund I, Neovius M. Weight loss and heart failure: a Nationwide study of gastric bypass surgery versus intensive lifestyle treatment. Circulation [Internet]. 2017 Apr 25;135:1577–85.
19. Ashrafian H, le Roux CW, Darzi A, Athanasiou T. Effects of bariatric surgery on cardiovascular function. Circulation [Internet]. 2008 Nov 11;118:2091–102.
20. Antonopoulos AS, Tousoulis D. The molecular mechanisms of obesity paradox. Cardiovasc Res [Internet]. 2017 Jul 1;113:1074–86.
21. McCloskey CA, Ramani GV, Mathier MA, Schauer PR, Eid GM, Mattar SG, et al. Bariatric surgery improves cardiac function in morbidly obese patients with severe cardiomyopathy. Surgery for Obesity and Related Diseases: Official Journal of the American Society for Bariatric Surgery [Internet]. 2007;3:503–7.
22. Aggarwal R, Harling L, Efthimiou E, Darzi A, Athanasiou T, Ashrafian H. The effects of bariatric surgery on cardiac structure and function: a systematic review of cardiac imaging outcomes. Obes Surg [Internet]. 2016 May;26:1030–40.
23. Sjöström L, Peltonen M, Jacobson P, Sjöström CD, Karason K, Wedel H, et al. Bariatric surgery and long-term cardiovascular events. JAMA [Internet]. 2012 Jan 4;307:56–65.
24. Sellers D, Srinivas C, Djaiani G. Cardiovascular complications after non-cardiac surgery. Anaesthesia [Internet]. 2018 Jan;73(Suppl 1):34–42.
25. van Noord C, Eijgelsheim M, Stricker BHC. Drug- and non-drug-associated QT interval prolongation. Br J Clin Pharmacol [Internet]. 2010 Jul;70:16–23.
26. Masoomi H, Buchberg B, Reavis KM, Mills SD, Stamos M, Nguyen NT. Factors predictive of venous thromboembolism in bariatric surgery. Am Surg [Internet]. 2011 Oct;77:1403–6.
27. Finks JF, English WJ, Carlin AM, Krause KR, Share DA, Banerjee M, et al. Predicting risk for venous thromboembolism with bariatric surgery: results from the Michigan bariatric surgery collaborative. Ann Surg [Internet]. 2012 Jun;255:1100–4.
28. Wells PS, Anderson DR, Rodger M, Forgie M, Kearon C, Dreyer J, et al. Evaluation of D-dimer in the diagnosis of suspected deep-vein thrombosis. The New England Journal of Medicine [Internet]. 2003 Sep 25;349:1227–35.
29. Di Nisio M, Squizzato A, Rutjes AWS, Büller HR, Zwinderman AH, Bossuyt PMM. Diagnostic accuracy of D-dimer test for exclusion of venous thromboembolism: a systematic review. Journal of Thrombosis and Haemostasis: JTH [Internet]. 2007 Feb;5:296–304.
30. National Clinical Guideline Centre (UK). Venous thromboembolic diseases: The management of venous thromboembolic diseases and the role of thrombophilia testing. Guidance: National Institute for Health and Clinical Excellence; 2012.
31. Wells PS, Anderson DR, Rodger M, Ginsberg JS, Kearon C, Gent M, et al. Derivation of a simple clinical model to categorize patients probability of pulmonary embolism: increasing the models utility with the SimpliRED D-dimer. Thromb Haemost [Internet]. 2000 Mar;83:416–20.
32. Blachere H, Latrabe V, Montaudon M, Valli N, Couffinhal T, Raherisson C, et al. Pulmonary embolism revealed on helical CT angiography: comparison with ventilation-perfusion radionuclide lung scanning. AJR American Journal of Roentgenology [Internet]. 2000 Apr;174:1041–7.

33. Landesberg G. Monitoring for myocardial ischemia. Best Pract Res Clin Anaesthesiol [Internet]. 2005 Mar;19:77–95.
34. Thygesen K, Alpert JS, Jaffe AS, Chaitman BR, Bax JJ, Morrow DA, et al. Fourth universal definition of myocardial infarction (2018). Kardiologia polska [Internet]. 2018;76:1383–415.
35. Landesberg G, Beattie WS, Mosseri M, Jaffe AS, Alpert JS. Perioperative myocardial infarction. Circulation [Internet]. 2009 Jun 9;119:2936–44.
36. Landesberg G, Mosseri M, Zahger D, Wolf Y, Perouansky M, Anner H, et al. Myocardial infarction after vascular surgery: the role of prolonged stress-induced, ST depression-type ischemia. J Am Coll Cardiol [Internet]. 2001 Jun 1;37:1839–45.
37. Devereaux PJ, Goldman L, Cook DJ, Gilbert K, Leslie K, Guyatt GH. Perioperative cardiac events in patients undergoing noncardiac surgery: a review of the magnitude of the problem, the pathophysiology of the events and methods to estimate and communicate risk. CMAJ: Canadian Medical Association journal = journal de l'Association medicale canadienne [Internet]. 2005 Sep 13;173:627–34.
38. Writing Committee for the VISION Study Investigators, Devereaux PJ, Biccard BM, Sigamani A, Xavier D, Chan MTV, et al. Association of postoperative high-sensitivity troponin levels with myocardial injury and 30-day mortality among patients undergoing noncardiac surgery. JAMA [Internet]. 2017 Apr 25;317:1642–51.
39. Ponikowski P, Voors AA, Anker SD, Bueno H, Cleland JGF, Coats AJS, et al. ESC guidelines for the diagnosis and treatment of acute and chronic heart failure: the task force for the diagnosis and treatment of acute and chronic heart failure of the European Society of Cardiology (ESC). Developed with the special contribution. Eur J Heart Failure [Internet]. 2016;18:891–975.
40. Rodseth RN, Biccard BM, Chu R, Lurati Buse GA, Thabane L, Bakhai A, et al. Postoperative B-type natriuretic peptide for prediction of major cardiac events in patients undergoing noncardiac surgery: systematic review and individual patient meta-analysis. Anesthesiology [Internet]. 2013 Aug;119:270–83.
41. Massoure P-L, Camus O, Fourcade L, Simon F. Bilateral leg oedema after bariatric surgery: A selenium-deficient cardiomyopathy. Obes Res Clin Pract [Internet]. 2017;11:622–6.
42. Boldery R, Fielding G, Rafter T, Pascoe AL, Scalia GM. Nutritional deficiency of selenium secondary to weight loss (bariatric) surgery associated with life-threatening cardiomyopathy. Heart Lung Circ [Internet]. 2007 Apr;16:123–6.
43. Yahalom M, Koren O, Rozner E, Turgeman Y. Cardiomyopathy associated with zinc deficiency after bariatric surgery. The International Journal of Angiology: Official Publication of the International College of Angiology, Inc [Internet]. 2019 Jun;28:145–6.
44. Viegas F, Viegas C, França E, Kleuser K, de Barros F. Takotsubo syndrome as a cause of false acute abdomen in the early postoperative period after bariatric surgery-a report of two cases. Obes Surg [Internet]. 2016;26:2547–51.
45. Mahamid A, Mizrahi M, Gur C, Adar T. Exacerbation of left ventricular outlet obstruction in hypertrophic obstructive cardiomyopathy: an unexpected complication of gastric banding. J Surg Case Rep [Internet]. 2014 May;13:2014.
46. Sahloul M, Bowley D, Richardson M. Unique complication of laparoscopic adjustable gastric band? A misplaced band encircling the abdominal aorta. BMJ Case Rep [Internet]. 2018 Dec 31;11:e228082.
47. Dean K, Scott J, Eichhorn P. Aortoenteric fistula at the site of a marginal ulcer after Roux-en-Y gastric bypass. Am Surg [Internet]. 2018 Aug 1;84:e312–3.
48. LABS Writing Group for the LABS Consortium, Belle SH, Chapman W, Courcoulas AP, Flum DR, Gagner M, et al. Relationship of body mass index with demographic and clinical characteristics in the Longitudinal Assessment of Bariatric Surgery (LABS). Surgery for Obesity and Related Diseases: Official Journal of the American Society for Bariatric Surgery [Internet]. 2008;4:474–80.
49. Raftopoulos I, Martindale C, Cronin A, Steinberg J. The effect of extended post-discharge chemical thromboprophylaxis on venous thromboembolism rates after bariatric surgery: a prospective comparison trial. Surg Endosc [Internet]. 2008 Nov;22:2384–91.

50. Watson T, Fleisher L. Acute heart failure in the postoperative period. In: Mebazaa A, Gheorghiade M, Zannad FM, editors. Acute heart failure. London: Springer; 2008. p. 323–32.
51. Lee TH, Marcantonio ER, Mangione CM, Thomas EJ, Polanczyk CA, Cook EF, et al. Derivation and prospective validation of a simple index for prediction of cardiac risk of major noncardiac surgery. Circulation [Internet]. 1999 Sep 7;100:1043–9.
52. Poirier P, Alpert MA, Fleisher LA, Thompson PD, Sugerman HJ, Burke LE, et al. Cardiovascular evaluation and management of severely obese patients undergoing surgery: a science advisory from the American Heart Association. Circulation [Internet]. 2009 Jul 7;120:86–95.
53. Hamadi R, Marlow CF, Nassereddine S, Taher A, Finianos A. Bariatric venous thromboembolism prophylaxis: an update on the literature. Expert Rev Hematol [Internet]. 2019 Sep;12:763–71.
54. Obeid FN, Bowling WM, Fike JS, Durant JA. Efficacy of prophylactic inferior vena cava filter placement in bariatric surgery. Surgery for Obesity and Related Diseases: Official Journal of the American Society for Bariatric Surgery [Internet]. 2007;3:606–8. discussion 609–10
55. Schuster R, Hagedorn JC, Curet MJ, Morton JM. Retrievable inferior vena cava filters may be safely applied in gastric bypass surgery. Surg Endosc [Internet]. 2007 Dec;21:2277–9.
56. Birkmeyer NJO, Share D, Baser O, Carlin AM, Finks JF, Pesta CM, et al. Preoperative placement of inferior vena cava filters and outcomes after gastric bypass surgery. Ann Surg [Internet]. 2010 Aug;252:313–8.
57. Mahawar KK, Kumar P, Carr WR, Jennings N, Schroeder N, Balupuri S, et al. Current status of mini-gastric bypass. J Minimal Access Surg [Internet]. 2016;12:305–10.
58. Gagner M. The future of sleeve gastrectomy. Eur Endocrinol [Internet]. 2016 Mar;12:37–8.
59. Dawood MM, Gutpa DK, Southern J, Walia A, Atkinson JB, Eagle KA. Pathology of fatal perioperative myocardial infarction: implications regarding pathophysiology and prevention. Int J Cardiol [Internet]. 1996 Nov 15;57:37–44.

Neurological Complications After Bariatric Surgery

13

Ramen Goel, Amrit Nasta, and Madhu Goel

All answers lie in the neurons.

— Abhijit Naskar

13.1 Introduction

The term "complications" implies any deviation from the normal postoperative course. The incidence of complications is often used as an indicator for the quality of surgery. The occurrence of complications in bariatric surgery is not accepted by the patient, family, and the society because obesity is usually not perceived to be a disease. Though early postoperative complications like bleed, leak, etc. are commonly discussed, long-term issues like neurological complications are rarely discussed in bariatric forums. Mostly associated with nutritional deficiencies, neurological complications are often diagnosed late underscoring the importance of increasing awareness of this complication.

Patients with obesity suffer from malnutrition with 20–30% presenting with micro-nutrient deficiencies before surgery [1]. After surgery, these deficiencies can worsen because of inadequate intake, vomiting episodes, mal-absorption, lack of balanced diet, bacterial overgrowth, and reduced gastric acid. Despite guidelines for postoperative micro-nutrient supplementation, variations are prevalent in dietary practice followed by patients and even amongst bariatric clinicians. As more diversionary procedures are being performed, this requirement gains additional significance.

R. Goel (✉) · A. Nasta · M. Goel
Center of Metabolic Surgery, Wockhardt Hospital, Mumbai, India

A. G. Bhasker et al. (eds.), *Management of Nutritional and Metabolic Complications of Bariatric Surgery*,
https://doi.org/10.1007/978-981-33-4702-1_13

It is probably important to mention here that the systematic review and meta-analysis published in 2019 showed an overall improvement of peripheral neuropathy in patients undergoing bariatric surgery [2].

Epidemiology A large longitudinal bariatric series reported an incidence of 1.3% (133/9996) of neurological complications [3]. Abarbanel et al. [4] described that neurological complications developed 3–20 months after restrictive procedures in 4.6% of their 500 patients. The highest incidence, however, was recorded in a study from the Mayo Clinic that described 16% of peripheral neuropathy among patients undergoing bariatric surgery [5]. The incidence of neurological complications in another study of 592 sleeve gastrectomy was 1.18% after 4.6 ± 3.4 months [6]. There are no large scale studies reporting post-bariatric neurological complications from India.

Neurological Complications

- Encephalopathy
- Behavioral abnormalities
- Seizures
- Cranial nerve palsies
- Ataxia
- Myelopathy
- Plexopathies
- Peripheral neuropathy
- Mono-neuropathies: Carpal tunnel syndrome, Meralgia paresthetica
- Compartment syndromes
- Myopathy
- Myotonia

Based on the duration of onset after surgery, they can be classified as:

1. Early (within 1 year)
   - Compression injury of peripheral nerve/muscle: Brachial plexus injury, meralgia paresthetica
   - Encephalopathy: Wernicke's encephalopathy, Korsakoff's psychosis
   - Polyradiculopathy: Acute Guillian-Barre syndrome
2. Late (after 1 year)
   - Optic neuropathy.
   - Myelopathy: Subacute combined degeneration of the spinal cord
   - Peripheral neuropathy: Burning feet syndrome, Carpel tunnel syndrome
   - Myopathy

Pathophysiology of Neurological Complications

1. Mechanical injury to peripheral nerves and muscles: This risk is higher in patients with obesity during surgical positioning (steep head up) due to inadequate padding of pressure points, hyperextension of joints (brachial plexus

injury), injury during arterial line access, or mechanical retractors. There is also a risk of fatal rhabdomyolysis and myopathies associated with compression injury [5]. Additionally, loss of fat makes nerves more susceptible to compression in the postoperative period.
2. Neural inflammation and immunological mechanisms: There have been reports of inflammatory infiltrates in nerve biopsies from patients who had neurological complications after surgery (acute/subacute polyneuropathy or radiculoneuropathy) [3, 5]. In a setting of severe weight loss, a cachexia-like state with associated nutritional deficiencies may lead to inflammatory and immune-mediated neuropathy [5].
3. Nutritional: The most accepted etio-pathogenesis of neurological complications is vitamin and mineral deficiency due to inadequate intake (surgical restriction), hyperemesis, or reduced absorption from the intestine (surgical bypass) [5].

Proposed Mechanisms of Nutritional Deficiency

- Stomach: Loss of gastric acid and intrinsic factor, inadequate meal size, repeated emesis.
- Intestine: Reduced absorptive surface (duodenum is the main absorption site of calcium, iron, and vitamin B1), bacterial overgrowth.
- Others: Intolerance to certain foods (milk, rice, meats, fiber).

Specific Deficiencies

1. Thiamine (vitamin B1): Thiamine deficiency may occur within 3–6 months postoperatively but has been reported as early as 6 weeks [7, 8]. Vitamin B1 is obtained mainly from vegetables, whole-grain, and supplemented foods. The storage of vitamin B1 is only about 25–30 mg; thus, its stores can be depleted within 2–3 weeks The typical history is insufficient oral intake and repeated episodes of vomiting. As thiamine is mainly absorbed in the duodenum, deficiency can occur, even in restrictive procedures like sleeve gastrectomy, despite oral supplementation if emesis is present. Vitamin B1 deficiency can lead to depression of transketolase activity, reduced oxygen uptake, and lactic acidosis [9]. Impairment of cellular oxidative metabolism and reduction in thiamine-dependent enzymes results in selective neuronal cell death [10].

   Wernicke's encephalopathy and Korsakoff's syndrome have been associated with thiamine deficiency. The diagnostic criteria for Wernicke's encephalopathy require two of the following four features:
   (a) Dietary deficiency
   (b) Oculomotor abnormality (nystagmus)
   (c) Cerebellar dysfunction (ataxia) and
   (d) Confusion or mild memory impairment

   Peripheral neuropathy may also accompany Wernicke encephalopathy and has been referred to as "bariatric beriberi." It may occur earlier than Wernicke's encephalopathy and mainly affects the lower limbs with both sensory and motor deficits. Sometimes, it may progress rapidly over a few days mimicking Guillain-Barré syndrome. Permanent impairment of recent memory with confabulations, known as Korsakoff's syndrome, is also associated with thiamine deficiency.

Deficiency can be confirmed by measuring the vitamin B1 pyrophosphate effect in erythrocyte transketolase studies. A typical clinical picture with the features of encephalopathy, coupled with the response to administration of parenteral vitamin B1, is sufficiently diagnostic. Sometimes, a magnetic resonance imaging (MRI) of the brain may be required, which shows characteristic abnormalities-hyperintense signal abnormalities on T2-weighted images in the dorso-medial thalamic nuclei, periventricular gray matter, and mammillary bodies. Treatment consists in intravenous (IV) administration: 500 mg IV three times a day for 3 days, followed by 250 mg IV daily until improvement stops. This dose must be followed by an oral dose of 50–100 mg daily [10, 11]. Patients with history of bariatric surgery and repeated postoperative vomiting should be given preventive thiamine supplementation by 250 mg IM once a day. Ophthalmoplegia usually resolves in a few hours and confusion improves within a few days. Complete recovery is possible within 3–6 months of initiation of therapy if the symptoms are recognized early [12]. If thiamine deficiency is not discovered early, patients may be left with permanent deficits and mental status changes.

2. Cobalamin (vitamin B12): Vitamin B12 deficiency may appear several years after bariatric surgery, since sufficient liver stores compensate for the initial dietary insufficiency [13]. The absorption of vitamin B12 requires the intrinsic factor derived from gastric parietal cells, acidic gastric pH, and its absorption in the ileum, any of which may be affected by bariatric surgery [14]. Vitamin B12 plays a role in the synthesis of the myelin sheath and in methylation of RNA which slows RNA degradation, explaining the involvement of long axons in vitamin B12 deficiency. Subacute combined degeneration is seen, in which the peripheral nerves and posterior columns of the spinal cord are chiefly affected (demyelinated). Common neurologic symptoms include paresthesias, weakness, hyporeflexia, spasticity, ataxia, loss of position and vibratory sense, incontinence, loss of vision from optic neuropathy, dementia, psychosis, and altered mood [15]. Severe autonomic symptoms may also rarely occur [16]. The initiation of vitamin B12 supplementation within 6 months postoperatively is recommended. Oral crystalline vitamin B12 at a dose of at least 350 mcg/day has been shown to maintain normal plasma vitamin B12 levels [17]. Optimal dosing of oral, sublingual, or intranasal forms of B12 supplementation has not been well studied.
3. Other deficiencies: Low plasma folate levels are seen in upto 42% of patients undergoing gastric bypass surgery after 3 years. Folate deficiency with an accompanying peripheral neuropathy is a known phenomenon [18]. Oral folic acid supplementation (400–500 μg/day; recommended 1 mg daily) has been shown to be effective in maintaining levels within the reference range [17, 19]. However, isolated folate supplementation can lead to masking of an underlying B12 deficiency, and may cause progression of neurological damage.

Niacin deficiency or pellagra have been reported with restrictive procedures like vertical gastroplasty [20]. This syndrome is characterized by symmetrical rash on sun-exposed areas (casal collar) with desquamation. Other features include diarrhea, photosensitivity, glossitis, dementia, hallucinations, and encephalopathy.

Vitamin D deficiency after gastric bypass may present with symptomatic hypocalcemia. In a report by Marinella [21], patients developed carpo-pedal spasms, intermittent facial twitching, and ophthalmoplegia in association with hypocalcemia many years after gastric bypass surgery. This patient responded well to calcium supplementation. Myopathy has been linked to vitamin D deficiency and has been shown to improve with treatment (400–800 units per day) [22]. Higher daily dose (1000–2000 units) have also been frequently used today [22]. These doses may be recommended in more malabsorptive procedures like OAGB or DS with longer bypassed limbs. Reduced vitamin D levels are common in the general population and all patients undergoing bariatric procedures should be screened pre-operatively with 25-hydroxyvitamin D levels. They can subsequently be modified based on serum levels and bone densitometry. Recommended doses of elemental calcium after bariatric surgery range from 1200 to 2000 mg daily, along with supplementary vitamin D [17, 19].

In addition to vitamin D, patients undergoing Roux-en-Y gastric bypass may also be at risk of deficiency of another fat-soluble vitamin, vitamin E which is also associated with neurological manifestations. Low vitamin E levels have been found 6–12 months after surgery but may not be apparent for 5–10 years [21]. Common findings in patients with vitamin E deficiency include hyporeflexia, proximal myopathy, limb, and truncal ataxia, reduced vibration and position sense, ophthalmoplegia, ptosis, and dysarthria [23]. Saccadic eye movements (following a moving object) may be slow, and progressive gaze impairment may be noticed. Some patients with ophthalmoplegia also have medial rectus dysfunction and an associated nystagmus. Severe vitamin E deficiency has also been linked with polyradiculopathies, peripheral neuropathies, and sensory axonopathy. The recommended dose of vitamin E is 400 IU daily. The proposed supplementation in asymptomatic patients post-surgery is a standard multi-vitamin formulation rich in vitamin E [24].

Copper deficiency may lead to myelopathy after bariatric surgery that is clinically indistinguishable from vitamin B12 deficiency. Kumar [25] described a 49-year-old lady who developed myelopathy characterized by spastic ataxia, symmetrical lower limb hyper-reflexia, and loss of vibratory perception and of pinprick and touch sensations in feet 24 years after bariatric surgery. As vitamin B12 levels were normal, serum copper and ceruloplasmin levels were measured and were found to be reduced. Patients improved clinically after intravenous administration of copper (as cupric sulfate). Other features found in patients with copper deficiency include peripheral neuropathy, optic neuropathy, myopathy, demyelination, and myelo-opticoneuropathy (Tables 13.1 and 13.2).

Table 13.1 Neurological complication, etiology, and symptoms

Complication	Etiology/Deficiency	Symptoms
Wernicke's encephalopathy	Thiamine	Ophthalmoplegia or nystagmus, ataxia, and mental status changes
Korsakoff's psychosis	Thiamine	Severe memory loss, anterograde amnesia, retrograde amnesia, confabulations
Polyradiculoneuropathies	Thiamine	Pain in the lower limbs, weakness, ascending paralysis, areflexia
Optic neuropathy	Vitamin A, vitamin B6, B12, and copper	Blurred vision with central scotoma, night blindness
Myelopathy/subacute combined degeneration	Vitamin B12, vitamin E, copper, rarely folate	Disabling gait ataxia, spasticity in the legs, paresthesias, loss of proprioception and vibratory sensations in legs, limb weakness
Polyneuropathy	Vitamin B1, B12, B6 (pyridoxine), vitamin E, copper, and possibly vitamin D and folate	Symmetric, distal, sometimes painful paresthesias ("burning feet syndrome"), sometimes weakness, gait ataxia, loss of pinprick, vibratory, and temperature sensation
Mononeuropathy	Same as polyneuropathy	Carpal tunnel syndrome, ulnar neuropathy, radial neuropathy, peroneal neuropathy [foot drop] lateral femoral cutaneous neuropathy (meralgia paresthetica) Restless leg syndrome
Myopathy	Protein, copper, selenium, magnesium, Calcium & Vitamin D	Weakness, vague muscle pains

Table 13.2 Studies reporting neurological complications after bariatric surgery and their findings

Study	N	Procedures	Complication	Deficiency
Koffman et al. [3]	96	RYGB, VBG, adjustable band, BPD-DS	Peripheral neuropathy = 60 Encephalopathy = 30 Myopathy = 7	Thiamine in 27 (28.1%)
Abarbanel et al. [4]	23/500 (4.6%)	RYGB, VBG	Polyneuropathy = 12 Wernicke's = 2	Thiamine in 3(12%)
Thaisetthawatkul et al. [5]	71/435 (16%)	Restrictive and malabsorptive	Polyneuropathy = 27 Mononeuropathy = 39 Radiculopathy = 5	–
Tabbara et al. [6]	7/592 [1.2%]	Sleeve gastrectomy	Polyneuropathy = 5 Wernicke's = 2	Thiamine 2 (29%)
Landais A [12]	2	Sleeve gastrectomy	Severe axonal neuropathy = 1 Wernicke's = 1	Thiamine, Vit. B6
Juhasz-Pocsine et al. [13]	26	Restrictive and malabsorptive	Myelopathy, encephalopathy, and polyradiculopathy	Vit. B12, copper
Sen et al. [26]	7/635	Sleeve gastrectomy	Peroneal nerve entrapment neuropathy	–

Overview of Treatment of Neurological Complications

It is important to detect and treat neurological complications early as delayed treatment may lead to irreversibility and residual neurodeficit has also been reported [27].

It is prudent to start empirical therapeutic supplementation even before the test results are available since the vitamin B complex does not carry toxic effects.

13.2 Conclusion

Neurological complications after bariatric surgery are rare. They are often preceded by gastrointestinal symptoms like vomiting of prolonged duration, rapid weight loss, and a failure of compliance with vitamin supplementation and dietary follow-up. Re-hospitalization may be necessary, and a multidisciplinary team management including a bariatric physician and nutritionist is crucial to establish the diagnosis, provide appropriate treatment, and halter the progression of these neurological complications.

Key Points

- Neurological complications after bariatric surgery are preventable and rare but are often diagnosed late.
- They are often preceded by gastrointestinal symptoms.
- The most common cause of neurological complications are nutritional deficiencies.
- Hospitalization may sometimes be necessary.
- Multidisciplinary team management is crucial.

References

1. Frantz DJ. Neurologic complications of bariatric surgery: involvement of central, peripherical and enteric nervous system. Curr Gastroenterol Rep. 2012;14:367–72.
2. Aghili R, Malek M, Tanha K, Mottaghi A. The effect of Bariatric surgery on Peripheral polyneuropathy: a systematic review and meta-analysis. Obes Surg. 2019 Sep;29(9):3010–20.
3. Koffman BM, Greenfield J, Ali II, et al. Neurologic complications after surgery for obesity. Muscle Nerve. 2006;33(2):166–76.
4. Abarbanel JM, Berginer VM, Osimani A, et al. Neurologic complications after gastric restriction surgery for morbid obesity. Neurology. 1987;37(2):196–200.
5. Thaisetthawatkul P, Collazo-Clavell ML, Sarr MG. A controlled study of peripheral neuropathy after bariatric surgery. Neurology. 2004;63(8):1462–70.
6. Tabbara M, Carandina S, Bossi M, et al. Rare neurological complications after sleeve gastrectomy. Obes Surg. 2016;26:2843–8.
7. Kramer LD, Locke GE. Wernicke's encephalopathy. Complication of gastric plication. J Clin Gastroenterol. 1987;9(5):549–52.
8. Sola E, Morillas C, Garzon S, Ferrer JM, Martin J, Hernandez-Mijares A. Rapid onset of Wernicke's encephalopathy following gastric restrictive surgery. Obes Surg. 2003;13(4):661–2.
9. Dreyfus PM, Victor M. Effects of thiamine deficiency on the central nervous system. Am J Clin Nutr. 1961;9:414–25.

10. Ke ZJ, DeGiorgio LA, Volpe BT, Gibson GE. Reversal of thiamine deficiency-induced neurodegeneration. J Neuropathol Exp Neurol. 2003;62(2):195–207.
11. Sechi G. Prognosis and therapy of Wernicke's encephalopathy after obesity surgery. Am J Gastroenterol. 2008;103(12):3219.
12. Landais A. Neurological complications of bariatric surgery. Obes Surg. 2014;24:1800–7.
13. Juhasz-Pocsine K, Rudnicki SA, Archer RL, et al. Neurologic complications of gastric bypass surgery for morbid obesity. Neurology. 2007;68(21):1843–50.
14. Berger JR. The neurological complications of bariatric surgery. Arch Neurol. 2004;61(8):1185–9.
15. Lindenbaum J, Healton EB, Savage DG, et al. Neuropsychiatric disorders caused by cobalamin deficiency in the absence of anemia or macrocytosis. N Engl J Med. 1988;318(26):1720–8.
16. Puntambekar P, Basha MM, Zak IT, Madhavan R. Rare sensory and autonomic disturbances associated with vitamin B12 deficiency. J Neurol Sci. 2009;287(1–2):285–7.
17. Aills L, Blankenship J, Buffington C, Furtado M, Parrott J. ASMBS allied health nutritional guidelines for the surgical weight loss patient. Surg Obes Relat Dis. 2008;4(5):S73–S108.
18. Boylan LM, Sugerman HJ, Driskell JA. Vitamin E, vitamin B-6, vitamin B-12, and folate status of gastric bypass surgery patients. J Am Diet Assoc. 1988;88(5):579–85.
19. Heber D, Greenway FL, Kaplan LM, Livingston E, Salvador J, Still C. Endocrine and nutritional management of the post-bariatric surgery patient: an endocrine society clinical practice guideline. J Clin Endocrinol Metab. 2010;95(11):4823–43.
20. Lopez JF, Halimi S, Perillat Y. Pellagra-like erythema following vertical banded gastroplasty for morbid obesity [in French]. Ann Chir. 2000;125:297–8.
21. Marinella MA. Ophthalmoplegia: an unusual manifestation of hypocalcemia. Am J Emerg Med. 1999;17:105–6.
22. Banerji NK, Hurwitz LJ. Nervous system manifestations after gastric surgery. Acta Neurol Scand. 1971;47(4):485–513.
23. Sokol RJ. Vitamin E deficiency and neurologic disease. Annu Rev Nutr. 1988;8:351–73.
24. Rudnicki SA. Prevention and treatment of peripheral neuropathy after bariatric surgery. Curr Treat Options Neurol. 2010;12(1):29–36.
25. Kumar N, McEvoy KM, Ahlskog JE. Myelopathy due to copper deficiency following gastrointestinal surgery. Arch Neurol. 2003;60:1782–5.
26. Şen O, Karaca FC, Türkçapar A. Neurological complication after laparoscopic sleeve gastrectomy: foot drop. Obes Surg. 2019;30:957. https://doi.org/10.1007/s11695-019-04285-6.
27. Landais A. Neurological complications of bariatric surgery. Obes Surg. 2014 Oct;24(10):1800–7.

Musculoskeletal Complications After Bariatric Surgery

14

Sonja Chiappetta, Christine Stier, Mark Rice, Errichetta Napolitano, Giuseppina Casalino, and Vincenzo Bottino

It does seem incredible that a disease that can be diagnosed and can be successfully treated is not a major health issue. We must do all we can to prevent, treat and ultimately cure this painful and life restricting disease.

Baroness Julia Cumberlege, member House of Lords, former UK health minister, prominent osteoporosis advocate.

Abbreviations

AGB	Adjustable gastric banding
BIA	Bioelectrical Impedance Analysis
BMD	Bone mineral density
BMI	Body Mass Index
BPD	Biliopancreatic diversion
DEXA	Dual-energy X-ray absorptiometry
EOSS	Edmonton Obesity Staging System
OAGB	One-anastomosis gastric bypass
PTH	Parathyroid hormone

S. Chiappetta (✉) · M. Rice · E. Napolitano · G. Casalino · V. Bottino
Obesity and Metabolic Surgery Unit, Department of General Surgery, Ospedale Evangelico Betania, Naples, Italy

C. Stier
Obesity Center NRW, Sana Kliniken, Hürth, Germany

A. G. Bhasker et al. (eds.), *Management of Nutritional and Metabolic Complications of Bariatric Surgery*,
https://doi.org/10.1007/978-981-33-4702-1_14

RYGB Roux-en-Y gastric bypass
SG Sleeve gastrectomy
SHPT Secondary hyperparathyroidism

14.1 Introduction

Obesity is associated with weight-related disorders, and besides metabolic comorbidities, limitations of mobility and functional status impact patients' quality of life. Musculoskeletal complaints are common in most of the patients with obesity [1], and obesity is a risk factor for developing osteoarthritis, especially of the knee and hand [2]. Special attention should be given to sarcopenic obesity, which is a phenotype of low lean muscle mass and high adiposity, that is more common in the elderly. Moreover, it seems to be associated with a higher risk of type 2 diabetes mellitus, and thus represents a significant predictor of all-cause mortality among older people [3, 4].

Weight loss after surgery for obesity and weight-related diseases shows a substantial ameliorative impact on musculoskeletal pain and leads further to a reduction of disability derived from joint disease [5]. On the other hand, due to malnutrition and insufficient postoperative supplementation, musculoskeletal complications might occur after surgery for obesity. Especially, disorders of calcium and vitamin D metabolism, bone loss, and bone fractures are described as sequelae and complications in the literature [6]. Another complication is sarcopenia, a reduced lean muscle mass, which might occur after excessive weight loss and malnutrition [7].

The clinical guidelines of the European Association for the Study of Obesity (EASO) and the American Society for Metabolic and Bariatric Surgery (ASMBS) strongly recommend routine calcium and vitamin D supplementation after surgical weight loss procedures, especially gastric bypass procedures and biliopancreatic diversion. Both advocate regular monitoring of markers of bone mineral metabolism as an outcome measure to reduce the long-term risk of bone fractures [8]. In addition, dual-energy X-ray absorptiometry (DEXA) should be performed before surgery and biannually thereafter to monitor bone mineral density (BMD) [9].

Clinical practical recommendations support regular physical activity after surgery to preserve and build muscle mass. Patients should be advised to perform moderate aerobic physical activity to include a minimum of 150 min/week with the goal of increasing it to 300 min/week, including strength training 2–3 times/week [8].

14.2 Incidence/Prevalence

A high incidence (up to 90%) of vitamin D deficiency is described in patients with obesity prior to surgery and is reported variably in the follow-up but can occur in up to 100% post surgery [9]. Despite routine supplementation, vitamin D deficiency is particularly high after biliopancreatic diversion (BPD), Roux-en Y gastric bypass (RYGB), and one-anastomosis gastric bypass (OAGB). After restrictive procedures, such as sleeve gastrectomy (SG) or adjustable gastric banding (AGB), no significant decrease in vitamin D levels was observed [8].

Similarly, the prevalence of secondary hyperparathyroidism (SHPT) in people with morbid obesity is high before surgery and continues to increase with time, especially after gastric bypass. Wei et al. analyzed 1470 patients who underwent AGB, SG, RYGB, and OAGB regarding SHPT before and after surgery. In this study, the authors demonstrated an overall prevalence of 21% of SHPT prior to surgery and vitamin D level was the only independent predictor of SHPT before surgery. Procedure analysis showed the highest prevalence of SHPT at 1 and 5 years after surgery in OAGB (50.6% and 73.6%, respectively) and RYGB (33.2% and 56.6%, respectively). In comparison, significantly lower prevalence was seen after restrictive procedures (GB 25.8% and 38.5%; SG 17.8% and 41.7%). Serum PTH at 1 year after surgery correlated with decreased Body Mass Index (BMI) and weight loss. Multivariate analysis confirmed that age, gender, calcium level, and bypass procedure were independent predictors of SHPT after surgery [10].

Svanevik et al. studied 113 patients 2 years after surgery, who underwent either a standard or distal gastric bypass and the resulting relation to SHPT and bone turnover markers. They found a higher prevalence of SHPT after distal gastric bypass, without however resulting in a significant difference in the effect on bone turnover markers. Two years after standard as well as distal gastric bypass, a comparable increase in bone turnover markers was observed [11].

Alejo et al. examined 321 patients, who underwent BPD. They showed, that in the ninth year after surgery, SHPT increased to a maximum of 81.9% [12]. Pilkington et al. described a mixture of osteomalacia and SHPT in up to 54% and polyarthralgia in up to 13% after jejunoileal bypass [13].

Geoffroy et al. analyzed the incidence of reduction of BMD in 110 patients undergoing SG or gastric bypass. The authors found a clinically significant reduction in BMD in 62.1% of the patients at 6 months and 71.6% at 12 months after surgery. Four cases of osteopenia, one fracture, but no case of osteoporosis was observed. In the univariate analysis BMD loss was related to the reduction of BMI ($p < 0.01$), weight loss ($p < 0.01$), fat mass ($p < 0.01$), and lean mass ($p < 0.01$). In the multivariate analysis, a significant association was found between the reduction in BMD and the excess weight loss percentage ($p < 0.001$) [14].

Fracture risk after surgery was studied by Yu et al. in 15,032 patients undergoing either RYGB or AGB. RYGB patients were at increased risk of nonvertebral fracture (hazard ratio [HR] = 1.43, 95% confidence interval [CI] 1.13–1.81) compared to AGB patients. In fracture site-specific analyses, RYGB patients were at increased risk for hip (HR = 1.54, 95% CI 1.03–2.30) and wrist fractures (HR = 1.45, 95% CI 1.01–2.07). The risk of nonvertebral fracture after RYGB manifested after more than 2 years and increased in subsequent years, with the highest risk in the fifth year after surgery (HR = 3.91, 95% CI 1.58–9.64). The authors concluded, that RYGB is associated with a 43% increased risk of nonvertebral fracture compared to AGB, and that risk increases 2 years after surgery [15].

In a prospective observational study, Muschitz et al. compared the effects of RYGB and SG on bone metabolism and found an increased turnover and resulting BMD loss at all skeletal sites 2 years after both bariatric procedures [16].

In a retrospective case–control study with 12,676 patients undergoing bariatric surgery, Rousseau et al. analyzed fracture risk, age, and sex matched with 38,028 individuals with obesity and 126,760 controls with normal BMI. They found that the adjusted postoperative fracture risk was higher in the bariatric group than in the group with obesity (relative risk 1.38, 95% confidence interval 1.23–1.55) and control (1.44, 1.29–1.59) groups. An increase in fracture risk was significant only for BPD [17]. They also showed that "for the first time that risk of fracture is site specific and changes from a pattern associated with obesity (higher susceptibility for distal lower limb fracture and lower susceptibility for upper limb fracture) to a pattern in which risk of lower limb fracture is reduced but risk of fracture at sites typical of osteoporosis is increased (upper limb, clinical spine, pelvis, hip, femur)."

14.3 Adverse Sequelae Regarding Musculoskeletal Complications

- *Disorder of calcium/vitamin D metabolism* is a sequela after surgery for obesity, especially after gastric bypass and malabsorptive procedures [8].
- Weight loss after obesity and metabolic surgery is described as a combination of loss of fat, and *loss of muscle and bone mass* [6]. Optimal for weight loss might be a high ratio of lean/fat tissue mass, which means a reduction in fat mass while preserving lean mass (muscle and bone) [18]. However, some muscle loss is a constant accompaniment after surgery and in severe form may lead to sarcopenia.

14.4 Pathophysiology of the Enlisted Adverse Sequelae

Calcium absorption occurs preferentially in the duodenum and proximal jejunum and is facilitated by vitamin D and gastric acid. Vitamin D is absorbed both in the jejunum and ileum.

Therefore, calcium absorption decreases after bypass procedures, which result in reduced gastric acid production and which simultaneously bypass the major site of resorption, namely the duodenum and the proximal jejunum.

Depending on sun exposure, the most fraction of vitamin D is produced endogenously in the skin. In contrast, 25-hydroxy cholecalciferol and 1,25-dihydroxycholecalciferol are sourced from diet and are mostly absorbed in the jejunum and ileum. As a fat-soluble vitamin, vitamin D needs bile acids for its uptake. The influence on the gastrointestinal composition of bile acids after bypass surgery is not known, but a resulting influence may be assumed.

It seems to be clear that the prevalence of SHPT depends on sufficient vitamin D and calcium supplementation. Therefore, reduced calcium intake after restrictive procedures and calcium and vitamin D malabsorption in malabsorptive operations are the main cause for SHPT after surgery. The resulting most important consequence of coupled calcium and vitamin D deficiencies is bone demineralization with the risk of long-term fractures [8].

As already noted above, the real calcium alimentation is difficult to evaluate while already simultaneously elevated PTH increases bone metabolism and dissolves calcium from bone mass, thus maintaining calcium serum level homeostasis.

Bone health and obesity have a complex relationship. There is a growing body of counterintuitive observation that bone mineral density increases with obesity [19].

On the other hand, the prevalence of vitamin D deficiency is reported to be as high as 90% in patients with obesity [9]. It is mandatory to measure and correct vitamin D deficiency before surgery with an oral vitamin D load [20].

Weight loss with bariatric surgery may decrease bone mineral density due to decreased mechanical loading of bones during locomotion, and increased calcium loss resulting from a combination of elevated parathyroid hormone and reduced extra ovarian estrogen production, due to fat loss [21–23].

14.5 Diagnosis

The diagnosis of musculoskeletal complications after bariatric surgery is based on clinical and lab tests. Clinical signs and symptoms are leg cramping, tingling sensation, back pain, and weakness.

Monitoring the fat mass/fat-free mass with the help of a body composition analyzer (BCA machine) is also helpful in identifying sarcopenia and taking prompt action.

Lab tests include measurement of serum and 24 h urinary calcium, vitamin D, phosphorus, parathormone, and dual-energy X-ray absorptiometry (DEXA scan). Sometimes, it may be useful to measure osteocalcin and Urinary N- and C-telopeptide and cross-links type 1 collagen telopeptides that are indicators of bone resorption.

The normal range of Serum calcium should be 9–10.5 mg/dL in patients without renal disease and vitamin D (25(OH)D) should be >30 ng/mL (>75 nmol/L).

Luger et al. recommend 25(OH)D concentrations to be above 50 nmol/L at least during the first postoperative year to decelerate bone loss in patients undergoing OAGB [24].

14.6 Follow-Up

During follow-up, it is recommended to ensure musculoskeletal health, to [25]:

- Monitor adherence with physical activity recommendation
- Monitor 24-h urinary calcium excretion at 6 months and then annually
- Monitor 25-vitamin D and parathyroid hormone (PTH) after RYGB and BPD
- Perform (DEXA) biannually

Supplementation may be considered adequate, if levels for serum calcium, bone-specific alkaline phosphatase and/or osteocalcin, vitamin D, PTH, and 24-h urinary calcium excretion rates are normal.

Additionally, prior and post-surgery Bioelectrical Impedance Analysis (BIA) might help to measure body composition [26]. In our department, we implemented BIA measurement prior to surgery and during follow-up to control fat mass and fat-free mass. Figures 14.1, 14.2, and 14.3 show repeated BIA measurements during follow-up in patients after SG and OAGB.

14.7 Management

After surgery, the regular consumption of 1200–2000 mg/day of elemental calcium along with 2000–3000 IU of vitamin D is recommended [9]. Calcium citrate was preferred to calcium carbonate because it seemed to be better absorbed in the absence of gastric acid [20]. Today it is clear that both are equal [27]. Calcium carbonate should be taken with meals, while calcium citrate must be taken in between the meals.

Since this standard supplementation is frequently insufficient to maintain sufficient vitamin D levels in patients with malabsorption, much higher oral or parenteral doses may be required. Therefore, the adequacy of calcium and vitamin D supplementation should be evaluated in all patients, with regular controls of urinary calcium excretion and markers of bone mineral metabolism [8].

In post-bariatric patients with established osteoporosis, pharmacologic treatment with bisphosphonates may be considered. Before starting bisphosphonate treatment, vitamin D deficiency as well as calcium supplementation needs to be fully corrected in order to avoid severe hypocalcemia, hypophosphatemia, and osteomalacia [8, 20, 25]. Intravenous bisphosphonates are the preferred choice because of concerns about low absorption and the potential risk of anastomotic ulcer with oral bisphosphonates. Recommended intravenous drugs were zoledronate (5 mg once a year) or ibandronate (3 mg every 3 months), whereas oral bisphosphonates were alendronate (70 mg/week), risedronate (35 mg/week or 150 mg/month), and ibandronate (150 mg/month). The effectiveness of both intravenous and oral bisphosphonates in improving bone mineralization in bariatric patients were never proved [8, 20, 25].

14.8 Take-Home Message

Disorder of calcium and vitamin D metabolism is a typical sequelae after surgery for obesity and weight-related diseases, especially after gastric bypass and further malabsorptive procedures. Vitamin D deficiency should be corrected before surgery with an oral vitamin D load. Regular intake of calcium and vitamin D has to be maintained after surgery with at least 1200–2000 mg/day of elemental calcium along with 2000–3000 IU of vitamin D.

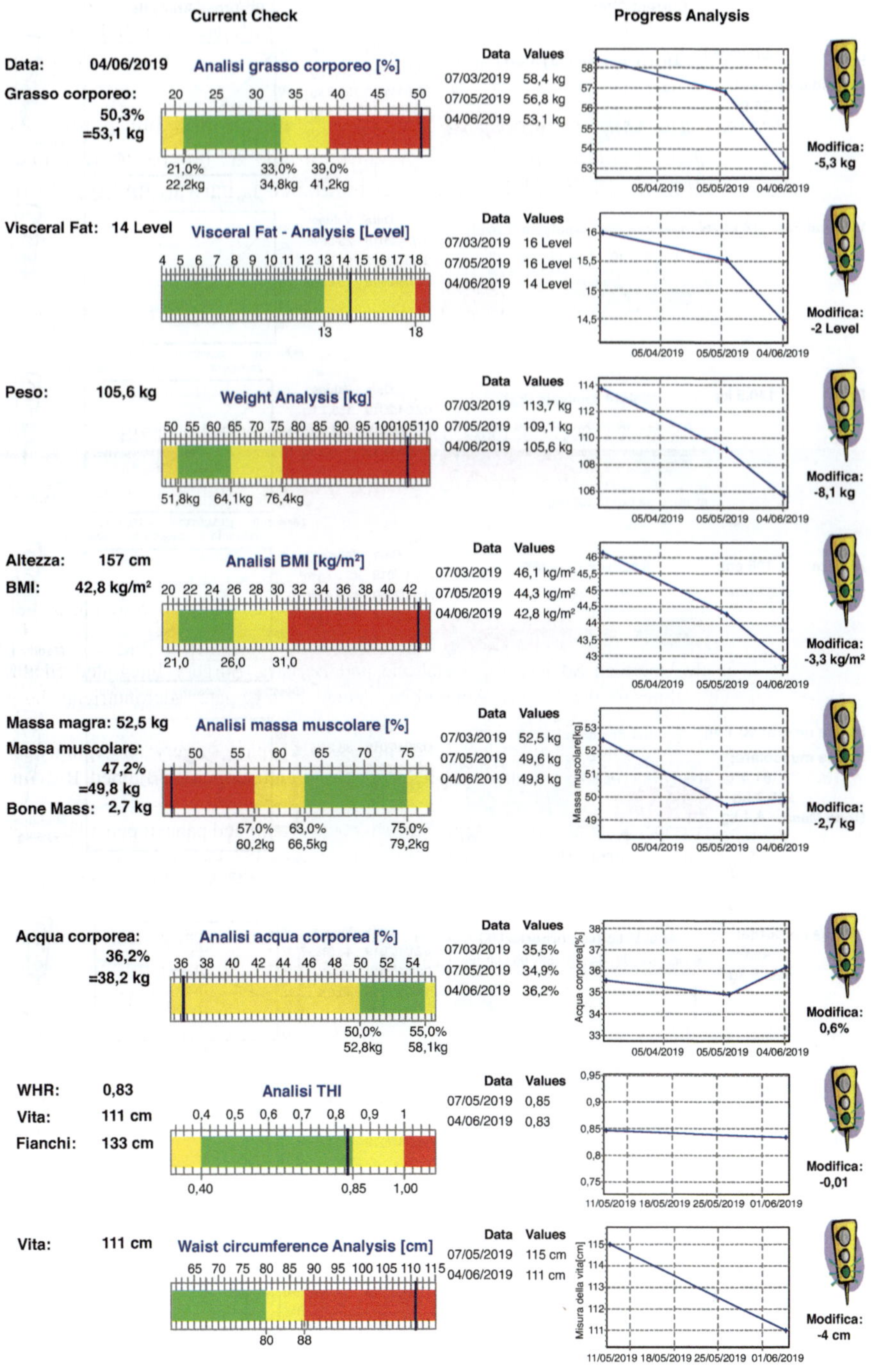

Fig. 14.1 A female, 39-year-old patient, 157 cm, 113.7 kg, BMI 46.1 kg/m², EOSS 1, underwent SG in date 24.04.2019. BIA shows fat mass, visceral mass, fat-free mass at 6-week follow-up

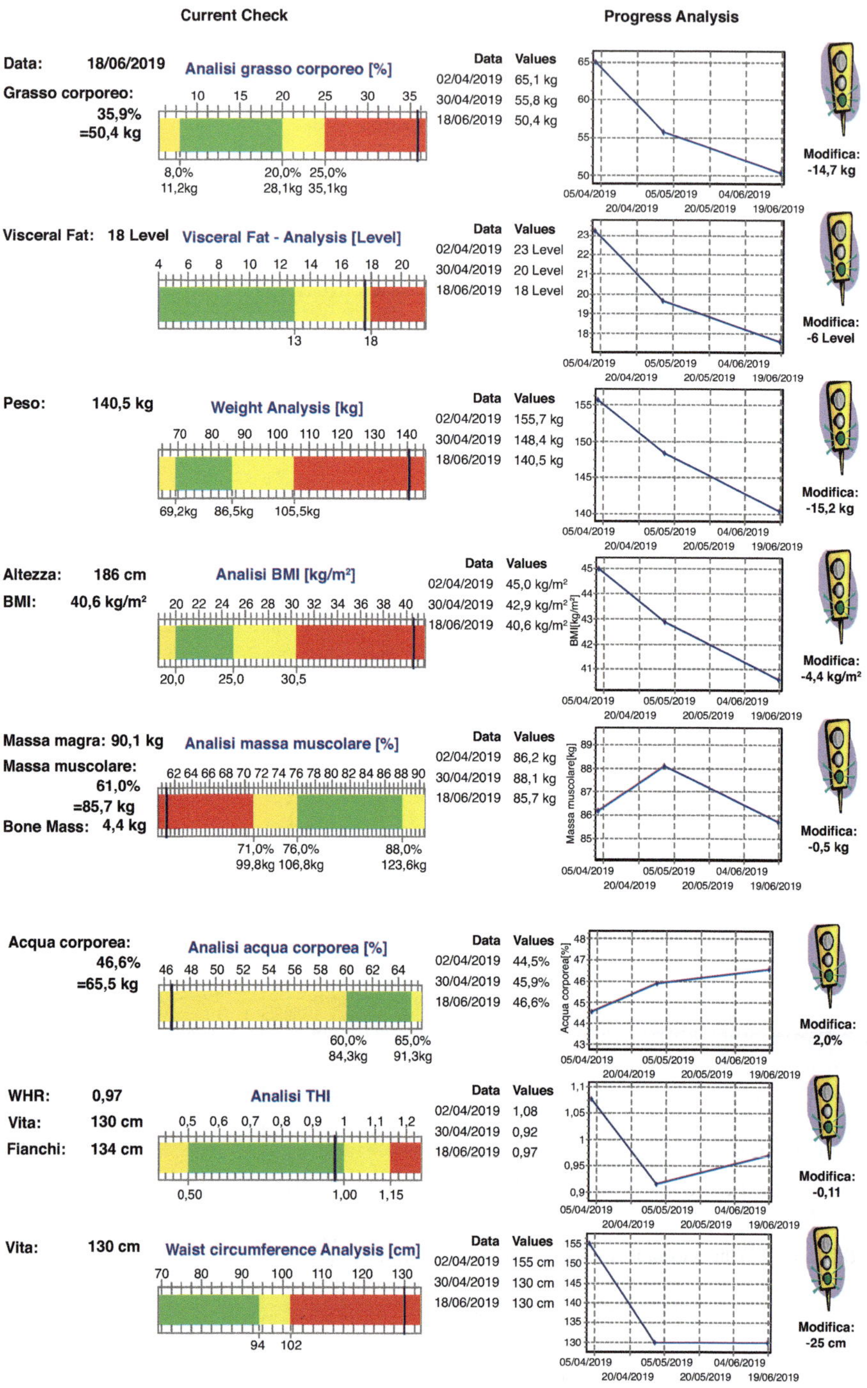

Fig. 14.2 A male, 27-year-old patient, 187 cm, 163 kg, BMI 46.6 kg/m², EOSS 2, underwent SG in date 20.03.2019. BIA shows fat mass, visceral mass, fat-free mass at 3-months follow-up

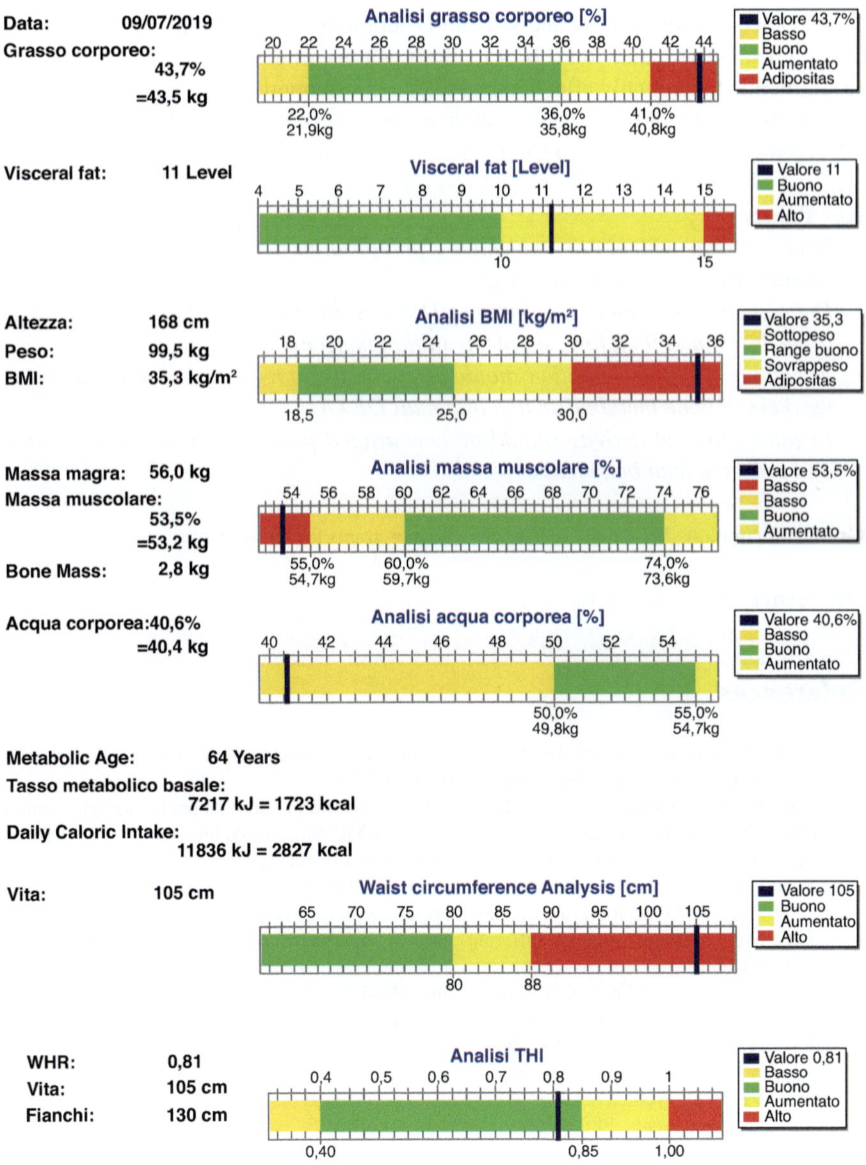

Fig. 14.3 A female, 49-year-old patient, 168 cm, 105 kg, BMI 37.2 kg/m^2, EOSS 2, underwent Mini-Gastric Bypass after inadequate response post AGB in date 06.06.2019. BIA shows fat mass, visceral mass, fat-free mass at 1-month follow-up

The adequacy of calcium and vitamin D supplementation should be evaluated in all patients, with regular controls of markers of bone mineral metabolism. DEXA is recommended biannually after surgery to detect osteoporosis.

Finally, regular physical activity after surgery preserves and builds muscle mass. BIA measurement might help follow the patients and to detect patients at risk.

Key Points

- *Many patients with obesity may have a preoperative deficiency of Vitamin D that should be assessed and corrected.*
- *Deficiencies of calcium and Vitamin D are to be expected after most bariatric procedures, and therefore, supplementation is necessary.*
- *Adequacy of supplementation should be evaluated at regular time intervals using markers of bone metabolism and biannual DEXA.*
- *Regular physical activity should be encouraged post surgery in order to build and preserve lean body mass.*

Grant Information We did not receive any funds or grants for this research.

Disclosure None declared.

References

1. Hooper MM, et al. Musculoskeletal findings in obese subjects before and after weight loss following bariatric surgery. Int J Obes. 2007;31:114–20.
2. Grotle M, et al. Obesity and osteoarthritis in knee, hip and/or hand: an epidemiological study in the general population with 10 years follow-up. BMC Musculoskelet Disord. 2008;9:132.
3. Khadra D, et al. Association between sarcopenic obesity and higher risk of type 2 diabetes in adults: a systematic review and meta-analysis. World J Diabetes. 2019;10:311–23.
4. Zhang X, et al. Association of sarcopenic obesity with the risk of all-cause mortality among adults over a broad range of different settings: a updated meta-analysis. BMC Geriatr. 2019;19:183.
5. De Luca M, et al. Indications for surgery for obesity and weight-related diseases: position statements from the international federation for the surgery of obesity and metabolic disorders (IFSO). Obes Surg. 2016;26:1659–96.
6. Pizzorno L. Bariatric surgery: bad to the bone, Part 1. Integr Med (Encinitas). 2016;15:48–54.
7. Voican CS, et al. Predictive score of sarcopenia occurrence one year after bariatric surgery in severely obese patients. PLoS One. 2018;13:e0197248.
8. Busetto L, et al. Practical recommendations of the obesity management task force of the European association for the study of obesity for the post-bariatric surgery medical management. Obes Facts. 2017;10:597–632.
9. Parrott J, et al. American society for metabolic and bariatric surgery integrated health nutritional guidelines for the surgical weight loss patient 2016 update: micronutrients. Surg Obes Relat Dis. 2017;13:727–41.
10. Wei JH, et al. High incidence of secondary hyperparathyroidism in bariatric patients: comparing different procedures. Obes Surg. 2018;28:798–804.
11. Svanevik M, et al. Bone turnover markers after standard and distal Roux-en-Y gastric bypass: results from a randomized controlled trial. Obes Surg. 2019;29(9):2886–95.

12. Alejo Ramos M, et al. Secondary hyperparathyroidism in patients with biliopancreatic diversion after 10 years of follow-up, and relationship with vitamin D and serum calcium. Obes Surg. 2019;29:999–1006.
13. Pilkington TR, et al. Musculo-skeletal abnormalities after jejunoileal bypass. Int J Obes. 1981;5:509–12.
14. Geoffroy M, et al. Impact of bariatric surgery on bone mineral density: observational study of 110 patients followed up in a specialized center for the treatment of obesity in France. Obes Surg. 2019;29:1765–72.
15. Yu EW, et al. Fracture risk after bariatric surgery: Roux-en-Y gastric bypass versus adjustable gastric banding. J Bone Miner Res. 2017;32:1229–36.
16. Muschitz C, et al. Sclerostin levels and changes in bone metabolism after bariatric surgery. J Clin Endocrinol Metab. 2015;100:891–901.
17. Rousseau C, et al. Change in fracture risk and fracture pattern after bariatric surgery: nested case-control study. BMJ. 2016;354:i3794.
18. Josse AR, et al. Increased consumption of dairy foods and protein during diet- and exercise-induced weight loss promotes fat mass loss and lean mass gain in overweight and obese premenopausal women. J Nutr. 2011;141:1626–34.
19. Shayganfar A, Ebrahimian S, Masjedi M, Daryaei S. A study on bone mass density using dual energy X-ray absorptiometry: does high body mass index have protective effect on bone density in obese patients. J Res Med Sci. 2020;25:4.
20. Allied Health Sciences Section Ad Hoc Nutrition Committee, Aills L, et al. ASMBS allied health nutritional guidelines for the surgical weight loss patient. Surg Obes Relat Dis. 2008;4:S73–108.
21. Hunter GR, et al. Weight loss and bone mineral density. Curr Opin Endocrinol Diabetes Obes. 2014;21:358–62.
22. Jensen LB, et al. Bone minerals changes in obese women during a moderate weight loss with and without calcium supplementation. J Bone Miner Res. 2001;16:141–7.
23. Villareal DT, et al. Bone mineral density response to caloric restriction-induced weight loss or exercise-induced weight loss: a randomized controlled trial. Arch Intern Med. 2006;166:2502–10.
24. Luger M, et al. Changes in bone mineral density following weight loss induced by one-anastomosis gastric bypass in patients with vitamin D supplementation. Obes Surg. 2018;28:3454–65.
25. Mechanick JI, et al. Clinical practice guidelines for the perioperative nutritional, metabolic, and nonsurgical support of the bariatric surgery patient—2013 update: cosponsored by American Association of Clinical Endocrinologists, The Obesity Society, and American Society for Metabolic & Bariatric Surgery. Obesity (Silver Spring). 2013;21(Suppl 1):S1–27.
26. Marra M, et al. Assessment of body composition in health and disease using bioelectrical impedance analysis (BIA) and dual energy X-ray absorptiometry (DXA): a critical overview. Contrast Media Mol Imaging. 2019;2019:3548284.
27. Ring Madsen L, et al. Effect of calcium citrate vs calcium carbonate on elevated parathyroid hormone after Roux-en-Y gastric bypass. A double-blinded, randomized trial. Clin Endocrinol. 2018;89:734–41.

Reproductive Complications After Bariatric Surgery in Males and Females

15

Ahmad Bashir, Ashraf Haddad, and Abdelrahman Nimeri

The reproduction of mankind is a great marvel and mystery. Had God consulted me in the matter, I should have advised him to continue the generation of the species by fashioning them of clay.

—Martin Luther

15.1 Female Reproductive System

Ahmad Bashir, Ashraf Haddad, and Abdelrahman Nimeri

15.1.1 Introduction

According to the World Health Organization, obesity has tripled since 1975. In 2016, more than 1.9 billion adults, 18 years and older, were overweight including more than 650 million obese adults. Furthermore; over 340 million children and adolescents aged 5–19 were overweight or obese in the same year [1].

A. Bashir · A. Haddad
Gastrointestinal Bariatric Medical Center (GBMC), Jordan Hospital, Amman, Jordan
e-mail: Ahmad.Bashir@gbmc-jo.com; Ashraf.haddad@gbmc-jo.com

A. Nimeri (✉)
Department of Surgery, Carolinas Medical Center, Atrium Health Weight Management, Charlotte, NC, USA
e-mail: Abdelrahman.Nimeri@atriumhealth.org

A. G. Bhasker et al. (eds.), *Management of Nutritional and Metabolic Complications of Bariatric Surgery*,
https://doi.org/10.1007/978-981-33-4702-1_15

The number of bariatric & metabolic surgeries (BMS) is on the rise worldwide [2]. It is conceivable that physicians of all specialties will be encountering young females of child bearing age with previous BMS. Therefore, it is of uttermost importance that we understand the long-term hormonal and reproductive implications of BMS.

15.1.2 Obesity and Infertility

Infertility affects one in seven couples [3], and in a significant proportion of these affected couples obesity is directly or indirectly associated with anovulation, subfertility, or infertility [3].

In addition, just being overweight with a body mass index (BMI) > 25 kg/m^2 has a negative impact on the hypothalamic-pituitary-gonadal axis, on gametogenesis, and the outcomes of assisted reproductive technology [4].

Gonadal dysfunction can be one of the most prevalent co-morbidities in morbidly obese and is present in up to 36% of women undergoing BMS [5]. Obesity also increases the rate of miscarriage regardless of the mode of conception [3].

The term "obesity associated gonadal dysfunction" OAGD was introduced in 2014 to describe patients in which the normal adipose tissue distribution and function (dictated by low androgen and high estrogen concentrations) is lost due to an imbalance favoring the increase in androgen levels leading to a change in adipose tissue distribution. This imbalance occurs due to obesity and visceral adiposity [6]. This leads to a vicious cycle of androgen excess, abdominal deposition of body and visceral fat. Further androgen production by the peripheral fat leads to gonadal dysfunction which can be ameliorated by weight loss [7]. However, the literature on the effect of BMS on womens' reproductive health outcomes is still limited [8].

In this chapter, we will discuss important topics pertaining to the reproductive health of young women undergoing BMS including postoperative hormonal changes, pregnancy after bariatric surgery, nutritional deficiencies, sexual functions, and pelvic floor disorders.

15.1.3 Sexual Dysfunction and Pelvic Floor Disorders

15.1.3.1 Effect of Surgery on Sexual Function

Obesity and its associated comorbidities increase the probability of sexual disorders [9]. Female sexual dysfunction can be widespread and is affected by biological, social, as well as psychological factors. In addition, female Functional Sexual Index (FSFI) is a validated self-report questionnaire to assess the level of sexual function. It has six domains which include desire, arousal, lubrication, orgasm, satisfaction, and pain [10]. The Sexual Quality of Life-Female scores is another questionnaire that assesses the impact of sexual dysfunction on quality of life [11]. These tools are used to measure sexual dysfunction in females.

Female sexual dysfunction is more commonly diagnosed in the obese population [9]. FSFI has been shown to strongly correlate with BMI. Both obesity and BMI have been shown to affect multiple sexual function parameters from FSFI including arousal, orgasm, satisfaction, and lubrication. Obesity and BMI did not affect desire and pain [12].

However; sexual dysfunction in females with obesity appears to be improved by marked weight reduction [12]. This improvement has been demonstrated in women after BMS as well [9]. Women who lose weight after surgery will feel more attractive, have higher self-esteem, and have decreased anxiety which will translate into better Sexual Quality of Life-Female scores that describe the emotional aspects of their sexual life. The desire and arousal domains of FSFI are significantly improved after BMS as well [13]. A key issue is the excessive hanging skin after BMS, which the majority of patients develop, and its negative effect on the benefits of surgery. Excessive skin can cause overall impairment in daily life and affect sexual function and intimacy as well. The associated depression and concerns regarding body image can contribute to weight regain. Thus; it is important to optimize body image issues to optimize the psychological and weight outcomes of BMS [14].

In conclusion, obesity increases the probability of sexual disorders and dysfunction. Sexual dysfunction is improved by both marked weight loss and after BMS.

15.1.3.2 Effect of Surgery on Pelvic Floor Disorders

Obesity is an established risk factor for pelvic floor disorders. The risk of developing urinary incontinence for example increases with increasing BMI across all BMI classes [15].

BMS improves pelvic floor disorders through multiple mechanisms. The decrease in intra-abdominal pressure that accompanies weight loss has been suggested as one factor. The resolution of comorbidities like diabetes and hypertension is another contributing factor [16].

Furthermore, surgery has been shown in multiple studies to significantly improve urinary incontinence, pelvic organ prolapse, and colorectal/anal symptoms but not necessarily fecal incontinence [16–18].

BMS has been reported to result in resolution of urinary incontinence in 52% of preoperatively incontinent patients [18]. Relative risk reduction of urinary incontinence of 67% and pelvic organ prolapse of 52% postoperatively has been reported [19].

The risk of pelvic floor disorders including urinary incontinence increases with obesity. BMS and its associated weight loss along with resolution of comorbidities such as diabetes and hypertension lead to improvement or resolution of pelvic floor disorders.

15.1.4 Hormonal Changes in Women After BMS

Multiple complex hormonal mechanisms contribute to female obesity besides genetic predisposition. Abdominal obesity can perpetuate a vicious cycle where abdominal adiposity leads to increased peripheral estrogen production through increased aromatase activity leading to androgen deficiency. This decreases muscle mass and increases abdominal adiposity. The fat cells cause a decrease in adiponectin levels and an increase in tumor necrosis factor alpha and interleukin 6 which will aggravate peripheral insulin resistance, obesity, and perpetuate the vicious cycle [5].

The exact hormonal changes and their effect on female reproductive function after BMS is not fully understood. However, few studies have described hormonal and menstrual changes after BMS.

A study assessing 4 years outcome of sex hormones after BMS revealed overall significant improvement in reproductive hormones. Testosterone and dehydroepiandosterone sulfate levels decreased over 4 years. Follicle stimulating hormone, leutinizing hormone, and sex hormone binding globulin levels all significantly increased after surgery. The exception was estradiol which did not change after BMS [20].

A second study following patients after RYGB with urinary progestin measurements at 12 months revealed that ovulatory frequency and luteal phase quality was not changed but the follicular phase was shorter. Biochemical hyperandrogenism improved with no change in the associated clinical features like sebum production, hirsutism, or acne. Thus ovulation rate and quality appears to be relatively unaffected by morbid obesity, body composition, caloric restriction after gastric bypass, or long-term weight loss [21].

One of the indicators of fertility and ovarian reserve is the Anti-Mullerian Hormone (AMH) and it represents the severity of polycystic ovary syndrome (PCOS). AMH is significantly higher in the PCOS patients in both women with or without obesity and is also positively related to testosterone, androstenedione, and dehydroepiandosterone [22]. After BMS, AMH levels decreases in patients whether or not they suffered from PCOS before surgery. However, those patients with preoperative PCOS had a higher chance of AMH levels normalizing postoperatively [22].

Obesity perpetuates a vicious cycle of hormonal imbalance and overall androgen deficiency. Postoperatively, BMS leads to improvement of reproductive hormones with no change in the ovulation frequency or ovum quality.

15.1.5 Pregnancy and Bariatric Surgery

15.1.5.1 Pregnancy Outcomes and Surgery-to-Conception Interval

BMS has positive effects on fertility. With these positive changes on fertility, inadvertent pregnancy despite adequate conventional contraception is possible after RYGB [23].

There is a lot of debate regarding the "Ideal" surgery-to-conception timing. Early conception during the time of rapid weight loss after BMS has been speculated to cause preterm delivery, fetal growth restriction, low birth weight, and congenital anomalies. In addition the weight gain of conception during time of maximal weight loss can hypothetically limit the maternal benefit of postoperative weight loss [24].

Two studies reported the outcomes of surgery-to-conception-interval on pregnancy following BMS. The first study compared early (≤18 months) versus late (>18 months) conception after RYGB. There was no difference in adverse obstetrical outcomes (preterm premature rupture of membranes, gestational diabetes, oligohydramnios, intrauterine growth restriction, pre-term or post-term delivery) or adverse newborn outcomes (Apgar score < 7, intensive care admission, or birth defects) [24].

A second study used the same time interval criteria to compare outcomes after SG. The study revealed that the late pregnancy group had higher gestational weight gain (11 vs. 8 kg), lower hemoglobin in early pregnancy (10 vs. 10.4 gm/dl), and after delivery (12.3 vs. 12.6 gm/dl). The same study showed that the other maternal and perinatal outcomes were similar between the two groups [25].

Several studies compared pregnancy outcomes after BMS with matched controlled pregnancies. The first studies examined the Swedish Medical Birth Register. In the Swedish study, pregnancies post-surgery were associated with lower risk of gestational diabetes and large for gestational age infants. In contrast, the rates of small for gestational age and short gestation were higher (although the risk of preterm birth was not significantly different) [26]. Similarly, a study examining birth certificates and maternally linked discharge data in Washington State reported higher risk of small for gestational age, prematurity, neonatal intensive care admission, and lower Apgar score. This study however, reported that a long surgery-to-conception interval of more than 4 years (not 18 months like the aforementioned studies) is actually associated with lower risk of prematurity, small for gestational age, and neonatal intensive care admission [27].

Other reported outcomes of post bariatric surgery conception included lower risks of macrosomic infants, lower risk of prolonged labor, and lower risk of cesarean section which has been reported by some authors while others reported that mothers with prior BMS who remained obese were most likely to undergo a cesarean section [27–29] (Table 15.1).

15.1.5.2 Gestational Diabetes and Oral Glucose Tolerance Test

Gestational diabetes is frequently encountered during pregnancy, and BMS performed before pregnancy significantly reduces the risk of gestational diabetes but the risk is still higher than the normal weight population [30]. In addition, the oral

Table 15.1 Change of maternal and neonatal risks after bariatric surgery*

Increased risk	Decreased risk	No significant risk	Controversial
Small for gestational age	Gestational diabetes	Preterm birth	Cesarean section
Short gestation	Large for gestational age		
Neonatal intensive care admission	Macrosomia		
Lower Apgar score	Prolonged labor		

*Risks compared to general population

glucose tolerance test used to diagnose gestational diabetes is challenging in pregnant women after BMS due to hypoglycemia during the test in up to half of the patients with previous BMS and it is likely to induce symptoms of dumping syndrome. RYGB and short surgery to conception interval are associated with higher risk of developing hypoglycemic symptoms. Interestingly; hypoglycemia symptoms did not correlate with gestational diabetes and patients who developed hypoglycemia had lower rates of gestational diabetes [31] An alternative screening methods for gestational diabetes for this patient population includes a non-fasting 50 gm glucose challenge test which seems to be better tolerated or daily capillary blood glucose measurements before and after meals for 3–7 days to be done between the 24 to the 28-week of pregnancy [30].

15.1.5.3 Nutritional Deficiencies and Birth Defects

The risk of birth defects after BMS have been suggested to either be increased secondary to nutritional deficiencies or decreased due to the effect of decreased maternal BMI [32].

All patients undergoing BMS should receive daily multivitamins with trace minerals as they are at risk for deficiency of vitamins including B12, B1, C, folate, A, D, K, irons, selenium, zinc, and copper [33]. These common postoperative deficiencies can be exacerbated by the effects of pregnancy like morning sickness, hyperemesis, reflux, and bloating [34]. It has been shown that BMS increases the risk of small for age infants and micro-nutrient deficiencies in the mother and the newborn [35, 36].

Compliance with vitamin supplementation after BMS is a significant concern. A single center study at a university in France followed 48 adult pregnant women who underwent BMS (AGB, SG & RYGB). In this French study, only 56.8% took vitamins preconception, 77.8% during the first trimester, 96.3% during the second trimester, and 100% during the last trimester. Nutritional deficiencies included Vitamins A, D, C, B1, B9, and selenium. Interestingly, and despite supplements vitamin A and C deficiencies increased throughout the third trimester [35].

Another study compared cord blood samples from newborns from RYGB mothers to newborns from non-obese mothers. The post RYGB neonates had higher chance of having lower concentrations of calcium, zinc, iron, and vitamin A. Currently, a comparison to the neonates of morbidly obese mother is lacking [36].

Apart from the aforementioned deficiencies, vitamin A levels seem to be negatively impacted by BMS, and when combined with pregnancy, the risk is greater [37]. This can lead to low retinol and b-carotene levels during pregnancy which might increase the risk for developing night blindness [37]. However, not all Vitamin A supplements are safe during pregnancy (retinol-based products are best avoided) [34].

It is advisable to wait at least 12 months or until the weight stabilizes postoperatively before pregnancy. In case of pregnancy, a multidisciplinary team approach is key to monitor nutrition. Adequate prenatal supplementation should start at the preconception phase as iron and vitamins A, B12, K, and folate deficiencies are associated with maternal and fetal complications especially because over-the-counter supplements might not provide the required amounts of certain micronutrients in this high-risk population [33, 34].

The final key issue to be discussed is whether BMS increases the risk of birth defects. Two major studies assessed the risk of birth defects in pregnant mothers after BMS. The first examined the Swedish Medical Birth Register from 2006 to 2011 (matched controlled study) and the second examined birth certificates and linked discharge data in Washington State from 1980 to 2013 (population based retrospective cohort study). Both studies did not find any significant difference in the risk of congenital malformations and birth defects after BMS [26, 27].

In conclusion, fertility improves after BMS. The "Ideal" surgery-conception interval seems to be between 12 and 18 months post-surgery or after weight stabilization. BMS is associated with lower risk of gestational diabetes, large for gestational age, macrosomia, cesarean section, and prolonged labor. BMS was not shown to increase the risks of birth defects, Vitamin supplementation should start preconception and continue throughout the pregnancy.

Key Points

1. *Obesity is a significant cause of female infertility/subfertility*
2. *The "Ideal" surgery-conception interval seems to be between 12 and 18 months post-surgery or after weight stabilization.*
3. *Obesity causes hypogonadism secondary to increased oestrogen suppression of pituitary, decreasing the production of LH and FSH*
4. *The decreased fertility in obesity is due to hypogonadism, decreased sexual function, as well as effects on fertilisation, and conception.*
5. *Bariatric surgery improves frequency of ovulation, oocyte quality, fecundity, and decreases the risk of Gestational diabetes mellitus, miscarriages and macrosomia. There is also a lower risk of prolonged labor and emergency LSCS after bariatric surgery*
6. *Studies have not found any significant difference in the risk of congenital malformations and birth defects after BMS*
7. *Common preoperative deficiencies may be exacerbated by pregnancy.*

15.2 Male Reproductive Complications

Ahmad Bashir, Ashraf Haddad, and Abdelrahman Nimeri

15.2.1 Introduction

Although obesity rates were more common in females, the CDC reports that this gap has almost disappeared with more pronounced and visible effects on their reproductive system [38]. Nevertheless, more females undergo bariatric and metabolic surgery (BMS). Male Obesity-Secondary Hypogonadism (MOSH) is well known, and its negative effects on fertility and erectile function are established in males [39] but may be understated in the bariatric patient population. There are very few reports on MOSH and its outcome after bariatric surgery. Most of the published studies report only the early outcomes. The number of studies reporting complications of bariatric surgery on reproductive system are scant, and generally, lack of improvement of preoperative sexual dysfunction in the presence of residual obesity or weight regain is more common than complications affecting the system directly after significant and maintained weight loss. In this segment of the chapter, we will discuss the effects of bariatric surgery on obesity related hypogonadism, sex hormone changes, sperm & seminal fluid, erectile dysfunction and sexual quality of life along with reported complications of bariatric surgery on reproductive system in males.

15.2.2 Male Obesity-Secondary Hypogonadism (MOSH)

MOSH in males is defined as a decrease in circulating Testosterone with low or reduced gonadotropin [40]. It affects 45–64% of patients suffering from obesity through direct and indirect effects [5, 39, 41]. We will look at the effects of obesity & bariatric surgery on sex hormones, sperm & seminal fluid, sexual dysfunction & quality of life secondary to these problems.

15.2.2.1 Sex Hormones

Obesity & age affect gonadal hormones as well as seminal quality in men [42]. In a large case-cohort study involving more than 2000 subjects, increasing BMI was associated with decrease in Testosterone, inhibin B & LH levels in males after adjusting for other comorbidities.

A recent systematic review on the effects of obesity and weight loss on sex hormone levels showed a decrease in total and free testosterone along with a decrease in Sex Hormone-Binding Globulin (SHBG) with increasing obesity [43]. It was previously thought that the decrease in SHBG was the reason for decrease in TT. However, FT is also reduced in males suffering from obesity. This meta-analysis included comparative studies analysing the effect of low-calorie diet (LCD) or bariatric surgery (BS) on sex hormones levels before and after weight loss, including 11 randomized controlled trials (RCTs) (9 LCD, 2 BS). Overall, with successful weight loss TT & FT, SHBG, and Gonadotropins (LH and FSH) increased. Circulating estrogen decreased with weight loss. The changes were proportional to the weight loss, especially in young non-diabetic patients. BS was associated with a greater improvement due to higher persistent weight loss, more so after Biliopancreatic Diversion (BPD). Decrease in fat mass leading to less estrogen production by adipose tissue and thus reducing the negative feedback on HPA axis has been suggested as the mechanism for the above changes. Other mechanisms suggested are: Central Leptin resistance, Insulin resistance, and decreased production of SHBG [39]. In a paper by Calderon et al., TT & FT levels were inversely related to both glucose and HOMA-IR, with glucose being the only variable inducing variability in both TT & FT.

Calderon et al. [41] studied the effect of three surgery types on the change in sex hormones: gastric bypass, sleeve gastrectomy and adjustable gastric banding. All types were successful in inducing improvement in sex hormones measured. Only SHBG was significantly higher in gastric bypass as opposed to other types. FT increase correlated with a decrease in fasting blood sugar. No statistical significance was found in other hormone changes, glycemic resolution or weight loss in a short follow-up period of 6 months.

When comparing the levels after bariatric surgery between the froup with obesity and a lean control group over 6–16 years, Rosenblatt et al. [44] demonstrated that changes in hormones after bariatric surgery (ORYGB and LRYGB) are sustained. TT, FT & SHBG were all significantly higher in bariatric group compared to obese controls and not statistically different from lean controls. LH & FSH were greater in bariatric group with normal LH/FSH ration. BMI correlated with levels of TT & FT in all three groups. Persistent or recurrent obesity led to decreased levels of hormones compared to patients maintaining weight loss.

15.2.2.2 Sperm and Seminal Fluid

It may expected that spermatogenesis and seminal fluid would be affected in obesity, given the changes in sex hormones.

Paasch et al. [42], compared a large population from an infertility clinic to a set of controls for sex hormones and sperm analysis. The two groups were matched for hormonal imbalances, and differed only in weight. They found an inverse U-shaped curve distribution of Total Sperm Count (TSC) and Total Sperm Count with normal morphology (TCN). Both underweight and subjects with obesity had lower counts than normal BMI or BMI in the overweight range. Motility did not appear to be affected by BMI. Age affected motility greater than BMI. However, in the age group 20–30 years, BMI inversely correlated with motility and therefore impacted fertility.

In another study, Samavat et al. [45] matched patients with obesity seeking surgical weight loss, with lean controls. In addition to the semen analysis, they also looked at acrosome reaction (AR), zona pellucida (ZP) binding and their actual timings as these determine fertility more accurately. They found a statistically significant difference in the volume and immotile fraction (50.2% vs. 37.4% respectively in patients with obesity versus lean subjects). Azoospermia was only present in patients with obesity (0% in lean subjects vs. 13% in obese group). Oligospermia & asthenozoospermia were more common in the group with obesity. Due to above findings, only 57% of the patients in group with obesity were able to complete the AR & ZP testing, while 76% of lean subjects did it. Spermatozoa in group with obesity had reduced ability to respond to respond to proper stimuli, & instead had a higher percentage of spontaneous AR without ZP binding, lacking the proper timing to bind, thus the reduced fertility.

A meta-analysis by Campbell et al. [46] studied more than 30 papers with greater than 115 thousand participants. Infertility, assisted reproduction & non-viable pregnancy were more common in couples with a male suffering from obesity. Routine parameters in semen analysis did not differ significantly: Sperm concentration, morphology & ejaculate volume. Progressive motility was slightly reduced in subjects with obesity that was only significant in the clinical setting using WHO criteria. However, on further testing of DNA fragmentation, low mitochondrial membrane potential (MMP), and change in seminal fluid factors: neoprotein, interleukin-8, alpha-glucosidase, were significantly more common in subjects with obesity compared to normal weight. These cause the increased paternal infertility in patients with obesity through higher concentration of reactive oxygen species (ROS). All these factors coupled together reduce fertilization, impair embryonic development & increase loss of viable pregnancy.

The number of studies looking at the effects of bariatric surgery on semen quality are few. di Frega et al. [47] have reported complete arrest of spermatogenesis proven by testicular biopsy on six patients who underwent RYGB despite normal hormonal assays & previous fertility, with all presenting within 1–2 years from the operation.

Sermondade et al. [48] reported three cases: 2 RYGB, 1 LSG, suffering from primary infertility with no abnormalities found in their partners. Despite successful weight loss, their semen analysis within the first year showed drastic worsening: reduction in concentration, progressive motility and percentage of spermatozoa. One normalized after 2 years of follow-up, rest had not yet reached 2 years at the time of publication.

In a case series of six patients, Lergo et al. [49] reported that semen concentration reduced in the first month, but continued to increase slowly till it normalized by 12 months.

El Baridis et al. [50] studied 46 patients who underwent LSG up to 1 year after surgery. Semen parameters improved only in patients with oligospermia or azoospermia. Azoospermia improved in 46% of patients, 10% of oligospermia worsened or remained unchanged, 58% improved but not significantly, with only 32% almost normalizing.

Samavat et al. [51] compared patients who underwent bariatric surgery (LRYGB 23 subjects) with matched controls with obesity (eight patients awaiting bariatric surgery) who were under lifestyle intervention. At 6 months, repeat analysis showed a decrease in the prevalence of hypogonadism from 74 to 9% on hormonal assay in the surgery group. Patients with normal seminal analysis increased from 26 to 39% in the surgery group. An increase in sperm count, improved progressive motility and decreased DNA fragmentation were observed after BS.

Recently, Carette et al. [52] in BARISPERM multicenter prospective study, added to the conflicting results. 46 patients (20 LRYGB, 26 LSG) with no history of infertility were followed up to 1 year. Total sperm counts continued to decrease from 6 months to 1 year, to the point that oligospermia increased from 17.4% preoperatively to 21.7%, with decrease in the total spermatozoa (15.4–12.4%). DNA fragmentation also worsened, with no change in motility or vitality of spermatozoa. No correlation was found between vitamin and pollutant levels in blood to these findings, as hypothesized by the previous studies to cause this temporary worsening.

Reis et al. [53] randomized 20 patients to Biliopancreatic diversion (BPD) versus lifestyle controls. At 20 months of follow up, they found no significant difference in all seminal fluid parameters between the surgical and control groups. This study represents the longest term follow up after bariatric surgery we currently have. The parameters studied were sperm concentration, motility, morphology, volume, and vitality.

Given the evidence, bariatric surgery has shown some worrisome effects on sperm and seminal fluid in the early period after surgery. The reversibility of these early changes in the long-term remains unclear. There is a need for larger well designed trials with long term follow-up.

15.2.2.3 Erectile Dysfunction (ED) and Sexual Quality of Life

1. ED is generally defined as persistent inability to attain and maintain a penile erection adequate for satisfactory sexual performance. Sexual function in men encompasses several domains: desire or drive, erection, ejaculation and overall satisfaction. Erectile or sexual dysfunction diagnosis relies on the literature on patients' feedback from several questionnaires, which could pose a response bias. The questionnaires available to address sexual function are, The Brief Male Sexual Inventory (BSFI): developed by O'leary et al. [54], The International Index of Erectile Function (IIEF): developed by Rosen et al. [55], The Sexual Health Inventory for Men (SHIM): developed also by Rosen et al. [56], only for diagnosing the severity of erectile dysfunction (ED) and others like: Sexual Quality of Life-Male Questionnaire (SQOL-M): developed by Abraham et al. (J Sex Med 2008 referenced in [57]). In addition, sexual function questionnaire (SFQ), and impact of weight on quality of life-lite (IWQOL-Lite) have been used as well to study sexual function after bariatric surgery [58].

Depending on the tools applied to diagnose Ed and SD, the reported outcomes vary considerably.

Obesity increases the incidence of erectile dysfunction and decreases overall sexual health. In Massachusetts Male Aging Study [59], ED was present in 22% of individuals with BMI > 30 kg/m^2 as opposed to 13% in individuals with normal weight.

The theory behind the increased incidence is an endothelial dysfunction in the release of nitric oxide that would cause a decreased blood flow in the corpus cavernosum, decreasing the ability for erection. This dysfunction is not only caused by the hormonal disturbances mentioned above, but also by the increased pro-inflammatory markers present in obesity. In an OLETF rat model study by Choi et al. [60], obese rats who showed less mean intracavernous pressure, less endothelial Nitric Oxide Synthase (eNOS), & neuronal NOS (nNOS). Rats who underwent bariatric surgery showed more cavernosal smooth muscle/collagen ratio with increase in eNOS and nNOS that was statistically significant.

Weight loss in most studies appears to contribute to improving ED & sexual health in the short-term. In more than one RCT utilizing lifestyle and diet intervention, an increase in IIEF scores occurred [61, 62].

Dallal et al. [63], compared 97 patients who underwent RYGB with normal population controls. Using BSFI, they found that all domain scores of sexual function were significantly lower in the surgery group preoperatively, the higher the weight the less the scores were before the intervention. At a mean of 19 months follow up

(6–45 months) post RYGB, all domain scores improved with statistical significance. The amount of weight loss correlated with the improvement in scores. All scores approached those of reference controls except ejaculatory function and overall sexual satisfaction.

However, Ranasinghe et al. (BJUI 2010 [64]), studied 34 males who underwent Laparoscopic Gastric Banding (LGB), and found significant worsening in erectile index and orgasmic function utilizing IIEF, despite significant weight lost over a mean of 22 months follow up. The overall score did not differ over the period of follow up and more males were started on medical treatment for ED. Interestingly 83% of the subjects had ED on preoperative questionnaire, a percentage higher than any reported study.

Kun et al. [65] confirmed the improvement of ED in 39 Chinese patients undergoing LRYGB over 1 year follow up after surgery utilizing IIEF. They also studied the cavernosal intima/media thickness with the cavernosal peak systolic velocity through doppler imaging and found the thickness to decrease by 45%, while PSV increased by 61%.

Rosenblatt et al. [44] provided the longest term (6–16 years) evidence available for sexual function after bariatric surgery (RYGB). Using IIEF, total scores in the 3 groups (BS, Obese controls, lean controls) did not differ. Bariatric surgery group had better ED scores compared to obesity controls, but not to lean controls. ED was still present in 54.5%, 78.6%, 35.7% of bariatric, obesity & lean groups respectively, while overall satisfaction was 31.8%, 7.1% and 42.9% in the same order, respectively. They attributed some of these results to relapsing obesity in some individuals.

Janik et al. [57] compared 30 patients undergoing eit'her LSG or LRYGB, followed up over 18 months, with 32 controls with obesity. 56% of the surgery group had ED. That number decreased to 20%, with none having severe ED scores compared to 16% preoperatively. Overall sexual satisfaction with sexual desire improved, while intercourse satisfaction worsened and orgasmic function remained unchanged. SQOL-M scores significantly improved postoperatively, and improvement occurred in 8/11 items, with strong correlation to IIEF scores. On multivariate analysis of the entire two groups, age and history of no bariatric surgery were the only two major risks for ED in their analysis.

One should also be aware of the effects of certain mineral deficiencies on sexual function. Mahawar et al. [66] reviewed Zinc deficiency after RYGB, and noted that impotence with skin rash, hair loss can be due this mineral deficiency. Zinc blood levels of patients with impotence should be investigated and replaced orally daily for up to 4 weeks, as they respond to such treatment in 83% of the time. Refractory deficiencies require intravenous replacement.

In the largest, most recent multicenter Longitudinal Assessment of Bariatric Surgery (LABS-2) trial published till present on sexual function, Steffen et al. [58], followed up 470 men with 59.9% follow up at 5 years after bariatric surgery. Overall, improvements were significant in overall satisfaction, sexual desire and physical limitations to sexual activity. Despite these improvements, and although better than the preoperative state, there was a deterioration in sexual desire and activity between years 1 and 5. Lower depressive symptoms were associated with better improvements, however, use of antidepressant medication was associated with deterioration in one or more domains of sexual function.

15.2.3 Conclusion

Overall, there is a strong evidence that bariatric surgery improves the sexual hormonal homeostasis that seems to be sustained long term. However, it does seem to correlate with the degree of weight lost, and this improvement decreases with weight regain. Sperm and seminal fluid quality tends to worsen in the short term, without any solid mid or long-term evidence to suggest reversal or improvements of these changes. The overall quality of sexual function, especially erectile dysfunction, appears to improve. There is still a further need for larger and more long-term studies to know the sustainability of these improvements.

Key Points

1. There is limited literature on effect of bariatric surgery on male reproductive system.
2. *There is a high prevalence of MOSH in obesity attributed to decrease in SHBG, FT, TT, FSH and LH secondary to suppression of pituitary by increased circulating estrogen.*
3. *Most studies report improvement in MOSH after surgical and non-surgical weight loss proportional to the amount of weight loss. Weight regain corroborates with relapse of hypogonadism.*
4. *Some literature suggests worsening of semen and sperm quality in the form of oligospermia and azoospermia after bariatric surgery. Long-term literature evidence is not available to know for sure if this is a reversible complication.*
5. *ED is more prevalent in population with obsity. Increased inflammatory cytokines reducing the release of endothelial NO have been implicated.*
6. *Most studies report an improvement in sexual function and sexual disorders after BS. The conflicting reports may be attributed to multiple factors affecting sexual function (interpersonal relationships, attraction to the partner, stress, health, medications)*

References

1. World Health Organization. Obesity and overweight factsheet. https://www.who.int/news-room/fact-sheets/detail/obesity-and-overweight.
2. Angrisani L, Santonicola A, Iovino P, et al. IFSO worldwide survey 2016: primary, endoluminal, and revisional procedures. Obes Surg. 2018;28(12):3783–94. https://doi.org/10.1007/s11695-018-3450-2.
3. Talmor A, Dunphy B. Female obesity and infertility. Best Pract Res Clin Obstet Gynaecol. 2015;29(4):498–506. https://doi.org/10.1016/j.bpobgyn.2014.10.014.

4. Glenn T, Harris AL, Lindheim SR. Impact of obesity on male and female reproductive outcomes. Curr Opin Obstet Gynecol. 2019;31(4):201–6. https://doi.org/10.1097/GCO.0000000000000549.
5. Escobar-Morreale HF, Santacruz E, Luque-Ramírez M, Botella Carretero JI. Prevalence of 'obesity-associated gonadal dysfunction' in severely obese men and women and its resolution after bariatric surgery: a systematic review and meta-analysis. Hum Reprod Update. 2017;23(4):390–408. https://doi.org/10.1093/humupd/dmx012.
6. Escobar-Morreale HF, Alvarez-Blasco F, Botella-Carretero JI, Luque-Ramírez M. The striking similarities in the metabolic association of female androgen excess and male androgen deficiency. Hum Reprod. 2014;29(10):2083–91. https://doi.org/10.1093/humrep/deu198.
7. Escobar-Morreale HF, San Millán JL. Abdominal adiposity and the polycystic ovary syndrome. Trends Endocrinol Metab. 2007;18(7):266–72.
8. Broughton DE, Moley KH. Obesity and female infertility: potential mediators of obesity's impact. Fertil Steril. 2017;107(4):840–7. https://doi.org/10.1016/j.fertnstert.2017.01.017.
9. Pichlerova D, Bob P, Zmolikova J, et al. Sexual dysfunctions in obese women before and after bariatric surgery. Med Sci Monit. 2019;25:3108–14. https://doi.org/10.12659/MSM.913614.
10. Rosen R, Brown C, Heiman J, et al. The Female Sexual Function Index (FSFI): a multidimensional self-report instrument for the assessment of female sexual function. J Sex Marital Ther. 2000;26(2):191–208.
11. Symonds T, Boolell M, Quirk F. Development of a questionnaire on sexual quality of life in women. J Sex Marital Ther. 2005;31(5):385–97.
12. Esposito K, Ciotola M, Giugliano F, et al. Association of body weight with sexual function in women. Int J Impot Res. 2007;19(4):353–7.
13. Janik M, Bielecka I, Paśnik K, Kwiatkowsk A, et al. Female sexual function before and after bariatric surgery: a cross-sectional study and review of literature. Obes Surg. 2015;25:1511–7. https://doi.org/10.1007/s11695-015-1721-8.
14. Ramalho S, Bastos A, Silva C, et al. Excessive skin and sexual function: relationship with psychological variables and weight regain in women after bariatric surgery. Obes Surg. 2015;25:1149–54. https://doi.org/10.1007/s11695-014-1514-.
15. Hannestad YS, Rortveit G, Daltveit AK, Hunskaar S. Are smoking and other lifestyle factors associated with female urinary incontinence? The Norwegian EPINCONT Study. BJOG. 2003;110(3):247–54.
16. Lian W, Zhengl Y, Huang H, Chen L, Cao B. Effects of bariatric surgery on pelvic floor disorders in obese women: a meta-analysis. Arch Gynecol Obstet. 2017;296:181–9. https://doi.org/10.1007/s00404-017-4415-.
17. Leshem A, Shimonov M, Amir H, Gordon D, Groutz A. Effects of bariatric surgery on female pelvic floor disorders. Urology. 2017;105:42–7. https://doi.org/10.1016/j.urology.2017.03.003.
18. Shimonov M, Groutz A, Schachter P, Gordon D. Is bariatric surgery the answer to urinary incontinence in obese women? Neurourol Urodyn. 2017;36(1):184–7. https://doi.org/10.1002/nau.22909.
19. Montenegro M, Slongo H, Juliato CRT, et al. The impact of bariatric surgery on pelvic floor dysfunction: a systematic review. J Minim Invasive Gynecol. 2019;26(5):816–25. https://doi.org/10.1016/j.jmig.2019.01.013.
20. Legro RS, Dodson WC, Gnatuk CL, et al. Effects of gastric bypass surgery on female reproductive function. J Clin Endocrinol Metab. 2012;97(12):4540–8. https://doi.org/10.1210/jc.2012-2205.
21. Chiofalo F, Ciuolil C, Formichi C, et al. Bariatric surgery reduces serum anti-mullerian hormone levels in obese women with and without polycystic ovarian syndrome. Obes Surg. 2017;27:1750–4. https://doi.org/10.1007/s11695-016-2528-y.
22. Sarwer DB, Wadden TA, Spitzer JC, et al. 4-year changes in sex hormones, sexual functioning, and psychosocial status in women who underwent bariatric surgery. Obes Surg. 2018;28(4):892–9. https://doi.org/10.1007/s11695-017-3025-7.

23. Vilallonga R, Himpens J, van de Vrande S. Long-term (7 years) follow-up of Roux-en-Y gastric bypass on obese adolescent patients (<18 Years). Obes Facts. 2016;9(2):91–100. https://doi.org/10.1159/000442758.
24. Wax JR, Cartin A, Wolff R, et al. Pregnancy following gastric bypass for morbid obesity: effect of surgery-to-conception interval on maternal and neonatal outcomes. Obes Surg. 2008;18:1517–21. https://doi.org/10.1007/s11695-008-9647-z.
25. Rottenstreich A, Levin G, Kleinstern G, et al. The effect of surgery-to-conception interval on pregnancy outcomes after sleeve gastrectomy. Surg Obes Relat Dis. 2018;14(12):1795–803. https://doi.org/10.1016/j.soard.2018.09.485.
26. Johansson K, Cnattingius S, Näslund I, et al. Outcomes of pregnancy after bariatric surgery. N Engl J Med. 2015;372(9):814–24. https://doi.org/10.1056/NEJMoa1405789.
27. Parent B, Martopullo I, Weiss NS, et al. Bariatric surgery in women of childbearing age, timing between an operation and birth, and associated perinatal complications. JAMA Surg. 2017;152(2):128–35. https://doi.org/10.1001/jamasurg.2016.3621.
28. Costa MM, Belo S, Souteiro P, Neves JS, et al. Pregnancy after bariatric surgery: maternal and fetal outcomes of 39 pregnancies and a literature review. J Obstet Gynaecol Res. 2018;44(4):681–90. https://doi.org/10.1111/jog.13574.
29. Belogolovkin V, Salihu HM, Weldeselasse H, et al. Impact of prior bariatric surgery on maternal and fetal outcomes among obese and non-obesemothers. Arch Gynecol Obstet. 2012;285(5):1211–8. https://doi.org/10.1007/s00404-011-2134-0.
30. Benhalima K, Minschart C, Ceulemans D, et al. Screening and management of gestational diabetes mellitus after bariatric surgery. Nutrients. 2018;10(10):E1479. https://doi.org/10.3390/nu10101479.
31. Rottenstreich A, Elazary R, Ezra Y, et al. Hypoglycemia during oral glucose tolerance test among post-bariatric surgery pregnant patients: incidence and perinatal significance. Surg Obes Relat Dis. 2018;14(3):347–53. https://doi.org/10.1016/j.soard.2017.11.031.
32. Benjamin RH, Littlejohn S, Mitchell LE. Bariatric surgery and birth defects: a systematic literature review. Paediatr Perinat Epidemiol. 2018;32(6):533–44. https://doi.org/10.1111/ppe.12517.
33. Shankar P, Boylan M, Sriram K. Micronutrient deficiencies after bariatric surgery. Nutrition. 2010;26(11–12):1031–7. https://doi.org/10.1016/j.nut.2009.12.003.
34. Slater C, Morris L, Ellison J, Syed AA. Nutrition in pregnancy following bariatric surgery. Nutrients. 2017;9(12):E1338. https://doi.org/10.3390/nu9121338.
35. Hazart J, Le Guennec D, Accoceberry M, et al. Maternal nutritional deficiencies and small-for-gestational-age neonates at birth of women who have undergone bariatric surgery. J Pregnancy. 2017;2017:4168541. https://doi.org/10.1155/2017/4168541.
36. Gascoin G, Gerard M, Sallé A, et al. Risk of low birth weight and micronutrient deficiencies in neonates from mothers after gastric bypass: a case control study. Surg Obes Relat Dis. 2017;13(8):1384–91. https://doi.org/10.1016/j.soard.2017.03.017.
37. Cruz S, Machado S, Cruz S, et al. Comparative study of the nutritional status of vitamin A in pregnant women and in women who became pregnant or did not after Roux-en-Y gastric bypass. Nutr Hosp. 2018;35(2):421–7. https://doi.org/10.20960/nh.1302.
38. Meldrum D. Introduction: obesity and fertility. Fertil Steril. 2017;107(4):0015–282. https://doi.org/10.1016/j.fertnstert.2017.02.110.
39. Calderón B, Gómez-Martín JM, Vega-Piñero B, Martín-Hidalgo A, Galindo J, Luque-Ramírez M, Escobar-Morreale HF, Botella-Carretero JI. Prevalence of male secondary hypogonadism in moderate to severe obesity and its relationship with insulin resistance and excess body weight. Andrology. 2016;4:62–7. https://doi.org/10.1111/andr.12135.
40. Hofstra J, Loves S, van Wageningen B, Ruinemans-Koerts J, Jansen I, de Boer H. High prevalence of hypogonadotropic hypogonadism in men referred for obesity treatment. Neth J Med. 2008;66:103–9.
41. Calderón B, Galdón A, Calañas A, Peromingo R, Galindo J, García-Moreno F, Rodriguez-Velasco G, Martín-Hidalgo A, Vazquez C, Escobar-Morreale HF, Botella-Carretero JI. Effects

of bariatric surgery on male obesity-associated secondary hypogonadism: comparison of laparoscopic gastric bypass with restrictive procedures. Obes Surg. 2014;24(10):1686–92. https://doi.org/10.1007/s11695-014-1233-y.

42. Paasch U, Grunewald S, Kratzsch J, Glander HJ. Obesity and age affect male fertility potential. Fertil Steril. 2010;94(7):2898–901. https://doi.org/10.1016/j.fertnstert.2010.06.047.
43. Corona G, Rastrelli G, Monami M, Saad F, Luconi M, Lucchese M, Facchiano E, Sforza A, Forti G, Mannucci E, Maggi M. Body weight loss reverts obesity-associated hypogonadotropic hypogonadism: a systematic review and meta-analysis. Eur J Endocrinol. 2013;168(6):829–43. https://eje.bioscientifica.com/view/journals/eje/168/6/829.xml
44. Rosenblatt A, et al. Sexual hormones and erectile function more than 6 years after bariatric surgery. Surg Obes Relat Dis. 2013;9(5):636–40. https://doi.org/10.1016/j.soard.2012.06.010.
45. Samavat J, Natali I, Degl'Innocenti S, Filimberti E, Cantini G, Di Franco A, Danza G, Seghieri G, Lucchese M, Baldi E, Forti G, Luconi M. Acrosome reaction is impaired in spermatozoa of obese men: a preliminary study. Fertil Steril. 2014;102(5):1274–1281.e2. https://doi.org/10.1016/j.fertnstert.2014.07.1248.
46. Campbell JM, Lane M, Owens JA, Bakos HW. Paternal obesity negatively affects male fertility and assisted reproduction outcomes: a systematic review and meta-analysis. Reprod BioMed Online. 2015;31(5):593–604. https://doi.org/10.1016/j.rbmo.2015.07.012.
47. di Frega AS, Dale B, Di Matteo L, Wilding M. Secondary male factor infertility after Roux-en-Y gastric bypass for morbid obesity: case report. Hum Reprod. 2005;20(4):997–8.
48. Sermondade N, Massin N, Boitrelle F, Pfeffer J, Eustache F, Sifer C, Czernichow S, Lévy R. Sperm parameters and male fertility after bariatric surgery: three case series. Reprod BioMed Online. 2012;24(2):206–10. https://doi.org/10.1016/j.rbmo.2011.10.014.
49. Legro RS, Kunselman AR, Meadows JW, Kesner JS, Krieg EF, Rogers AM, Cooney RN. Time-related increase in urinary testosterone levels and stable semen analysis parameters after bariatric surgery in men. Reprod BioMed Online. 2015;30(2):150–6. https://doi.org/10.1016/j.rbmo.2014.
50. El Bardisi H, Majzoub A, Arafa M, AlMalki A, Al Said S, Khalafalla K, Jabbour G, Basha M, Al Ansari A, Sabanegh E Jr. Effect of bariatric surgery on semen parameters and sex hormone concentrations: a prospective study. Reprod BioMed Online. 2016;33(5):606–11. https://doi.org/10.1016/j.rbmo.2016.08.008.
51. Samavat J, Cantini G, Lotti F, Di Franco A, Tamburrino L, Degl'Innocenti S, Maseroli E, Filimberti E, Facchiano E, Lucchese M, Muratori M, Forti G, Baldi E, Maggi M, Luconi M. Massive weight loss obtained by bariatric surgery affects semen quality in morbid male obesity: a preliminary prospective double-armed study. Obes Surg. 2018;28(1):69–76. https://doi.org/10.1007/s11695-017-2802-7.
52. Carette C, Levy R, Eustache F, Baron G, Coupaye M, Msika S, Barrat C, Cohen R, Catheline JM, Brugnon F, Slim K, Barsamian C, Chevallier JM, Bretault M, Bouillot JL, Antignac JP, Rives-Lange C, Ravaud P, Czernichow S. Changes in total sperm count after gastric bypass and sleeve gastrectomy: the BARIASPERM prospective study. Surg Obes Relat Dis. 2019;15(8):1271–9. https://doi.org/10.1016/j.soard.2019.04.019.
53. Reis LO, Zani EL, Saad RD, Chaim EA, de Oliveira LC, Fregonesi A. Bariatric surgery does not interfere with sperm quality—a preliminary long-term study. Reprod Sci. 2012;19(10):1057–62. https://doi.org/10.1177/1933719112440747.
54. O'Leary MP, Fowler FJ, Lenderking WR, Barber B, Sagnier PP, Guess HA, Barry MJ. A brief male sexual function inventory for urology. Urology. 1995;46(5):697–706.
55. Rosen RC, Riley A, Wagner G, Osterloh IH, Kirkpatrick J, Mishra A. The international index of erectile dysfunction (IIEF): a multidimensional scale for assessment of erectile dysfunction. Urology. 1997;49:822–30.
56. Rosen RC, Cappelleri JC, Smith MD, et al. Development and evaluation of an abridged, 5-item version of the International Index of Erectile Function (IIEF-5) as a diagnostic tool for erectile dysfunction. Int J Impot Res. 1999;11:319–26.

57. Janik MR, Bielecka I, Kwiatkowski A, Janik PE, Drazba T, Bujok J, Stanowski E, Paśnik K. Cross-sectional study of male sexual function in bariatric patients. Wideochir Inne Tech Maloinwazyjne. 2016;11(3):171–7.
58. Steffen KJ, King WC, White GE, Subak LL, Mitchell JE, Courcoulas AP, Flum DR, Strain G, Sarwer DB, Kolotkin RL, Pories W, Huang AJ. Changes in sexual functioning in women and men in the 5 years after bariatric surgery. JAMA Surg. 2019;154(6):487–98. https://doi.org/10.1001/jamasurg.2018.1162.
59. Feldman HA, Johannes CB, Derby CA, Kleinman KP, Mohr BA, Araujo AB, McKinlay JB. Erectile dysfunction and coronary risk factors: prospective results from the Massachusetts male aging study. Prev Med. 2000;30(4):328–38.
60. Choi YS, Lee SK, Bae WJ, Kim SJ, Cho HJ, Hong SH, Lee JY, Hwang TK, Kim SW. Bariatric surgery improves the cavernosal neuronal, vasorelaxation, and contraction mechanisms for erectile dysfunction as result of amelioration of glucose homeostasis in a diabetic rat model. PLoS One. 2014;9(8):e104042. https://doi.org/10.1371/journal.pone.0104042.
61. Esposito K, Giugliano F, Di Palo C, Giugliano G, Marfella R, D'Andrea F, D'Armiento M, Giugliano D. Effect of lifestyle changes on erectile dysfunction in obese men. A randomized controlled trial. JAMA. 2004;291(24):2978–84.
62. Moran LJ, Brinkworth GD, Martin S, Wycherley TP, Stuckey B, Lutze J, Clifton PM, Wittert GA, Noakes M. Long-term effects of a randomised controlled trial comparing high protein or high carbohydrate weight loss diets on testosterone, SHBG, erectile and urinary function in overweight and obese men. PLoS One. 2016;11(9):e0161297. https://doi.org/10.1371/journal.pone.0161297.
63. Dallal RM, Chernoff A, O'Leary MP, Smith JA, Braverman JD, Quebbemann BB. Sexual dysfunction is common in the morbidly obese male and improves after gastric bypass surgery. J Am Coll Surg. 2008;207(6):859–64. https://doi.org/10.1016/j.jamcollsurg.2008.08.006.
64. Groutz A, Gordon D, Schachter P, Amir H, Shimonov M. Effects of bariatric surgery on male lower urinary symptoms and sexual function. Neurourol Urodyn. 2017;36(3):636–9. https://doi.org/10.1002/nau.22980.
65. Kun L, Pin Z, Jianzhong D, Xiaodong H, Haoyong Y, Yuqian B, Hongwei Z. Significant improvement of erectile function after Roux-en-Y gastric bypass surgery in obese Chinese men with erectile dysfunction. Obes Surg. 2015;25(5):838–44. https://doi.org/10.1007/s11695-014-1465-x.
66. Mahawar KK, Bhasker AG, Bindal V, Graham Y, Dudeja U, Lakdawala M, Small PK. Zinc deficiency after gastric bypass for morbid obesity: a systematic review. Obes Surg. 2017;27(2):522–9. https://doi.org/10.1007/s11695-016-2474-8.

Hair Skin and Nail Related Complications After Bariatric Surgery

16

Rinky Kapoor, Sapna Vadera, Shiva Ram Male, and Debraj Shome

> *You can trace every sickness, every disease and every ailment to a mineral deficiency.*
>
> *—Dr. Linus Pauling.*

16.1 Introduction

Obesity is a major global public health issue. Apart from leading to multiple chronic health diseases, increasing morbidity, and decreasing quality of life, obesity also results in reduced overall life expectancy [1]. At present, bariatric surgery is the most effective treatment option for morbid obesity [2] and multiple surgical procedures are currently available including laparoscopic adjustable gastric banding (LAGB), laparoscopic Roux-en-Y gastric bypass (RYGB), laparoscopic sleeve gastrectomy (LSG), single-anastomosis gastric bypass and laparoscopic biliopancreatic diversion with (BPD-DS) or without (BPD) duodenal switch [3, 4].

R. Kapoor
Department of Dermatology, Cosmetic Dermatology and Dermato-Surgery, The Esthetic Clinics, Mumbai, India
e-mail: rinky.kapoor@theestheticclinic.com

S. Vadera · D. Shome (✉)
Department of Facial Plastic Surgery & Facial Cosmetic Surgery & Director, The Esthetic Clinics, Mumbai, India
e-mail: debraj.shome@theestheticclinic.com

S. R. Male
Optometry and Vision Sciences, School of Medical sciences, University of Hyderabad, Hyderabad, India

A. G. Bhasker et al. (eds.), *Management of Nutritional and Metabolic Complications of Bariatric Surgery*,
https://doi.org/10.1007/978-981-33-4702-1_16

Post any bariatric procedure, it is of prime importance to prevent nutritional deficiencies, prescribe appropriate supplementation, screen, and recognize the symptoms of deficiencies, and treat them appropriately if they emerge postoperatively [5]. Studies have also shown that adhering to a regular nutritional follow-up not only contributes to weight reduction post-surgery but helps in preventing further weight regain [5–7].

This is a review of current literature relating to hair, skin, and nail related complications in bariatric patients and how to prevent and treat them.

16.2 Incidence and Prevalence

As per WHO statistics, 2014, 13% of the world's adult population (>600 million people) were categorized as obese. Obesity is also on the rise in the adolescent population. Although less common compared to adults, the incidence of bariatric surgery has significantly increased amongst adolescents with severe obesity, rising fivefold between 1997 and 2003 [5]. It has also been reported in literature that complications related to Hair, Skin, and Nails are higher in adolescents suffering from obesity. Increased incidence of obesity is noted in individuals suffering from androgenetic alopecia (which occurs before 35 years of age) [8]. These adolescent bariatric patients require a close follow-up, specifically due to the non-adherence to recommended supplementation and also because of the anticipated longer life span with altered digestive physiology compared to adult bariatric patients [9].

16.3 Pathophysiology

16.3.1 Obesity and Pre-existing Nutritional Deficiencies

Obesity is usually considered as a state of overnutrition; however it has been recognized as a major risk factor for several nutrient deficiencies, including lower levels of antioxidants and certain fat-soluble vitamins. A wider variety of pre-existing nutritional deficiencies have been identified in morbidly obese adults undergoing bariatric surgery. This is due to a high intake of calorie-rich processed foods with poor nutritional quality. This is more common in developed countries, where there is an abundance of relatively cheap, energy-dense, but nutrient-poor food. On an average, 27–30% of the daily caloric intake of an American children and adults is composed of low-nutrient density food, accompanied by sweeteners and desserts contributing 18–24% of the total diet [10, 11]. The unprocessed nutrient-dense foods like fruits and vegetables, whole grains, dairy products, fish and protein sources, nuts, and legumes contribute to the bulk of vitamins and minerals obtained from a non-supplemented diet. The increase in the intake of nutrient-poor food contributes proportionately to the decrease in the intake of unprocessed, nutrient-dense foods [10].

Diets rich in fats (more than 30% of total caloric intake) are associated with decreased intake of folate, vitamins A, and vitamin C [12]. Similarly, increased intake of sweetened beverages also correlates with lower intake of milk, and therefore calcium and fortified vitamin D. The additional factors leading to Vitamin D3 deficiency include reduced physical activity, leading to decreased sun exposure, increased storage of vitamin D3 in excess adipose tissue, ethnicity, and skin tone [13].

Bariatric surgery is a further contributory to nutritional deficiencies in morbidly obese adolescents and adults [5, 14]. Although surgery can exacerbate pre-existing nutrient deficiencies, preoperative screening related to vitamin deficiencies has not been the norm in the majority of weight loss surgery (WLS) practices [13]. Screening is important because it is common for patients who present for WLS to have at least one vitamin or mineral deficiency preoperatively [13].

16.3.2 Pathophysiology of Metabolic Complications Post-Bariatric Surgery

All types of bariatric surgery lead to the reduction in total calorie intake, especially in the first 6 months postoperatively. These disorders are derived not only from inadequate food intake but also from the changes in the digestive system's anatomy and high levels of oxidative stress that interferes with the absorptive process. This can contribute to the decreased intake of all macronutrients and micronutrients, resulting in clinical deficiencies eventually [15–17].

One of the commonest fears of bariatric surgery patients is postoperative hair loss. Other issues related to skin and nails may arise long-term. For this reason, nutrition can have a great impact on hair, skin, and nail health because when forced to make a choice, the body will shift nutritional stores to vital organs like the brain and heart and away from the hair, skin, and nails [18].

16.3.3 Bariatric Surgery and Hair

16.3.3.1 Hair Growth Cycle

For most of our lives, hair growth and hair loss is a constant process. Human hair follicles have two states, anagen; a growth phase and telogen; a dormant or resting phase. All hair begins their life in the anagen phase, grows for some period of time, and then shifts into the telogen phase which lasts for about 100–120 days. Following this, the hair will fall out. At any given point of time, about 90% of hair are in the Anagen phase (in a growing phase) and 10% are in the Telogen phase (in a dormant or resting phase). This means that normally loss of hair is very less compared to hair growth, preventing noticeable hair loss [19–21].

However, specific types of stress can result in a shift of a much greater percentage of hairs into the telogen phase. The factors known to result in this shift or telogen effluvium include; high fever, severe infection, major surgery, acute physical trauma, chronic debilitating illness (such as cancer or end-stage liver disease), hormonal disruption (such as pregnancy, childbirth, or discontinuation of estrogen therapy), acute weight loss, crash dieting, anorexia, low protein intake, iron or zinc deficiency, heavy metal toxicity, some medications (such as beta-blockers, anticoagulants, retinoid, and immunizations). The most common type of hair loss after weight loss surgery is a diffuse loss known medically as telogen effluvium, which can have both nutritional and non-nutritional aspects [19–22].

16.3.3.2 Weight Loss Surgery and Hair Loss Association

Two major consequences of bariatric surgery include nutritional deficiencies and rapid weight loss. These alone are likely to account for much of the hair loss seen after surgery. In the absence of a nutritional issue, hair loss will continue until all hair that has shifted into the telogen phase has fallen out. There is no way of switching them back to the anagen phase. The hair loss rarely lasts for more than 6 months in the absence of a dietary cause as the hair follicles are not damaged in telogen effluvium, hair should then regrow. For this reason, most doctors can assure their weight loss surgery patients that with time and patience, and keeping up good nutritional intake, their hair will grow back. Discrete nutritional deficiencies are known to cause and contribute to telogen effluvium. One would be more suspicious of a nutritional contribution to post-bariatric surgery hair loss, only if hair loss continued for more than 1 year after surgery, hair loss started more than 6 months after surgery, patients' present with eating difficulty and/or has not complied with supplementation and also demonstrated low values of ferritin and zinc [23, 24].

The micronutrients whose absence may lead to hair-related complications (Figs. 16.1, 16.2 and 16.3) include Vitamins (A, B2, B5, B6, B9, C, D, E, K) Biotin, Copper, Iron, Selenium, Zinc, and Proteins. All the hair-related manifestations related to the abovementioned micronutrients post-Bariatric Surgery have been mentioned in Table 16.1 [16, 25].

16.3.4 Bariatric Surgery and Skin

16.3.4.1 Obesity and Its Effect on Skin

Obesity is known for its effects on the skin. It is associated with altered structure and content of collagen, greater transepidermal water loss, increased skin infections, and poor wound healing. Moreover, most obese patients suffer from acne and hirsutism, due to increased androgen production secondary to elevated insulin levels. Furthermore, certain dermatoses such as psoriasis, keratosis pilaris, seborrheic dermatitis, lichen sclerosis, scleroderma, livedo reticularis, granular parakeratosis, and others have also been attributed to obesity. Interestingly, various cutaneous complications have been reported in association with bariatric surgery for morbid obesity as well as a change in the course of many dermatoses from the previous studies [26]. Also, morbidly obese person suffers from several nutritional deficiencies often resulting in Nutritional Deficiency Dermatoses. As mentioned earlier, nutritional deficiencies are further increased following bariatric surgery owing to

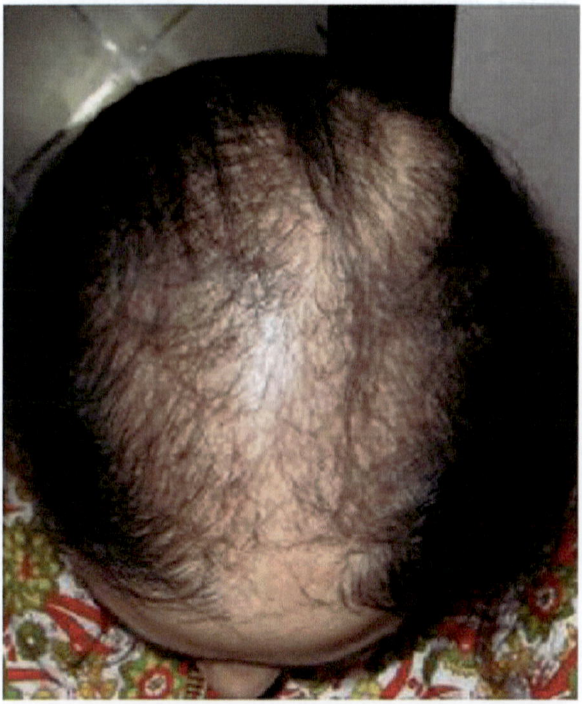

Fig. 16.1 Brittle hair due to deficiency of vitamin A or retinol

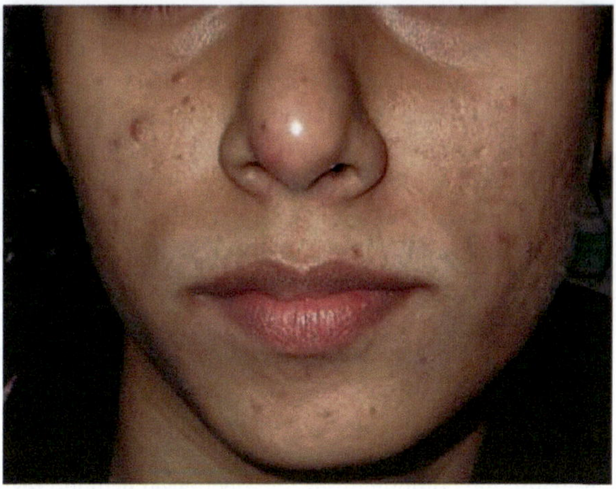

Fig. 16.2 Patient with acne due to deficiency of vitamin A or retinol

the restrictive, malabsorptive, or combined nature of the procedures [27]. Previous studies by Xanthakos, S. A. reported that out of 170 patients, 69% of patients were deficient in vitamin A (retinol) and 63% were deficient in vitamin D (calciferol), 4 years post-surgery [25].

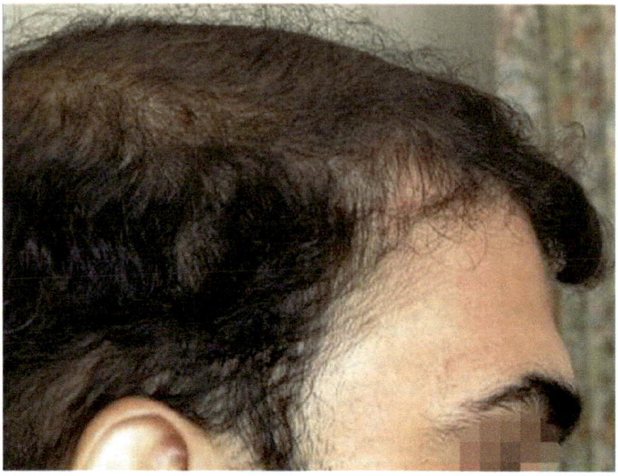

Fig. 16.3 Patient with alopecia having biotin deficiency

The micronutrients whose absence may lead to cutaneous manifestations include: Vitamins (A, B2, B5, B6, B9, C, D, E, K) Biotin, Copper, Iron, Selenium, Zinc, and Proteins. All the cutaneous manifestations related to the abovementioned micronutrients post-Bariatric Surgery have been mentioned in Table 16.1 [16, 25].

As a result of such anticipated deficiency, post-bariatric patients are routinely prescribed dietary supplements like milk, fruits, and rich polysaccharide foods as well as additional supplements like retinoic acid, biotin, protein, zinc, and copper to compensate for what they may lack later [28].

16.3.4.2 Weight Loss Surgery and Dermatologic Complications

After BS, there is a decrease in the concentration of heparan sulfate and perlecan and increase in type III collagen in patients' skin. Heparan sulfate is the main component of the nucleus where it is attached to various proteins. It is also present on the cell surface and extracellular matrix-like basement membrane. It plays a major role in biological activities like cell proliferation, hemostasis, inflammation, and angiogenesis to name a few. Perlecan is a prime component of the basement membrane where it interacts with growth factors such as vascular endothelial growth factor (VEGF)-A, and is considered essential for epidermal formation [29–31].

Type III is an immature collagen and is associated with poor healing capacity. Studies have shown, damage in the components of extracellular matrix specifically collagen and elastin fibers after bariatric surgery. Xing et al. in his immunofluorescence study demonstrated an increase in the expression of type III collagen in the skin of patients after bariatric surgery. All these changes lead to a higher rate of dermatologic complications and decreased esthetic results [29].

Apart from the above mentioned issues, bariatric surgery leads to large amount of redundant skin after surgery. This shows negative effects in almost 90% of the patients. This further adds to the functional problem, dermatosis, difficulty in maintaining hygiene, and most importantly the esthetic outcome [15, 16, 31].

Table 16.1 Nutrient deficiency and skin, hair, and nail related manifestations

Nutrient	Manifestations related to deficiency		
	Skin	Hair	Nails
Vitamin A or retinol	Xeroderma, acne, and keratotic follicular papules (in the anterolateral surface of thighs and arms, can also involve the extensor areas of the upper and lower limbs, shoulders, abdomen, dorsal region, buttocks, and neck), phrynoderma	Brittle hair	
Vitamin B2 or riboflavin	Mucositis, lip and angular cheilitis, glossitis, xerosis, seborrheic dermatitis, erythroderma scrotal, vulvar eczema, and toxic epidermal necrolysis.	Hair dandruff	
Vitamin B3 or niacin	Cheilitis, glossitis, Pellagra, photosensitive dermatitis in symmetric areas		
Vitamin B5 or pantothenic acid	Purpura, seborrheic dermatitis, angular stomatitis, and glossitis. Burning feet syndrome.	Leukotrichia (whitening of hair) Hair dandruff	
Vitamin B6 or Pyridoxine	Glossitis, oral mucosa ulceration, lip and angular cheilitis, Seborrheic dermatitis, photosensitive pellagra-like lesions	Hair dandruff	
Vitamin B9 or folic acid and B12 or cobalamin	Lip or angular cheilitis, Hunter's glossitis; mucocutaneous hypo- and hyperpigmentation		
Vitamin C or ascorbic acid	Poor wound healing, perifollicular petechiae, ecchymosis, keratosis pilaris purpura, scurvy (gingivitis, bleeding gums, keratosis pilaris), Sjögren-like syndrome	Brittle hair	
Vitamin D	Atopic dermatitis, acne, skin infections, psoriasis, autoimmune cutaneous diseases and skin cancer.		
Vitamin E	Atopic dermatitis, acne		
Vitamin K	Purpura, petechiae, ecchymosis, hematoma		
Biotin	Glossitis, keratosis pilaris, periorificial dermatitis, seborrheic dermatitis and erythroderma	Alopecia, hair dandruff, depigmented hair	

(continued)

Table 16.1 (continued)

Nutrient	Manifestations related to deficiency		
	Skin	Hair	Nails
Copper	Delayed wound healing Hypopigmentation of skin	Hypopigmentation of hair, thinning of hair and alopecia	Hypopigmentation of nails
Iron	Pallor, glossitis	Alopecia	Koilonychias (spoon-shaped nails) Onychorrhexis (ridges across the length of the nail Brittle nails
Selenium	Delayed wound healing, psoriasis, skin cancer		
Zinc	Acrodermatitis enteropathica (alopecia, acral, and periorificial symmetric, erosive and eczematous rash), delayed wound healing, stomatitis, psoriasiform dermatitis, blepharitis, angular cheilitis, vitiligo-like lesions	Dry, brittle hair and thinning hair	Paronychia (tender bacterial or fungal infection at the base of finger or toe nail) Beau lines (horizontal and vertical depression on the nail beds)
Protein	Aged appearance, erythematous, or hypopigmented lesions most evident in flexure Areas; hyperchromic lesions with smooth, fissured, or erosive surface; brittle, slow Growing nails, onychomadesis; follicular hyperkeratosis, pale extremities accompanied By edema; dry, brittle, dull, and thin hair, with brownish-red color before becoming Grayish-white, flag signal with alternating dark and light stripes in the hair Angular cheilitis, xerophthalmia, stomatitis, vulvovaginitis		Beau lines (horizontal and vertical depression on the nail beds)

16.3.4.3 Psoriasis and Bariatric Surgery

Some skin diseases associated with Obesity often show improvement post-Bariatric Surgery. Psoriasis is one of the chronic inflammatory disorders of the skin, which is more frequent and severe in obese patients. Several studies have reported and explained improvement in psoriasis after bariatric surgery. In a report by Farias, M. M et al. almost two-third of patients with psoriasis reported a postoperative improvement in psoriasis after undergoing weight loss surgery. It is postulated that the improvement is secondary to increased levels of glucagon-like peptide-1 (GLP-produced by the intestine. The level of GLP-1 may increase up to 20 times after gastric bypass surgery. Also, as this hormone is not hypersecreted after a purely restrictive gastric reduction, so the treatment with gastric band does not lead to the improvement of the disease [32].

16.3.4.4 Necrobiosis Lipoidica and Bariatric Surgery

Diabetes mellitus type 2 (DM2) is one of the most important comorbidities associated with obesity. It is a known fact that DM2 shows improvement after Bariatric Surgery and hence the latter is often called as "a metabolic surgery." Necrobiosis lipoidica (NL) is a dermatosis condition most often associated with diabetes and is characterized by single or multiple atrophic, granulomatous and erythematous-brownish lesions located commonly in the pretibial region. Although the precise etiology remains unknown. Reports from the literature suggest remission of NL post-bariatric surgery [33].

16.3.5 Bariatric Surgery and Nails

The nail unit is the invagination of the epidermis into the dermis. It mostly consists of a fully keratinized structure called as the nail plate and the tissues surrounding it. It is formed as a result of maturation and differentiation of the epithelial nail matrix cells, firmly attaching itself to the nail bed, and partially contributing to its formation. The nail bed is the structure upon which the nail rests. The blood-filled vascular network that is visible through the translucent plate, makes the nail bed appear pink in color. One-fifth of the thin horny layer which forms the ventral nail plate is produced by the nail bed keratinization. One of the most important functions of the fingernails is to enhance tactile discrimination and fine movements. Toe nails help in protecting the distal toes and contribute to pedal biomechanics. Apart from this, the nails have a significant contribution towards the esthetic appearance of the hand and foot [22, 34].

After bariatric surgery, malabsorption, lack of micronutrients, and lack of nutrition affect the health and beauty of nails. Nails start developing problems with the color, shape, texture, or thickness of the fingernails or toenails. One can see the horizontal and transverse depressions in the nail plate called as the Beau lines. These lines can occur after illness, injury to the nail, eczema around the nail, during chemotherapy for cancer, or because of the lack of proper nutrition. The appearance of these lines immediately after a bariatric surgery can be attributed to the deficiency of proteins and zinc in the postoperative phase. Beau lines are often confused with vertical ridges called as *Onychorrhexis* which are present across the length of the nail. Onychorrhexis and brittle nails are often a normal result of aging. They are seen in conditions like Raynaud's disease and hypothyroidism. The presence of brittle nails after a bariatric surgery indicates the deficiency of Iron. The deficiency of iron is also reflected in the form of Koilonychias. It results in thinning and upward curving of nail accompanied by raised ridges, giving a typical appearance of Spoon.

All nail related findings and the nutrients contributing to its appearance have been mentioned in chart 1 [35, 36].

16.4 Diagnosis

- Androgenetic Alopecia/Telogen effluvium might already be present and can aggravate postoperatively. Hair pull test can be done to diagnose this. To perform this test, the investigator grasps around 50–60 hairs between the thumb, the index, and the middle fingers as close to the scalp skin as possible. The hairs are pulled gently but firmly from proximal to distal ends. The test is considered positive if three or more hair are pulled out.
- Each bariatric unit has its own protocol for preoperative and postoperative screening of vitamins and minerals. Serum levels of vitamin D3 and B12 and calcium levels are commonly assessed.
- A low threshold for investigation of vitamins like thiamine and trace minerals like copper and zinc depending on clinical manifestations of hair/skin/nail complications.

16.5 Management

16.5.1 Nutritional Supplementation After Bariatric Surgeries

The nutritional care post any bariatric patient is a fine balance between bariatric diet protocols and individual postoperative dietary tolerances. The prime role of the dietician in postoperative bariatric care should be the establishment of a proper bariatric diet protocol based on individual tolerances, lifestyles, and nutritional requirements [35]. The main focus of the nutritional care after bariatric surgery should be to provide adequate energy and to support postoperative tissue healing and preservation of lean body mass during rapid weight loss. Although the protocols are surgeon specific, it may vary as per the progression of diet stages.

However, there are certain common nutritional goals [37]:

- Maximize weight loss and absorption of nutrients
- Maintain adequate hydration
- Avoid vomiting and dumping syndrome

16.5.2 Role of Dermatologist

The role of dermatologist is very crucial in maintaining the esthetics and skin health of the patient in the postoperative phase. For tackling and managing the hair, skin, and nail related issues in the post-surgical phase, the dermatologist must keep a track of the below-mentioned points [38]:

1. Anamnesis data: type of surgery performed (restrictive or not), current nutritional therapy, general symptoms (e.g., weakness, diarrhea, vomiting, neurological disorders, bleeding) history of recurrent cutaneous infections.
2. Physical exam data: complete examination of the skin, mucosa and hair and nails.
3. Educational sessions with the patient explaining to them the importance of personal hygiene cares on redundant skin.
4. Routine prescriptions of moisturizers for hydration of skin, since there are many deficiencies that can lead to xeroderma.
5. The recommended level of micronutrient supplementation has been discussed in another chapter previously.

16.5.2.1 Hair Fall Treatment

1. Topical Minoxidil:

   Minoxidil is a piperidinopyrimidine derivative which is available in the concentration of 2% and 5% solution. Although the role of Minoxidil in telogen effluvium is not clearly understood, it is considered to have mitogenic, nonhormonal effect on the epidermal cells which in turn prolongs the survival time. It prolongs the anagen phase and stimulates telogen hairs to re-enter anagen. It also enlarges miniaturized hair follicles. Topical minoxidil is less likely to fasten the regrowth in cases of acute TE because of an isolated or treatable inciting factor. However, it works well in cases of chronic TE where it maintains hair density and encourages new hair regrowth. Minoxidil 2% is applied twice daily or 5% minoxidil applied once daily to the entire scalp in women, and 5% is applied twice daily in men. Results are visible only after 6–12 months of use. Also, prior to initiating topical minoxidil, the patient should be informed about the increased hair shedding within 2–8 weeks of initiating treatment. As the dormant telogen follicles which are stimulated to re-enter anagen push out old club hair. Patients often perceive this as worsening of their condition which often leads to the cessation of the treatment. This positive sign indicates anagen induction with earlier "molting" of telogen hairs from the follicles [10, 39].
2. Platelet-Rich Plasma:

   Platelet-rich plasma (PRP) is an autogenous, liquid, platelet concentrate which is extracted from a patient's own peripheral blood by a centrifugation process. Because of the autologous nature of the blood the risk of hypersensitivity or immunogenic reactions and disease transmission is significantly reduced. The platelets and growth factors found in the PRP slurry are in 1.2- to 9-fold higher in concentration per volume, when compared with a patient's whole blood. When injected, the platelets release alpha granules containing multiple growth factors, including platelet-derived growth factor (PDGF), epidermal growth factor (EGF), transforming growth factor-ß (TGF-ß), vascular endothelial growth factor (VEGF), basic fibroblast growth factor (bFGF) and insulin-like growth factor-1 (IGF-1).

   These growth factors (GFs) stimulate hair regrowth by multiple pathways including Wnt/β-catenin signaling and activation of extracellular signal-regulated kinase and protein kinase B (Akt) signaling. As a consequence, PRP increases dermal papilla proliferation and cell survival and also upregulates the telogen-anagen transition.

There are multiple methods through which PRP can be obtained, but none of them is standardized till date. Usually, blood is drawn by venipuncture in a tube containing anticoagulant (sodium citrate or EDTA). The tube is then centrifuged for one or two cycles. After which three distinct layers are obtained (from top to bottom): platelet-poor plasma (PPP); buffy coat (BC), rich in platelets and white blood cells; and red blood cells. At times, a second cycle is recommended using PPP and BC. The second centrifugation results in a final product with a higher concentration of platelets—PRP. Depending on the protocol, PPP plus BC (one cycle) or PRP (two cycles) can be used for hair loss treatment.

Despite the plethora of literature on PRP, there is no fixed validated protocol regarding its centrifugation process. There are no guidelines to define the amount of solution to be injected per session or the total number of sessions required. Moreover, the entire procedure is cumbersome and its tedious to draw patient's blood at every visit, further adding to the cost of the treatment [40, 41].

16.5.3 Emerging Treatments

16.5.3.1 QR678

To overcome the disadvantages of PRP, a recombinant, bioengineered, hair growth factor formulation (QR 678) hair growth factor was formulated. (US patent no. 9,700,504 and India patent no. 310925, Indian FDA approval 2019). A QR Code is a code used in medicine derived from "Quick Response" and the number 678 in Morse Code signifies "there is no answer." Hence, the formulation was named as QR 678 which signifies "Quick Response to a disease which earlier had no answer," i.e., to alopecia. It consists of IGF-1, bFGF, VEGF, Keratinocyte Growth Factor (KGF), copper tripeptide, and thymosin β4 suspended in a sterile injectable vehicle. Vascular Endothelial Growth Factor (VEGF) is for angiogenesis & vascular permeability that will help maintain the blood supply around the hair follicle during the anagen growth phase, Basic Fibroblast Growth Factor (bFGF) has been found to promote hair growth by inducing the anagen phase in resting hair follicles and has been considered to be a potential hair growth-promoting agent. Insulin-like Growth Factor-1 (IGF-1) is useful in preventing the follicle from developing catagen-like status, Keratinocyte Growth Factor (KGF), Thymosin β4 influences follicle stem cell growth, migration, differentiation, and amp; protease production and amp; Copper tripeptide 1 promotes the growth of human hair follicles [42].

Studies by Kapoor and Shome have shown 8–12 sessions of QR678 have significantly contributed in arresting the hair fall and have shown marked improvement in the growth of hair [42].

Approx. 1.5 ml QR678 at each visit is injected on the scalp skin of the patients. On an average 60–70 tiny, intradermal injections are administered through a nappage technique using an insulin syringe at 1 cm apart with a volume of 0.02 ml per injection covering the visible areas of hair thinning and alopecia. A total of eight sessions are done at an interval of 3 weeks [42].

The effect of 8–10 sessions of QR678 in male and female patients with androgenetic alopecia and telogen effluvium post-bariatric surgery are shown in Figs. 16.4 and 16.5.

16.6 Take-Home Message

Patients undergoing weight loss surgery may have hair loss, skin, and nail related changes commonly after surgery due to the lower intake and inadequate absorption of protein, iron, biotin, zinc, vitamin B12, and essential fatty acids. These changes are often distressing for the patient. Unfortunately, early hair loss post-surgery is not preventable as it is most likely caused by surgery and rapid weight loss. However, loss of hair in the later phases post-bariatric surgery is indicative of nutritional deficiency and is a very important indicative sign.

Although adequate supplementation of these patients in order to prevent complications from evolving is of prime importance, the role of counseling and educating them in the postoperative phase cannot be overlooked. Clinicians must increase

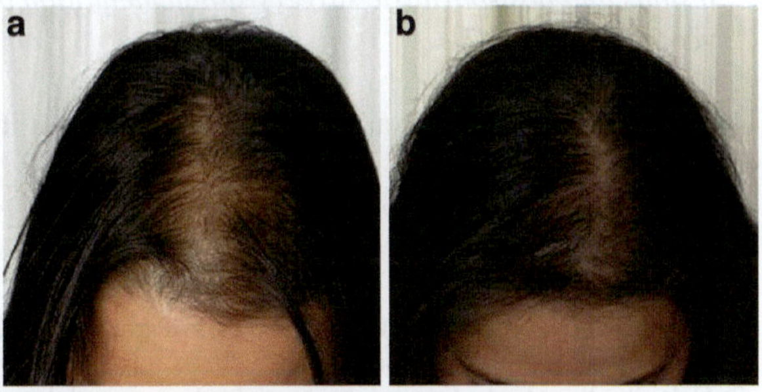

Fig. 16.4 Patient 1—Known case of Androgenetic alopecia, treated with QR 678 after bariatric surgery. (**a**) Preoperatively. (**b**) After eight sessions of QR678 (8 months postoperatively)

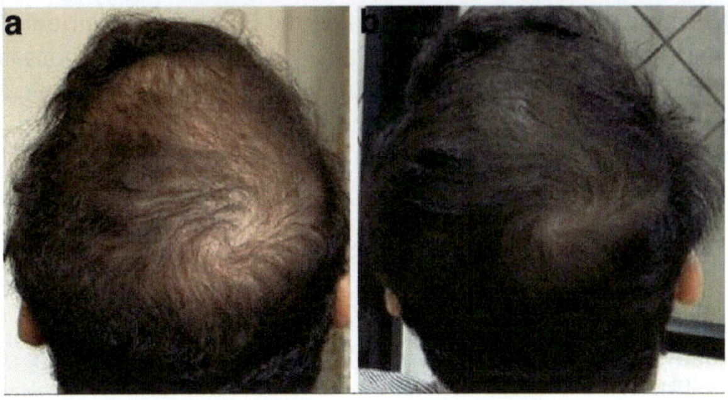

Fig. 16.5 Patient 2—Patient with male pattern hair loss—Improved after bariatric surgery followed by QR 678. (**a**) Preoperatively. (**b**) After 10 sessions of QR678 (10 months postoperatively)

their understanding of the presentation and treatment of macronutrient and micronutrient deficiencies that can arise after bariatric surgery. Recognition of these postoperative disorders will remain an ongoing educational process in these patients.

Key Points

1. *Obesity itself is associated with various hair/skin/nail manifestations as it is a state of malnutrition, and these may be exacerbated post-bariatric surgery.*
2. *Hair loss is to be expected 3–6 months after bariatric surgery due to telogen effluvium. This is usually self-limiting and in case of persistence beyond 6 months, or hair loss for more than a year, or in association with poor eating/non-compliance with supplementation, one must rule out micronutrient and vitamin deficiencies.*
3. *A number of treatment options are available in case of excessive hair loss such as topical minoxidil, platelet-rich plasma (PRP), and novel treatments like QR678.*
4. *Redundant skin is a consequence of excessive weight loss and hence almost always occurs post-bariatric surgery. Maintenance of hygiene is of prime importance as dermatoses may develop in skin folds.*
5. *Certain skin-related pathologies like psoriasis and necrobiosis lipoidica show improvement post-bariatric surgery.*
6. *Micronutrient and vitamin deficiencies can present as hair/skin/nail related lesions and post-bariatric surgery supplementation and follow-up is vital to prevent these.*

Conflict of Interests The authors state no conflict of interests.

References

1. World Health Organization. Obesity and overweight [Internet]. http://www.who.int/mediacentre/factsheets/fs311/en/. Accessed 4 Sep 2016.
2. Colquitt JL, et al. Surgery for weight loss in adults. Cochrane Database Syst Rev. 2014;8:CD003641.
3. Mechanick JI, et al. Clinical practice guidelines for the perioperative nutritional, metabolic, and nonsurgical support of the bariatric surgery patient—2013 update: cosponsored by American Association of Clinical Endocrinologists, The Obesity Society, and American Society for Metabolic & Bariatric Surgery. Obesity (Silver Spring). 2013;S1–27.
4. Lee WJ, Lin YH. Single-anastomosis gastric bypass (SAGB): appraisal of clinical evidence. Obes Surg. 2014;24:1749.
5. Schilling PL, et al. National trends in adolescent bariatric surgical procedures and implications for surgical centers of excellence. J Am Coll Surg. 2008;206:1.
6. Bloomberg RD, et al. Nutritional deficiencies following bariatric surgery: what have we learned? Obes Surg. 2005;15:145.
7. Fujioka K. Follow-up of nutritional and metabolic problems after bariatric surgery. Diabetes Care. 2005;28:481.
8. Otberg N, et al. Androgenetic alopecia. Endocrinol Metab Clin North Am. 2007;36:379.
9. Rand CS, Macgregor AM. Adolescents having obesity surgery: a 6-year followup. South Med J. 1994;87:1208.

10. Kant AK. Reported consumption of low-nutrient density foods by American children and adolescents: nutritional and health correlates, NHANES III, 1988 to 1994. Arch Pediatr Adolesc Med. 2003;157:789.
11. Kant AK. Consumption of energy-dense, nutrient-poor foods by adult Americans: nutritional and health implications. The third National Health and Nutrition Examination Survey, 1988–1994. Am J Clin Nutr. 2000;72:929.
12. Hampl JS, Betts NM. Comparisons of dietary intake and sources of fat in low- and high-fat diets of 18- to 24-year-olds. J Am Diet Assoc. 1995;95:893.
13. Keller KL, et al. Increased sweetened beverage intake is associated with reduced milk and calcium intake in 3- to 7-year-old children at multi-item laboratory lunches. J Am Diet Assoc. 2009;109:497.
14. Santry HP, et al. Trends in bariatric surgical procedures. JAMA. 2005;294:1909.
15. Neff KJH, Roux CW. Bariatric surgery. J Clin Pathol. 2013;66:90.
16. Hng KN, Ang YS. Overview of bariatric surgery for the physician. Clin Med. 2012;12:435.
17. Bavaresco M, et al. Nutritional course of patients submitted to bariatric surgery. Obes Surg. 2008. [Epub ahead of print].
18. Ruiz T, et al. Hair loss in females after sleeve gastrectomy: predictive value of serum zinc and iron levels. Am Surg. 2014;80:466.
19. Neve H, et al. Reversal of hair loss following vertical gastroplasty when treated with zinc sulphate. Obes Surg. 1996;6:63.
20. Updegraff TA, Neufeld NJ. Protein, iron, and folate status of patients prior to and following surgery for morbid obesity. J Am Diet Assoc. 1981;78:135.
21. Behrns KE, et al. Prospective evaluation of gastric acid secretion and cobalamin absorption following gastric bypass for clinically severe obesity. Dig Dis Sci. 1994;39:315.
22. Rushton DH. Clin Exp Dermatol. 2002;27:396–404.
23. Moize V, et al. Obese patients have inadequate protein intake related to protein intolerance up to 1 year following Roux-en-Y gastric bypass. Obes Surg. 2003;13:23.
24. Mock DM, et al. Nutrition in health and disease, vol. 459. 9th ed. Baltimore: Williams & Wilkins; 1999.
25. Xanthakos SA. Nutritional deficiencies in obesity and after bariatric surgery. Pediat Clin. 2009;56:1105.
26. Halawi A, et al. Bariatric surgery and its effects on the skin and skin diseases. Obes Surg. 2013;23:408.
27. Folope V, et al. Carences nutritionnelles liées à la chirurgie de l'obésité. Gastroentérologie clinique et biologique. 2007;31:369.
28. Mohapatra S, et al. Malnutrition in obesity before and after bariatric surgery, Disease-a. https://doi.org/10.1016/j.disamonth.2019.06.008.
29. Singh D, et al. Prognostication for body contouring surgery after bariatric surgery. Eplasty. 2012;12:e46.
30. Mitchell JE, et al. The desire for body contouring surgery after bariatric surgery. Obes Surg. 2008;18:1308.
31. Aldaqal SM, et al. Post-bariatric surgery satisfaction and body-contouring consideration after massive weight loss. N Am J Med Sci. 2013;5:301.
32. Jacob R, Vitamin C. In: Shils M, Olson J, Shike M, Ross AC, editors. Modern nutrition in health and disease, vol. 467. Philadelphia: Lippincott; 2000.
33. Dixon JB, et al. Bariatric surgery for type 2 diabetes. Lancet. 2012;379:2300.
34. Rossi A, et al. Hair and nail structure and function. J Appl Cosmetol. 2003;21:1.
35. Greg R. Growing beautiful fingernails after gastric bypass surgery. 2011. https://ezinearticles.com/expert/Greg_Race/529680. Accessed 27 Jul 2019.
36. Thibault R, et al. Twelve key nutritional issues in bariatric surgery. Clin Nutr. 2016;35:12. https://doi.org/10.1016/j.clnu.2015.02.012.
37. Bosnic G. Nutritional requirements after bariatric surgery. Crit Care Nurs Clin North Am. 2014;26:255.

38. Manzoni AP, Weber MB. Skin changes after bariatric surgery. Anais brasileiros de dermatologia. 2015;90:157.
39. Sinclair R. Telogen Effluvium. Alopecia. 2018;25:83.
40. Santos LD, Shapiro J. What's new in hair loss. Dermatol Clin. 2019;37:137.
41. Badran KW, Sand JP. Platelet-rich plasma for hair loss: review of methods and results. Facial Plast Surg Clin. 2018;26:469.
42. Kapoor R, Shome D. Intradermal injections of a hair growth factor formulation for enhancement of human hair regrowth–safety and efficacy evaluation in a first-in-man pilot clinical study. J Cosmetic Laser Therapy. 2018;20:369.

Ophthalmological Complications After Bariatric Surgery

17

Wee-Min Teh, Pek-Hwi Tan, and Reynu Rajan

17.1 Introduction

Bariatric surgery can have a profound impact on eye health. Without discounting the many beneficial effects of bariatric surgery [1, 2] it is important that we acknowledge the risk of developing ophthalmological complications with the potential to affect almost every component of the eye—the ocular surface (including conjunctiva and cornea), lens, retina, and optic nerve. The surgeon and multidisciplinary team must remain vigilant regarding early detection and prompt treatment of ocular complications brought about by the various perioperative factors such as prolonged duration of uncontrolled diabetes, drastic improvement of blood sugar level postoperatively, and nutritional deficiency following bariatric surgery. In this chapter, we will focus primarily on the ophthalmological complications of bariatric surgery with special interest on diabetic retinopathy, followed by ophthalmological complications brought about by nutritional deficiencies including hypovitaminosis.

W.-M. Teh
Department of Ophthalmology, Chang Gung Memorial Hospital, Taoyuan, Taiwan

Department of Ophthalmology, Hospital Melaka, Melaka, Malaysia

P.-H. Tan
Department of Ophthalmology, Hospital Tuanku Ja'afar, Seremban, Negeri Sembilan, Malaysia

R. Rajan (✉)
Department of Surgery, Faculty of Medicine, Universiti Kebangsaan Malaysia Medical Centre (UKMMC), The National University of Malaysia, Kuala Lumpur, Malaysia

A. G. Bhasker et al. (eds.), *Management of Nutritional and Metabolic Complications of Bariatric Surgery*,
https://doi.org/10.1007/978-981-33-4702-1_17

17.2 Bariatric Surgery and Diabetic Retinopathy

Diabetic retinopathy (DR) is a leading cause of vision loss in adults aged 20–74 years [3]. In 2010, of an estimated 285 million people worldwide afflicted with diabetes, more than one-third of them had signs of DR, and a third of these patients already had sight-threatening DR [defined as severe non-proliferative DR, proliferative DR, or the presence of diabetic macular edema (DME)] [4]. Among the well-established risk factors for the development of DR in cohort studies include the duration of diabetes, HbA1c levels, blood pressure, obesity, cholesterol level, and nephropathy [5–8].

The effect of bariatric surgery on weight and glycemic control has been well-documented. It has also shown a great superiority over medical therapy in inducing remission of type 2 diabetes in obese patients [1, 2]. However, glycemic levels that achieve a dramatic normalization within a short period of time may result in a paradoxical progression of DR in certain groups of patients. This is especially so if these individuals had longstanding diabetes which was poorly controlled, and if they already had preexisting DR [9, 10]. Studies as early as 30 years ago demonstrated this phenomenon of paradoxical early aggravation of DR, also known as "early worsening of diabetic retinopathy" (EWDR) when young type 1 diabetic patients with a long history of poorly controlled diabetes were initiated on intensive insulin treatment [11–13]. While this phenomenon was transient and limited in some, in others, more aggressive treatment with retinal laser photocoagulation was necessary to stem the damage that had occurred.

There are a few possible explanations for this early worsening of DR. Firstly, DR progression is not only dictated by hyperglycemia. Poor retinal perfusion as a result of microvascular damage leads to ischemia, oxidative stress, and inflammation. Kowluru found that in diabetes-induced rats, the initiation of euglycemia within 2 months of induction could reverse the increases in both retinal oxidative and nitrative stress [14]. However, reversal was only partial or even none when there was a delay of more than 2 and 6 months, respectively. The findings suggest that retinal proteins are oxidized or nitrosylated early (less than 2 months) in the disease course and are resistant to reversal after a short duration of hyperglycemia. This may contribute to the progression of DR even after the normalization of glycemic levels. Another possible explanation is the proposed theory of "the point of no return" that may occur early in the course of retinopathy, and after which disease progression is no longer influenced by a return to euglycemic state [12]. The changes in DR following bariatric surgery are unpredictable. Concerns regarding the rapid and substantial decrease in blood glucose levels that occur after surgery stem from prior knowledge of the effects of intensive medical treatment on DR progression as elaborated above. On top of that, episodes of postoperative postprandial hypoglycemia (PPH) may add to the damage on the retina.

Varadhan et al. conducted a small, retrospective, pilot study ($n = 22$) in 2012 to determine the effect of two bariatric surgical procedures (vertical sleeve gastrectomy and Roux-en-Y gastric bypass) on DR [15]. Retinal images were obtained preoperatively and at 6 and 12 months after surgery. Among those without preoperative DR (n = 15), two (13%) developed DR. Meanwhile, those in the preexisting DR group (n = 7) had two cases each of the progression and regression of DR, respectively. In effect, 16 out of 22 patients (73%) did not have any change in their DR status while 18% had either new onset or progression of DR.

In a prospective case-control study by Miras et al. [16], DR progression or improvement did not differ over a 12-month period between medically (n = 25) and surgically (n = 56) treated patients (P = 0.67 and P = 0.70 respectively). Meanwhile, the STAMPEDE (Surgical Therapy and Medication Potentially Eradicate Diabetes Efficiently) trial was a prospective randomized trial comparing the metabolic parameter outcomes of 150 obese type 2 diabetic patients who underwent either bariatric surgery or intensive medical therapy [17]. Ophthalmic examination of these patients revealed that DR evolution and visual acuity were stable in most patients (87%) at 2 years even though there was a larger reduction in the mean HbA1c levels in the bariatric surgery group (mean change −2.7%) compared to the medical treatment group (mean change −1.1%) [18].

17.3 Patients with No DR Prior to Bariatric Surgery

In patients without any DR changes preoperatively, most of them continue to maintain this status. Thomas et al. [19] in their observational study of 148 type 2 diabetic patients showed that up to 85% of patients without preoperative DR remained as such after their surgery, while a meta-analysis of four case-control studies (n = 148) by Cheung et al. [20] in 2015 showed an even higher proportion (92.5%) of patients who remained free of DR after bariatric surgery.

17.4 Patients with Preoperative DR

In general, DR did not progress in the majority of patients with preexisting DR prior to surgery. Cheung's [20] meta-analysis revealed that 57% of patients remained stable with no progression, while a retrospective observational study including 318 type 2 diabetic patients showed an even higher percentage (73%) of patients with no progression [21]. In fact, Murphy et al.'s [21] study showed that DR improvement was seen in 11% of their patients, while the meta-analysis by Cheung et al. [20] recorded 19.2% of patients who improved on their DR severity after bariatric surgery.

However, EWDR following bariatric surgery was up to 20% of patients with preexisting DR. About 16% were found to have worsening of DR severity in a retrospective observational study [21] while a meta-analysis including four case-control studies showed that progression occurred in 23.5% of patients with preoperative DR [20]. Compared with patients without preoperative DR, the odds ratio for progression was 2.77 (95% CI: 1.10–6.90; P = 0.03) in the meta-analysis [20]. However, this meta-analysis did have its weaknesses and limitations, as rightly pointed out by Pontiroli [22]. Table 17.1 summarizes the key features, outcomes, and risk factors for diabetic retinopathy in bariatric surgery patients.

Table 17.1 Diabetic retinopathy and bariatric surgery

Author (year)	Patients' baseline characteristics	Eye examination	Patients' DR outcomes after surgery	HbA1c changes during postoperative period	Risk factors associated with DR progression
Thomas (2014) [19]	Pilot observational study (Wales, UK) in 148 T2D obese with Bs during 1998–2012, including 40 with available HbA1c 2 years before and after surgery No preoperative DR: 65% ($n = 26$); minimal: 22.5% ($n = 9$); moderate: 2.5% ($n = 1$); severe NPDR: 10% ($n = 4$)	Before, 1 year after Bs	*No preoperative DR* ($n = 26$): no postoperative DR in 85% ($n = 22$), 1 or 2 microaneurysms in 4 *Minimal non-proliferative DR before Bs* ($n = 9$): regression in 56% ($n = 5$); stability in 44% ($n = 4$)	Reduction in: HbA1c = 1.8 ± 1.6%, fasting glucose = 3.3 ± 5.0 mmol/L after Bs	Higher preoperative blood glucose, greater HbA1c decreases in postoperative period with versus without DR progression ($P < 0.05$)
Murphy (2015) [21]	Retrospective observational study in 318 T2D with Bs during 2001–2012: 69% no DR preoperatively; 19% minimal; 8.5% mild or moderate; 4% severe DR	Before, after Bs	DR onset: 17% Stable DR: 73% DR progression: 16% Regression: 11%	Reduction of 3.9 ± 1.7% postoperatively HbA1c ≤ 6.5% (28% post surgery)	Progression to moderate to-severe NPDR: magnitude of HbA1c reduction, baseline NPDR, male gender
Schauer (2014) [17] Singh (2015) [18]	STAMPEDE: randomized prospective study of effects of Bs versus intensive medical treatment on metabolic parameters in 150 obese T2D Baseline HbA1c: 9.3%	Before, 2 years after Bs	No change in DR evolution in 86.5% at 2 years	Mean changes in HbA1c from baseline to 2 years: Medical therapy: −1.1; Bs: ~2.7–2.8	
Cheung (2015) [20]	Systematic review and meta-analysis of four case-control studies ($n = 148$). No randomized controlled trial No preoperative DR ($n = 80$), preoperative DR ($n = 68$)		*No preoperative DR* no DR: 92.5 ± 7.4%; progression: 7.5 ± 7.4% *Preoperative DR* stability in 57 ± 19%; progression in 24 ± 19%; regression in 19 ± 13%		Increased risk (OR: 2.77, 95% CI: 1.10–6.9; $P = 0.03$) with preoperative DR versus without DR

Miras (2015) [16]	Prospective case-control study in 83 obese T2D with Bs (bypass): 56 with complete ophthalmological data (17 no DR, 32 minimal-to-moderate, 6 severe NPDR, 1 PDR) versus 25 medical treatment (9 no DR, 9 minimal-to-moderate, 2 severe NPDR, 1 PDR)	Before, 1 year after Bs	*Bs patients:* 44 (78%) stable DR, 6 (11%) improvement, 6 (11%) worsening: 1 laser treated (moderate NPDR before Bs), 5 without DR before Bs *Medical patients*: 81% stable; 5% improvement; 14% worsening (1 laser photocoagulation)		No significant difference between Bs and medical patients in DR worsening ($P = 0.70$) or improvement ($P = 0.67$) after Bs
Amin (2016) [23]	Retrospective study of 152 T2D patients with Bs during 2005–2012 versus 155 usual medical treatment matched for age, HbA1c, duration of monitoring 106 patients: no DR at baseline Follow-up: 3.0 ± 1.9 years	Before, after Bs	*No DR at baseline* ($n = 106$): 2 (1.9%) severe NPDR *Background NPDR at baseline* ($n = 41$): 5 (12.2%) severe NPDR *No maculopathy before surgery* ($n = 143$): 8 (5.6%) developed maculopathy after Bs		Less severe DR and maculopathy in Bs versus medical patients: 5.7% (8/141) vs. 12.1% (12/99) $P = 0.075$; 5.6% (8/143) vs. 15.4% (16/104), $P = 0.01$, respectively
Chen (2017) [10]	Retrospective observational study of 102 T2D with Bs surgery during 2009–2015: 68% no DR, 30% moderate NPDR, 1% severe NPDR, 1% PDR Follow-up: 4 years	Before, every year after Bs	DR onset in 19%, stable DR in 70%, improvement in 11% at 1 year postoperatively New maculopathy in 6%	7.7–6.3%	Young age, male gender, high preoperative HbA1c, preoperative DR

Adapted from: Feldman-Billard [24]
Bs bariatric surgery, *T2D* type 2 diabetes, *NPDR* non-proliferative diabetic retinopathy, *PDR* proliferative diabetic retinopathy

17.5 Ophthalmology Referral for Diagnosis, Monitoring, and Treatment

Seeing that DR changes do occur after bariatric surgery, it is important for patients to be seen by the eye physician for preoperative assessment of DR. The International Clinical Diabetic Retinopathy and Diabetic Macular Edema Disease Severity Scale classification (Table 17.2) is widely used for the diagnosis and staging of DR severity [25].

Thereafter, the interval of follow-up visits should be determined by the severity of DR. Other risk factors for early worsening of DR should also be considered when determining the interval. These factors include higher preoperative blood glucose, greater HbA1c decreases in the postoperative period [19], male gender [10, 21], and younger age [10]. A simple algorithm below may be a helpful guide for the treating physician to monitor the compliance to ophthalmic follow-up and treatment (Fig. 17.1):

Table 17.2 Classification of diabetic retinopathy severity

Retinopathy stage	Findings on ophthalmoscopy
No apparent retinopathy	No abnormalities
Mild non-proliferative DR (NPDR)	Microaneurysms only
Moderate NPDR	More than just microaneurysms but less than severe NPDR
Severe NPDR	Any of the following: 1. More than 20 intraretinal hemorrhages in each of four quadrants 2. Definite venous beading in two or more quadrants 3. Prominent intraretinal microvascular abnormalities in one or more quadrants AND no signs of proliferative retinopathy
Proliferative DR (PDR)	One of the following: 1. Neovascularization 2. Vitreous/preretinal hemorrhage

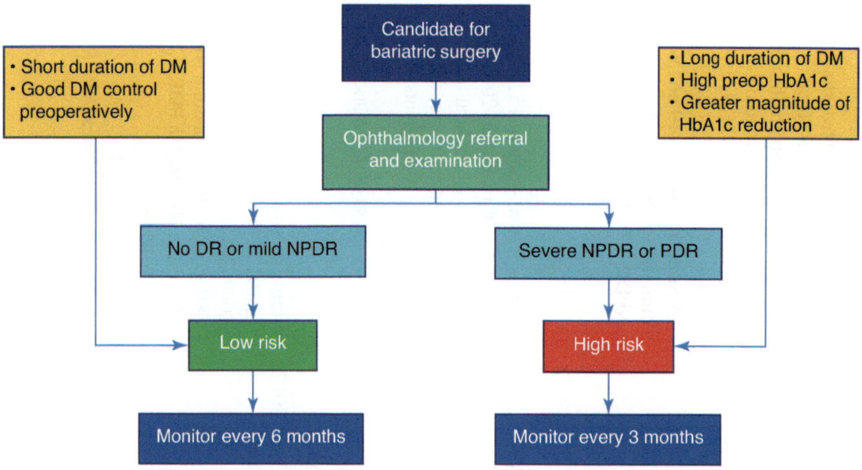

Fig. 17.1 Algorithm for ophthalmological monitoring in patients undergoing bariatric surgery

17.6 Ocular Complications Due to Nutritional Deficiencies

Bariatric surgery causes gastrointestinal anatomical and physiological alterations. After surgery, dietary modifications also occur. This can result in nutritional deficiency. The commonest nutritional deficiency is hypovitaminosis A. Other nutrients affected include vitamins B_{12}, B_1, C, D, E, K, folate, and minerals such as iron, selenium, zinc, and copper [26]. From these nutrients, those which have an impact on the normal function of the eye are vitamins A, E and B_1, and copper [27].

Some of the nutritional deficiencies and their associated eye findings/conditions are summarized below:

- Vitamin A: nyctalopia (night blindness), conjunctival xerosis with Bitot's spot, corneal xerosis, corneal ulceration, and keratomalacia
- Vitamin E: pigmentary retinopathy [28]
- Vitamin B_1 (thiamine): nystagmus, ophthalmoplegia (parts of the major syndrome of Wernicke's encephalopathy)
- Copper: optic neuropathy [29, 30]

Hypovitaminosis A is the most frequently documented vitamin deficiency after BPD-DS. One report found that the prevalence of vitamin A deficiency was up to 52% for patients 1 year after surgery and going up to as high as 69% for patients 4 years after BPD-DS [31]. More worryingly, many of these patients reported non-compliance with the dietary changes and supplements intake. This indicates the need for parenteral supplementation of vitamin A in a select group of patients.

While ocular complications such as conjunctival and corneal xerosis manifest as dry eye symptoms which can usually be managed with artificial tears supplementation, the more serious complications of nyctalopia and corneal ulceration can lead to permanent blindness. Nyctalopia occurred in 2.8% of patients who underwent biliopancreatic diversion (BPD) surgery [32].

17.7 Pathophysiology of Vitamin A Deficiency

Hypovitaminosis A can occur in bariatric patients via three mechanisms: impairment of metabolism, malnutrition, and malabsorption [33]. Vitamin A metabolism impairment can happen prior to the bariatric surgery due to non-alcoholic fatty liver disease (NAFLD), which occurs in 71–88% of obese patients [34]. NAFLD causes oxidative stress in the liver, which can be negated by vitamin A due to its antioxidant properties. Vitamin A is consumed in the evolution of NAFLD to reduce oxidative stress. This is evidenced by the inverse correlation between the severity of NAFLD and vitamin A levels in the liver [34]. Vitamin A metabolism can also be impaired by bariatric surgery. The surgery increases oxidative stress in the postoperative period. Thus, it can interfere with vitamin A absorption, processing, storage, and consumption [35].

Malnutrition can occur after bariatric surgery due to decrease in the dietary intake of micronutrients like carotenoids and retinol. This may be aggravated further by the traditional dietary advice of a low-fat diet after gastric bypass surgery, which further limits the absorption of fat-soluble vitamin (A, D, E, and K) [35]. Bariatric surgery, in effect, causes malabsorption of various nutrients. Its nonselective nature is the cause of various malabsorption syndromes, including that of vitamin A. This is because the food bypasses the duodenum and first portion of the jejunum, where most of the selective absorption processes take place [35].

17.8 Diagnosis of Vitamin A Deficiency

The diagnosis can be made by assessing the serum concentrations of retinol and/or retinol-binding protein (RBP) [36]. The normal levels of serum retinol are between 20 and 80 μg/dL. A diagnosis of VAD can be made with a concentration of serum retinol below 10 μg/dL. However, certain factors such as infection, protein status, adequacy of other nutrients, and organ diseases can affect serum retinol levels [36]. However, quantification of serum retinol is expensive, due to the utilization of high-performance liquid chromatography (HPLC). Furthermore, retinol is unstable when exposed to heat or light.

Serum RBP concentration assessment, on the other hand, is easier, cheaper, and requires less amount of serum (10–20 μL). It can be obtained via finger prick. However, not all RBP in the serum are complexed with retinol. The binding of RBP to retinol is influenced by certain factors such as the presence and degree of acute phase response, protein-energy malnutrition, liver disease, chronic renal failure, and acute stressful situation [36]. Thus, more studies are needed to establish serum RBP concentration as a useful marker for the diagnosis of vitamin A deficiency [37].

17.9 Treatment of Vitamin A Deficiency

According to treatment guidelines by the American Society for Metabolic and Bariatric Surgery (ASMBS), an oral regime of 10,000–25,000 international unit (IU) of vitamin A daily is suggested, until clinical improvement is seen (usually takes between 1 and 2 weeks). However, oral therapy is indicated only if there was no corneal involvement. In cases where the cornea is affected, vitamin A should be administered at 50,000–100,000 IU intramuscularly for 2 days, followed by 50,000 IU intramuscularly for 2 weeks [38].

Care should be taken to check for coexisting iron and copper deficiencies during the treatment for hypovitaminosis A, as these two mineral deficiencies can impair the resolution of vitamin A deficiency. Treatment with high-dose Vitamin A above 50,000 IU daily for a period longer than 3 months can lead to toxicity. Clinical manifestation includes dry and scaly skin, hair loss, mouth sores, painful hyperostosis, anorexia, and vomiting. Other serious complications are hypercalcemia, increased intracranial pressure, hepatomegaly, and cirrhosis [38].

The prognosis of vitamin A deficiency after treatment is generally good. Night blindness is the first symptom to resolve in 1–3 days. Conjunctival and corneal xerosis will take a couple of weeks to resolve. Corneal ulceration will often result in cornea scarring. Large corneal ulcers and localized keratomalacia can spread to involve the entire cornea, causing a painful blind eye.

17.10 Thiamine (B1) Deficiency and Wernicke's Encephalopathy

The body's store of vitamin B1 can be rapidly depleted in about 4–6 weeks, leading to one of the more commonly known syndromes of Wernicke's encephalopathy (WE). This is an acute neuropsychiatric condition due to an initially reversible biochemical brain lesion caused by overwhelming metabolic demands on brain cells that have depleted intracellular thiamine [39]. It is characterized by the triad of confusion, ataxia, and nystagmus. A review by Singh et al. in 2007 identified 37 cases of Wernicke's encephalopathy after bariatric surgery [40]. The onset of symptoms occurred between 2 and 78 weeks after various types of bariatric procedures, with most patients presenting within 12 weeks. Failure to recognize the signs of WE can be disastrous, as inappropriate treatment results in death or permanent brain damage.

17.10.1 Pathophysiology of WE

Thiamine is a coenzyme that plays a central role in cerebral metabolism. It acts as a cofactor for several enzymes involved in the Krebs cycle and the pentose phosphate pathway. Deficiency leads to decreased levels of alpha-keto-glutarate, acetate, citrate, acetylcholine, and accumulation of lactate and pyruvate. This results in metabolic imbalances leading to neuronal cell death.

17.10.2 Diagnosis of WE

It is a clinical diagnosis, with at least two of the following features required to make the diagnosis:

1. Dietary deficiency of thiamine
2. Eye signs
3. Altered mental status
4. Cerebellar dysfunction

In the case of patients with a recent history of bariatric surgery, only one of the latter triad of ataxia, confusion, and ophthalmoplegia is sufficient to alert the treating physician of the diagnosis of WE. Serum thiamine and erythrocyte transketolase levels may not be readily available at all facilities; serum thiamine may even be normal in some instances.

17.10.3 Treatment

A prompt correction of the thiamine deficiency is the mainstay of treatment. Parenteral administration of thiamine is the most effective and rapid method of correction. Up to 500 mg of thiamine given once to thrice daily parenterally may be necessary. It cannot be over-emphasized the importance of administering thiamine before or together with glucose solutions, because glucose oxidation may further decrease thiamine levels and thus exacerbate the neurological symptoms of WE.

17.11 Vitamin E Deficiency and Pigmentary Retinopathy

The photoreceptor cells of the retina consist of outer segments that contain a high proportion of polyunsaturated fatty acids. They are therefore more susceptible to lipid peroxidation. Vitamin E is a potent antioxidant shown to be effective in retarding the intracellular accumulation of lipofuscin pigments, which are the end-products of lipid peroxidation. Lipofuscin deposition in the retina causes toxicity that may be responsible for the progressive deterioration of retinal pigment epithelium (RPE) cell function, which could lead to retinal degeneration.

The clinical symptoms of Vitamin E deficiency may manifest only after 10–20 years of malnutrition. In the eye, poor vision and visual field defects are likely the results of severe photoreceptor damage. Funduscopic examination may reveal pigmentary changes not dissimilar to retinitis pigmentosa (Fig. 17.2).

Unfortunately, visual recovery is usually not possible to even with normalization of the body's vitamin E levels as the damage to the photoreceptors are irreversible. Nevertheless, treatment may limit further damage and preserve residual vision.

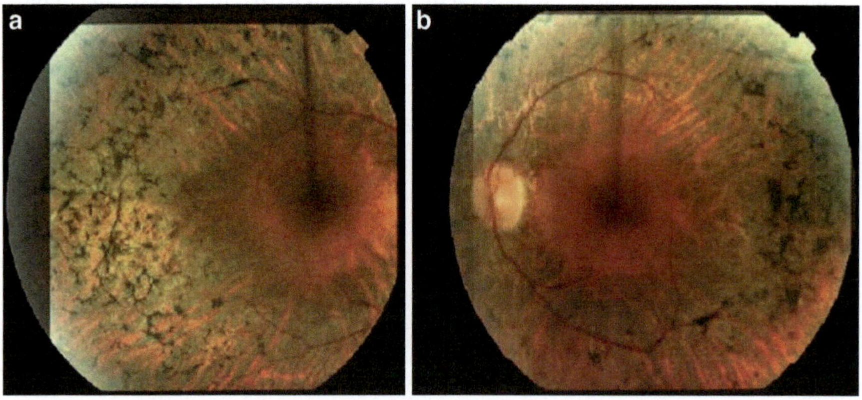

Fig. 17.2 Bony spicule-like hyperpigmentation (white arrows) of the peripheral retina seen in the right (**a**) and left (**b**) fundus. The optic disc in the left eye also has the pale and waxy appearance typical of retinitis pigmentosa (Adapted from Aslam A, Misbah SA, Talbot K, Chapel H. (2004) [41])

17.12 Optic Neuropathy Due to Copper Deficiency

Nutritional optic neuropathy can be caused by copper, B12, and/or thiamine deficiency following bariatric surgery [42]. Copper deficiency may take 3 years (and up to over 20 years) after bariatric surgery to be symptomatic [43]. Eye symptoms include an enlarged blind spot and progressive vision loss bilaterally. Examination shows sectoral or generalized pallor of the optic disc and poor vision. Fortunately, treatment with copper supplementation may reverse the symptoms experienced.

17.13 Take-Home Message

With the global increase in the prevalence of obesity and metabolic syndrome showing no signs of slowing down in the near future, the demand for bariatric surgery is also expected to continue to increase. With more and more surgeons showing interest in performing bariatric surgery, it is vital that their training incorporates a fair share of emphasis on early detection and management of complications including that related to nutritional deficiencies following bariatric surgery. Ophthalmological complications remain underdiagnosed and less spoken about as compared to the other more obvious potential complications such as leak and bleed. If neglected, ophthalmological complications could result in chronic visual impairment or worse, permanent blindness. Concerted multidisciplinary team effort by the surgeon, endocrinologist, eye physician, and dietitian is key to reducing this risk. Patient education should aim to empower the patient to want to take responsibility for their own health, adhere to follow-up plan, and show compliance to nutritional advice including consumption of vitamins following surgery.

References

1. Gloy VL, et al. Bariatric surgery versus non-surgical treatment for obesity: a systematic review and meta-analysis of randomised controlled trials. BMJ. 2013;347:f5934.
2. Ribaric G, et al. Diabetes and weight in comparative studies of bariatric surgery vs conventional medical therapy: a systematic review and meta-analysis. Obes Surg. 2014;24:437–55.
3. Cheung N, et al. Diabetic retinopathy. Lancet. 2010;376(9735):124–36.
4. Yau JW, et al. Global prevalence and major risk factors of diabetic retinopathy. Diabetes Care. 2012;35(3):556–64.
5. Xu J, et al. Ten-year cumulative incidence of diabetic retinopathy. The Beijing Eye Study 2001/2011. PLoS One. 2014;9(10):e111320.
6. Jin P, et al. The 5-year onset and regression of diabetic retinopathy in Chinese type 2 diabetes patients. PLoS One. 2014;9(11):e113359.
7. Kajiwara A, et al. Gender differences in the incidence and progression of diabetic retinopathy among Japanese patients with type 2 diabetes mellitus: a clinic-based retrospective longitudinal study. Diabetes Res Clin Pract. 2014;103(3):e7–10.
8. Salinero-Fort MA, et al. Four-year incidence of diabetic retinopathy in a Spanish cohort: the MADIABETES study. PLoS One. 2013;8(10):e76417.

9. Silva RA, et al. Severe worsening of diabetic retinopathy following bariatric surgery. Ophthalmic Surg Laser Imag Retina. 2013;44 Online(6):E11-4.
10. Chen Y, et al. Does bariatric surgery prevent progression of diabetic retinopathy? Eye. 2017;31:1131–9.
11. van Ballegooie E, et al. Rapid deterioration of diabetic retinopathy during treatment with continuous subcutaneous insulin infusion. Diabetes Care. 1984;7:236–42.
12. Lauritzen T, et al. Effect of 1 year of near-normal blood glucose levels on retinopathy in insulin-dependent diabetics. Lancet. 1983;1:200–4.
13. Dahl-Jørgensen K, et al. Rapid tightening of blood glucose control leads to transient deterioration of retinopathy in insulin dependent diabetes mellitus: the Oslo study. Br Med J (Clin Res Ed). 1985;290:811–5.
14. Kowluru RA. Effect of reinstitution of good glycemic control on retinal oxidative stress and nitrative stress in diabetic rats. Diabetes. 2003;52(3):818–23.
15. Varadhan L, et al. Bariatric surgery and diabetic retinopathy: a pilot analysis. Obes Surg. 2012;22:515–6.
16. Miras AD, et al. Type 2 diabetes mellitus and microvascular complications 1 year after Roux-en-Y gastric bypass: a case-control study. Diabetologia. 2015;58:1443–7.
17. Schauer PR, et al. Bariatric surgery versus intensive medical therapy for diabetes – 3-year outcomes. N Engl J Med. 2014;370:2002–13.
18. Singh RP, et al. Effect of bariatric surgery versus intensive medical management on diabetic ophthalmic outcomes. Diabetes Care. 2015;38:e32–3.
19. Thomas RL, et al. Does bariatric surgery adversely impact on diabetic retinopathy in persons with morbid obesity and type 2 diabetes? A pilot study. J Diabetes Complications. 2014;28:191–5.
20. Cheung D, et al. The impact of bariatric surgery on diabetic retinopathy: a systematic review and metaanalysis. Obes Surg. 2015;25:1604–9.
21. Murphy R, et al. Progression of diabetic retinopathy after bariatric surgery. Diabet Med. 2015;32:1212–20.
22. Pontiroli AE, Ceriani V. Does bariatric surgery influence diabetic retinopathy? Obesity surgery. 2015;25(6):1066.
23. Amin AM, et al. The impact of bariatric surgery on retinopathy in patients with type 2 diabetes: a retrospective cohort study. Surg Obes Relat Dis. 2016;12:606–12.
24. Feldman-Billard S, et al. Early worsening of diabetic retinopathy after rapid improvement of blood glucose control in patients with diabetes. Diabetes Metab. 2018;44(1):4–14.
25. Wilkinson CP, et al. Proposed international clinical diabetic retinopathy and diabetic macular edema disease severity scales. Ophthalmology. 2003;110(9):1677–82.
26. Shankar P, et al. Micronutrient deficiencies after bariatric surgery. Nutrition. 2010;26(11–12):1031–7.
27. Parrish CR. Severe micronutrient deficiencies in RYGB patients: rare but potentially devastating. Pract Gastroenterol. 2011;100:13–27.
28. Rino Y, et al. Vitamin E deficiency begins within 6 months after gastrectomy for gastric cancer. World J Surg. 2014.
29. Naismith RT, et al. Acute and bilateral blindness due to optic neuropathy associated with copper deficiency. Arch Neurol. 2009;66(8):1025–7.
30. Pineles SL, et al. Combined optic neuropathy and myelopathy secondary to copper deficiency. Surv Ophthalmol. 2010;55(4):386–92.
31. Slater GH, et al. Serum fat-soluble vitamin deficiency and abnormal calcium metabolism after malabsorptive bariatric surgery. J Gastrointest Surg. 2004;8:48–55.
32. Scopinaro N, et al. Biliopancreatic diversion. World J Surg. 1998;22(9):936–46.
33. Lee WB, et al. Ocular complications of hypovitaminosis A after bariatric surgery. Ophthalmology. 2005;112(6):1031–4.
34. Chaves GV, et al. Association between liver vitamin A reserves and severity of nonalcoholic fatty liver disease in the class III obese following bariatric surgery. Obes Surg. 2014;24(2):219–24.

35. Zalesin KC, et al. Vitamin a deficiency after gastric bypass surgery: an underreported postoperative complication. J Obes. 2011;2011.
36. de Pee S, Dary O. Biochemical indicators of vitamin A deficiency: serum retinol and serum retinol binding protein. J Nutr. 2002;132(9 Suppl):2895S–01.
37. Guerreiro RA, Rui R. Ophthalmic complications of bariatric surgery. Obes Surg. 2015;25(1):167–73.
38. Allied Health Sciences Section Ad Hoc Nutrition Committee, Aills L, Blankenship J, et al. ASMBS allied health nutritional guidelines for the surgical weight loss patient. Surg Obes Relat Dis. 2008;4(5 Suppl):S73–108.
39. Thomson AD, Marshall EJ. The natural history and pathophysiology of Wernicke's encephalopathy and Korsakoff's psychosis. Alcohol Alcohol. 2006;41(2):151–8.
40. Singh S, Kumar A. Wernicke encephalopathy after obesity surgery: a systematic review. Neurology. 2007;68:807–11.
41. Aslam A, Misbah SA, Talbot K, Chapel H. Vitamin E deficiency induced neurological disease in common variable immunodeficiency: two cases and a review of the literature of vitamin E deficiency. Clin Immunol. 2004;112(1):24–9.
42. Moss HE. Bariatric surgery and the neuro-ophthalmologist. J Neuro-Ophthalmol. 2016;36(1):78.
43. Shah AR, Tamhankar MA. Optic neuropathy associated with copper deficiency after gastric bypass surgery. Retinal Cases Brief Rep. 2014;8(1):73–6.

Hematological Complications After Bariatric Surgery

18

Ariel Shuchleib, Diego Camacho, and Natan Zundel

Blood is a very special juice.

—Goethe

18.1 Introduction

Obesity is an epidemic that has been growing worldwide, its prevalence has more than doubled in the past 20 years, currently more than 35% of the US population is suffering from being overweight or obese. Bariatric and metabolic surgery are considered as the mainstay of treatment for obesity since it has demonstrated significantly better efficacy in decreasing weight and improving comorbidities as compared to lifestyle modification and medical management [1]. Nevertheless, despite all the advantages of surgery, there can be some short and long-term complications associated with bariatric procedures. In this chapter, we will focus on the hematological morbidity that can arise from surgical procedures.

Hematological complications could be acute like hemorrhage or venous thromboembolism or chronic that more frequently are related to vitamin or mineral deficiencies [2].

A. Shuchleib
ABC Medical Center, Anahuac University Mexico, Mexico City, Mexico

D. Camacho
Albert Einstein College of Medicine, The Bronx, NY, USA
e-mail: dicamacho@montefiore.org

N. Zundel (✉)
University at Buffalo, Buffalo, NY, USA

Jackson North Medical Center, Miami, FL, USA

A. G. Bhasker et al. (eds.), *Management of Nutritional and Metabolic Complications of Bariatric Surgery*,
https://doi.org/10.1007/978-981-33-4702-1_18

18.2 Hemorrhage

As surgery evolves and better techniques and hemostatic devices appear, postoperative bleeding incidence has been trending down in the immediate postoperative period. The advent of laparoscopic techniques has further decreased the incidence of hemorrhage in the surgical setting. However, the incidence will vary on the type of surgery being done and the presence or absence of a coagulopathy in the patient. Its calculated to be between 0 and 4.4% [3, 4]. Surgical bleeding could be categorized in two different ways, depending on location; intraabdominal or intraluminal, or according to the time of presentation as acute, early, late, and chronic [5]. Diagnosis and management of bleeding complications can be difficult and when it is severe it usually involves either an endoscopic or surgical intervention.

The nutritional component for bleeding will be addressed further in this chapter when vitamin K and vitamin C deficiencies are discussed.

18.3 Venous Thrombo-embolism

Surgery and obesity are two factors that are known to have a prothrombotic effect. Obesity leads to a constant proinflammatory state which leads to hypercoagulability in addition to fibrinolytic dysfunction. The hypercoagulable state is observed with increased platelet activation, elevated levels of fibrinogen, and coagulation factors VIII, IX, XI, and XII [6]. Samuels et al. compared a cohort of patients with obesity that underwent bariatric surgery with healthy subjects using TEG (thromboelastography) and tPA challenged TEG. They found that patients with obesity formed stronger clots much quicker and were more resistant to fibrinolysis than the controls. In their follow-up they also found that this situation improved but did not normalize completely after 6 months despite a significant weight loss [7].

The incidence of deep vein thrombosis (DVT) after bariatric surgery varies and it has been reported to be from 0.2% to 1.3% at 30 days and 0.42% at 90 days [2]. Diagnosis and management of DVT in the post-bariatric patients are the same as in the general population. Diagnosis is based on a duplex ultrasound and management is based on anti-coagulation, unless there is a suspected compromise from the limb, then thrombolysis or a vascular surgery intervention would be warranted.

Even though DVT prophylaxis is almost universally accepted for bariatric surgery, the exact dose of medication, duration, and timing for initiation of treatment has not been defined. In a recent study from Stony Brook University, authors analyzed data from almost 12,000 patients and as expected they found a higher rate of DVT in patients without any chemoprophylaxis compared with patients who received it (0.58 vs. 0.11%). They also found a higher incidence of transfusions in patients who got chemoprophylaxis preoperatively comparing to patients who got it only after surgery [8].

Porto-mesenteric vein thrombosis (PMVT) is an uncommon but potentially lethal entity and its incidence has been increasing slowly as laparoscopic procedures become more readily available. Its exact incidence is hard to find due to its uncommon occurrence or probably it is underreported in the literature. One of the few studies that states the incidence of this problem refers to approximately 1% incidence of PMVT in patients who had undergone a sleeve gastrectomy [9].

The exact pathophysiology of PMVT is not completely defined, however some factors have been attributed to the procedures and some to the patients. Some of the underlying factors related to the surgery are thought to be; transection of the short gastric vessels, aggressive dissection near the pylorus and behind the stomach along the splenic vein, and other general laparoscopic risk factors including increased intraabdominal pressure, carbon dioxide induced vasoconstriction, reverse Trendelenburg position, and dehydration post-surgery [10].

Diagnosis of PMVT is most often done with a CT scan of the abdomen with IV contrast on patients that present with abdominal pain, nausea, vomiting, or fever. Doppler ultrasound has a low sensitivity in the acute process; however, it can be used as a follow-up study to assess progression or resolution. Laboratory values are usually nonspecific and can include leukocytosis, elevation on the acute phase reactants, among others.

As in DVT, PMVT treatment is based on systemic anti-coagulation, on rare occasions, a thrombectomy or fibrinolysis has to be performed. It is important to start the treatment as soon as possible to have better chances of success on clot resolution and anti-coagulation therapy should be instituted for at least 3–6 months [11].

18.4 Mineral Deficiency

18.4.1 Iron Deficiency Anemia

This is one of the earliest nutritional deficiencies that occur after metabolic surgery, particularly on the patients who get a procedure with a malabsorptive component like the Roux en Y gastric bypass (RYGB) or the biliopancreatic diversion with or without duodenal switch (BPD/BPD-DS). Its incidence varies widely depending on the series reviewed and ranges from 6 to 50%. Iron deficiency anemia is more commonly seen in females, especially those who are premenopausal [12].

Patients can present with symptoms including fatigue, palpitations, anxiety, hair loss, pica among other usual symptoms related to anemia or sometimes it may be found on routine bloodwork done on postsurgical patients. To make the diagnosis, other than having microcytic anemia serum, iron, ferritin, transferrin levels, and total iron-binding capacity should be measured [2].

Multiple Factors Are Related to the Pathophysiology of This Disease:

- Decreased Consumption: Meat is a major source of iron and it has been shown that patients after a bariatric procedure consume significantly less red meat. Crowley et al. did a survey where they found out that less than 30% of the patients ingested the recommended daily allowance of iron [13].
- Decreased Gastric Acid: The first stages for the metabolism of iron requires acid to make it more soluble and facilitate its absorption by converting it from ferric

to the ferrous state. Any gastric procedure in which part of the stomach is excised or bypassed reduces the quantity of parietal cells and subsequently on the concentration of gastric acid. This leads to hampered absorption.
- Exclusion of the Duodenum: There are two forms of iron that are absorbed—heme iron (from certain foods like meat) and inorganic iron. Inorganic iron gets absorbed throughout the small bowel, however heme iron is mainly absorbed in the duodenum and proximal aspect of the jejunum. Any procedure that bypasses these regions like the RYGB, BPD, BPD-DS, decreases iron absorption significantly [12].

Screening of iron levels in patients that had a metabolic procedure should be done routinely, supplementation is advised on the patients with at least 18 mg/day but in menstruating females or patients with anemia at least 45–60 mg/day should be administered [14]. Most patients respond to oral supplementation however a few may need parenteral supplementation and in some extreme cases reversal of the procedure may have to be considered.

18.4.2 Copper Deficiency

Copper is a trace metal that is mainly absorbed in the duodenum and stomach and to a lesser extent in the rest of the small bowel. It is an important co-factor in enzymatic processes involved in hematopoiesis and catecholamine synthesis and is also a very important component of the vascular, skeletal, and the nervous systems.

Copper deficiency can reveal itself with hematological diseases like anemia, neutropenia, or myelodysplasia. Since copper deficiency can also be associated with a demyelinating neuropathy, it is not uncommon for it to be confused with a vitamin B12 deficiency. Copper also plays an important role in iron deficiency anemia since there are many copper-dependent enzymes like ceruloplasmin, hephaestin, and cytochrome-c oxidase that have important roles in the metabolism and transportation of iron [15].

Luckily it is not very common, but a few case reports of pancytopenia and myelodysplastic syndrome have been reported after bariatric surgery.

When a myelodysplastic syndrome develops usually secondary to copper deficiency, it most commonly presents as anemia with neutropenia, and less often as thrombocytopenia. Copper is a mineral required for the proper function of different metalloproteins including ceruloplasmin and cytochrome-C, which are required for the transport of iron. Its deficiency explains the anemia that is associated; however, the pathophysiology of the neutropenia and thrombocytopenia is not completely defined.

Some suggested etiologies are: Destruction of myeloid progenitors in the bone marrow, inhibition of differentiation, and egress of the cells out of the bone marrow [16].

The diagnosis of a copper deficiency may be difficult as it does not have too many clinical signs. Hypopigmentation of the skin, hair, and nails can be seen but the actual diagnosis can be made by measuring serum levels of ceruloplasmin and copper, these must be done in addition to the measurement of vitamin B12 and MDS levels in patients with neuropathy. Recommended copper supplementation is 1 mg/day for patients who have undergone a sleeve gastrectomy or gastric banding and 1–2 mg/day for patients who have undergone an RYGB or BPD+/-DS [14].

18.4.3 Calcium, Phosphorus, Zinc, Selenium, Chromium, and Magnesium Deficiencies

The trace elements mentioned in Table 18.1 serve as cofactors in many processes in the body, and their deficiency may lead to anemias. Table 18.1 summarizes their involvement.

18.5 Vitamin Deficiencies

18.5.1 Folic Acid and Vitamin B12

Anemia secondary to vitamin B12 and folate are less common than iron deficiency anemia since their supplementation is very efficient and vitamin B12 storage could take years to deplete. Absorption of vitamin B12 gets affected after bariatric/metabolic surgery. Its absorption requires hydrochloric acid as well as intrinsic factor, both of which are secreted by the parietal cells. Hydrochloric acid from the stomach helps the dissolution of the bound form of B12 complexes. This then binds to the intrinsic factor and this new complex gets absorbed in the terminal ileum.

Folate deficiency can be due to decreased intake, however, it could also be related to a B12 deficiency, since it plays a vital role in the conversion of the inactive methyl-tetrahydrofolic acid to active tetrahydrofolic acid.

The deficiency of either one of those vitamins leads to megaloblastic anemia. Folate deficiency can lead to neural tube defects in pregnant women and vitamin B12 deficiency can lead to weakness, neuropathy, and cognitive disfunction [2, 15].

Oral supplementation of B12 and folate is usually sufficient but, in some cases, parenteral administration of B12 may be required. The recommended dose for supplementation is 350–500 μg/day oral, disintegrating tablet, sublingual, liquid or

Table 18.1 Hematological implications of minerals and trace elements [2]

Mineral	Manifestation
Calcium	Iron deficiency anemia
Chromium	Iron deficiency anemia
Phosphorus	Anemia
Selenium	Anemia
Zinc	Anemia

nasal, or 1000 mcg/month IM. Folate supplementation is advised as 400–800 mcg on the general population and 800–1000 mcg to females on childbearing ages [14].

18.5.2 Vitamin K

Vitamin K deficiency is a very rare occurrence after bariatric surgery and is usually associated with the more malabsorptive procedures like the BPD+/-DS. The etiology for this deficit is fat mal-absorption. Since it is a fat-soluble vitamin, bacterial overgrowth, and modification of the gut microbiota also add to its deficiency.

The microbiota is very relevant in vitamin K deficiency since there are two types of vitamin K. K1 is the one that is ingested, and it comes mainly from leafy vegetables, and K2 is a product of the metabolism from the intestinal flora, particularly Bacteroides [17, 18].

Vitamin K plays a key role in the activation of some coagulation factors (II, VII, IX, X, protein C, and protein S) acting as an enzyme/co-factor. The clinical manifestations of a severe deficiency are related to hemorrhagic diathesis and symptoms include delay in blood clotting, mucosal bleeding, bleeding gums, nose bleeding, spontaneous internal bleeding, and heavy menstruation [17].

The diagnosis is usually made indirectly in patients with prolonged coagulation times, particularly INR. Direct measurement of vitamin K in the serum is not precise. Metabolites from it could be checked in the urine, however, those could also vary according to the renal function. Some other proteins could be studied, however, most laboratories do not have these tests, and variations in them could also be due to liver dysfunction.

Supplement recommendations after an RYGB, gastric sleeve, or band are 90–120 μg/day, and on patients that had a BPD, 300 μg/day should be given. In case treatment is needed on an acute setting of malabsorption, 10 mg parenterally should be given, but if the patient has a chronic malabsorption the recommended dose is 1–2 mg/day orally [14, 18].

18.6 Thiamine (B1), Riboflavin (B2), Niacin (B3), Pantothenic Acid (B5), Pyridoxine (B6), Biotin (B7), Vitamin A, Vitamin C, Vitamin D, Vitamin E

Deficiency of the rest of the vitamins either water soluble or fat soluble could have a very small hematologic component if there is a deficiency. It is summarized in Table 18.2.

Key Points

- *Fortunately, hematological complications are uncommon after bariatric surgery. In the acute setting bleeding and thrombosis are most commonly seen.*
- *DVT/PE and PMVT are uncommon but potentially lethal complications after bariatric surgery, in order to decrease their incidence prophylaxis must be given. Unfortunately, a universal protocol for it still does not exist.*

Table 18.2 Hematological implications of minerals and trace elements deficiency [2]

Vitamin	Manifestation
Thiamine (B1)	Megaloblastic anemia
Riboflavin (B2)	Normochromic normocytic anemia, megaloblastic anemia
Niacin (B3)	Anemia
Pantothenic (B5)	Anemia
Pyridoxine (B6)	Sideroblastic microcytic anemia
Biotin (B7)	Anemia
Vitamin A	Normocytic and normochromic anemia
Vitamin C	Bleeding disorder and anemia
Vitamin D	Anemia
Vitamin E	Anemia, hemolysis of RBC

- *If a thrombotic complication arises it is important to start the treatment as soon as possible to decrease morbidity and mortality.*
- *Long-term hematological complications are related to vitamin or mineral deficiencies, and hence it is very important to evaluate and supplement them lifelong after bariatric surgery.*
- *Routine blood work should be done at least once a year after surgery to detect deficiencies early on and prevent complications.*

References

1. Buchwald H, et al. Bariatric surgery: a systematic review and meta-analysis. JAMA. 2004;292(14):1724–37.
2. Al-Jafar H, et al. Potential hematology and nutritional complications of bariatric surgery. Ann Hematol Oncol. 2018;5(5):1209.
3. Mehran A, et al. Management of acute bleeding after laparoscopic Roux-en-Y gastric bypass. Obes Surg. 2003;13:842–7.
4. Chousleb E, et al. Routine abdominal drains after laparoscopic Roux-en-Y gastric bypass: a retrospective review of 593 patients. Obes Surg. 2004;14:1203–7.
5. Abraham F, et al. Postoperative bleeding in the bariatric surgery patient. ASMBS Textbook Bariatric Surg. 2014;9:241–7.
6. Rottenstreich A, et al. Assessment of the procoagulant potential after laparoscopic sleeve gastrectomy: a potential role for extended thromboprophylaxis. Surg Obes Relat Dis. 2018;14:1–7.
7. Samuels J, et al. Prospective assessment of fibrinolysis in morbid obesity: tissue plasminogen activator resistance improves after bariatric surgery. Surg Obes Relat Dis. 2019;15:1153–9.
8. Altieri MS, et al. Evaluation of VTE prophylaxis and the impact of alternate regimens on post-operative bleeding and thrombotic complications following bariatric procedures. Surgical Endoscopy. 2018;32:4805–12.
9. Alsina E, et al. Incidence of deep vein thrombosis and thrombosis of the portal-mesenteric axis after laparoscopic sleeve gastrectomy. J Laparoendosc Adv Surg Tech A. 2014;24(9):601–5.
10. Shaheen O, et al. PMVT after sleeve gastrectomy. Surg Obes Relat Dis. 2017;13:1422–33.
11. Rottenstreich A, et al. Abdominal thrombosis following bariatric surgery. Surg Obes Relat Dis. 2017;13:78–84.
12. Love AL, Billett HH. Obesity, bariatric surgery, and iron deficiency: true, true, true and related. Am J Hematol. 2008;83:403–9.
13. Crowley LV, et al. Late effects of gastric bypass for obesity. Am J Gastroenterol. 1984;79:850–60.

14. Parrott J, et al. American Society for Metabolic and Bariatric Surgery Integrated Health Nutritional Guidelines for the Surgical Weight Loss Patient 2016 Update: Micronutrients. Surg Obes Relat Dis. 2017 May;13(5):727–41.
15. Chen M, et al. Hematological disorders following gastric bypass surgery: emerging concepts of the interplay between nutritional deficiency and inflammation. Biomed Res Int. 2013;2013:205467.
16. Robinson SD, Cooper B, et al. Copper deficiency (hypocupremia) and pancytopenia late after gastric bypass surgery. Proc (Bayl Univ Med Cent). 2013;26(4):382–6.
17. Halder M, et al. Vitamin K: double bonds beyond coagulation insights into differences between vitamin K1 and K2 in health and disease. Int J Mol Sci. 2019;20(4):896.
18. Sherf-Dagan S, et al. Vitamin K–what is known regarding bariatric surgery patients: a systematic review. Surg Obes Relat Dis. 2019;15:1402–13.

Psychological Issues After Bariatric Surgery

19

Denise Ratcliffe

There is a reciprocal association over time between depression and obesity.

—Dr. Floriana S. Luppino

19.1 Introduction

As the number of people having bariatric surgery has increased there is more longitudinal data available about the physical and psychological changes and issues that may occur. Alongside this increase in the number of people having bariatric surgery, the psychological approach has evolved towards identifying and managing psychological issues amongst individuals before and after bariatric surgery. Initially the focus for bariatric psychology involved 'gate-keeping' access to surgery by attempting to identify specific psychological contraindications to surgery. However, given that the evidence supporting this approach is doubtful, and the physical benefits of bariatric surgery are compelling, the psychological approach has shifted towards identifying potential challenges and offering timely interventions in order to manage complications and challenges. This is a more nuanced approach towards psychological assessment and intervention, trying to balance potential risks and benefits, and planning ahead for potential challenges that may jeopardise weight or psychosocial outcomes. As a result of this shift towards a more collaborative, facilitative approach (partly because of the lack of clear and consistent evidence regarding psychological contraindications), more people with complex or comorbid

D. Ratcliffe (✉)
Phoenix Health, Chester, UK
e-mail: contact@drdeniseratcliffe.co.uk

A. G. Bhasker et al. (eds.), *Management of Nutritional and Metabolic Complications of Bariatric Surgery*,
https://doi.org/10.1007/978-981-33-4702-1_19

psychological issues are having bariatric surgery. There is also a greater awareness of the psychological issues that can arise following surgery—either pre-existing difficulties that are reactivated as a result of surgery or new difficulties that are related to the changes following surgery. The above factors mean that there is a greater need for post-operative assessment and support through the process as psychological difficulties emerge or recur.

It is important to carefully consider how we perceive and plan for psychological challenges and complications following surgery. We need to provide adequate psychological resources within the bariatric multidisciplinary team based on the pragmatic expectation that it is highly likely that some individuals will experience psychological challenges. This is partly because those seeking bariatric surgery have higher rates of psychological problems compared to (a) individuals not seeking treatment for their obesity and (b) the general population. Furthermore, bariatric surgery (and its concomitant changes in weight, eating, etc.) often has a marked psychosocial impact in different domains of an individual's life.

It is helpful to draw a distinction between post-operative psychological issues which are related to pre-existing mental health disorders (e.g. depression, binge eating, etc.) versus psychosocial adjustment issues which are a typical and expected part of the process. Much of the research has focused on post-operative psychological issues that are related to mental health diagnoses (e.g. depression, binge eating, etc.), partly because this lends itself to empirical research. There has recently been more focus on psychological factors that are transdiagnostic, e.g. impulsivity [1] and persistence [2]. In addition, it is important to pay attention to the more subtle, less measurable adjustment issues that may arise which can create significant tension and distress. There are some qualitative papers that have focused on this and give a useful clinical insight into the lived experience (both the positives and the challenges) of living with bariatric surgery [3].

Much of the research which has focused on the impact of psychological issues following bariatric surgery is that weight is often used as the primary outcome measure. This is not the only relevant domain of interest following bariatric surgery. It is important to consider the effect of psychological challenges post-surgery not just in terms of their impact on weight loss/kg, but also how they influence psychological functioning and quality of life [4]. Perhaps one of the reasons why the research has not identified clear psychological predictors of outcomes at least in the short term, is because the weight has been the primary outcome measure. Given the extremely powerful effects of bariatric surgery on weight loss, this is likely to obscure the detection of any other psychosocial factors. One of the reasons why this longer term follow-up data is important is that the physiological effects of surgery wane over time therefore creating more scope for psychological factors to emerge. Furthermore, as you will see in the literature reviewed in this chapter, when we focus on the psychosocial outcomes of surgery (as well as weight outcomes) then often problems tend to become more apparent. Although individuals may have lost a significant amount of weight, they may still have significant levels of distress that impact on their quality of life and functioning (and may in the longer term then start to impact on their weight trajectory).

In this chapter, we will start by briefly reviewing the literature on pre-operative psychological issues as it is important to understand the issues faced by the group seeking bariatric surgery to consider the impact these may have post-surgery. As mentioned previously, psychological difficulties following surgery can be conceptualised as being on a continuum in terms of severity, complexity, and consequences. These range from focusing on pre-existing mental health difficulties to the development of new mental health difficulties to adjustment problems that could be considered integral to the bariatric surgery process.

19.2 Pre-operative Psychological Difficulties

In order to think about the psychological challenges and complications that may occur after surgery, it is important to understand the context for these in terms of the population seeking bariatric surgery. We will briefly provide an overview of the type of mental health issues that are more frequently experienced by those seeking bariatric surgery. It is important to have some awareness of the psychological issues that are more prevalent amongst this cohort as this can influence the focus of pre-operative preparation and inform post-operative monitoring.

There are higher rates of premorbid psychological conditions and difficulties amongst individuals seeking bariatric surgery compared to both individuals living with obesity who are not seeking treatment and the general population. There is also a positive association between increased psychiatric disorders and BMI [5–7]. Past experience of mental health difficulties is the strongest predictor of future mental health difficulties. Therefore, it can be concluded that as the group of individuals seeking bariatric surgery has a history of greater premorbid psychological difficulties, they are more likely to have psychological difficulties in the future.

A number of studies have provided important information about the prevalence and type of psychological difficulties experienced by individuals seeking bariatric surgery. In one study, individuals were interviewed about their psychiatric history and current difficulties prior to bariatric surgery (but independently of the clinical assessment process) [6]. The authors found that 66% of individuals had a lifetime prevalence of psychiatric disorder and 38% met current diagnostic criteria. The most common difficulties were mood disorders with high rates of depression (45.5% lifetime, 10% current), anxiety (37.5% lifetime, 24% current), and binge eating disorder (27.1% lifetime, 16% current). Rates are higher amongst individuals seeking treatment compared to individuals living with obesity in the community. A recent meta-analysis confirmed that depression (19%) and BED (17%) were the most common psychiatric diagnoses individuals presented with at the time of surgery [8]. It is important to note that there is a bidirectional relationship between obesity and psychological difficulties, i.e. psychological difficulties may be a causal factor in obesity but obesity often creates psychological difficulties too [9].

There are also higher rates of childhood sexual, physical, and emotional abuse as well as emotional and physical neglect amongst adults who have bariatric surgery compared to the general population [10]. Furthermore, there is consistent evidence that adverse childhood experiences increase the risk of developing obesity [11].

Binge eating disorder (BED), defined as eating an unusually large amount of food within a short period of time coupled with a loss of control over eating, is common amongst those seeking bariatric surgery. It is noteworthy that binge eating disorder (BED) is often a proxy for other psychological conditions. Individuals with a lifetime history of eating disorder (primarily BED) were much more likely to meet diagnostic criteria for an additional psychiatric condition (mainly anxiety) compared to those without a lifetime history of disordered eating (84% vs. 45%) [5].

These high rates of psychological difficulties are one of the reasons why it is important to provide a psychological assessment for all individuals seeking bariatric surgery. The psychological assessment is an opportunity to identify unidentified or untreated difficulties, to consider how these may impact on the individual's ability to adjust and make necessary changes and to plan ahead so that the team and patient are aware of the specific challenges that an individual may face following surgery and to plan accordingly [12]. Whilst attempts should be made to clarify the true purpose of the psychological assessment (facilitative, rather than gatekeeping), issues may sometimes arise as patients may not be fully transparent about psychological difficulties pre-operatively due to concern that disclosing these will lead to being denied access to surgery. This means that some psychological difficulties are only revealed or become apparent post-surgery and it is important that there are adequate psychological resources available to respond promptly and effectively with unanticipated difficulties.

19.3 Post-operative Psychological Difficulties

In the following section, we will review the literature on changes to pre-existing mental health or psychological problems following surgery, both in terms of their impact on weight loss and also psychosocial outcomes. We will also consider how the nature of some of these difficulties may shift in their presentation (for example from binge eating to graze eating) and how new difficulties may arise (e.g. alcohol issues). The main post-operative psychological difficulties can be split into (a) eating difficulties (including BED and other eating disorders) (b) mental health and mood difficulties (c) suicidality and (d) alcohol problems. We will then focus our attention on psychosocial adjustment issues that are a usual, but often challenging, part of the bariatric process. These have often been overlooked in the literature as they do not lend themselves to quantitative research.

Before focusing on the psychological difficulties that may arise following surgery, it is important to preface this by highlighting the fact many people experience significant improvements in their psychological health following surgery. For example a large prospective study found that rates of psychiatric disorders decreased in the 3 years following surgery [13]. There is also some evidence that psychological improvements are tied in with, or contingent upon, weight loss so when weight loss plateaus or individuals experience weight regain, there is an increased risk of psychological difficulties returning [14, 15]. This is why it is important to focus on longitudinal data that goes beyond the typical 2-year follow-up period.

19.4 The Impact of Problematic Eating Behaviours Following Bariatric Surgery

As previously outlined, there are high rates of Binge Eating Disorder (BED) amongst individuals seeking bariatric surgery, and that this is often comorbid with other psychological conditions [16]. The diagnostic criteria for BED are not fully applicable to the eating behaviours of individuals who have had bariatric surgery. In particular, the criteria relating to classifying objective binges (i.e. eating a large volume of food in a short space of time) which may not be physically possible after surgery. The criteria which relate to experiencing a loss of control (LOC) whilst eating appear to be highly relevant as this is the characteristic that is strongly related to distress, functioning, and post-surgery outcomes [17].

Whilst rates of BED are high pre-operatively, most research studies have found that pre-operative BED does not predict weight loss following surgery [18]. However, those individuals who meet the criteria for preoperative binge eating disorder are at greater risk of experiencing difficulties with LOC eating post-operatively [19]. There is also consistent evidence that LOC eating and other problematic eating behaviours can be an emergent or new problem for a significant number of individuals (one study reported up to 40%) following surgery [20–22]. There is consistent evidence that experiencing post-operative LOC eating is associated with poorer weight loss [23, 24]. Furthermore, the numbers of individuals experiencing a recurrence or re-emergence of these difficulties increases as time elapses since surgery [24]. Conceicao et al. (2017) found evidence of different weight loss trajectories following surgery for those with problematic eating behaviours such as LOC or grazing behaviour. These data show that there was a deterioration of weight loss outcomes particularly around 20 months after surgery [20].

Longitudinal data has investigated changes in eating pathology with 3-year follow-up data from the longitudinal assessment of bariatric surgery-3 (LABS-3) Psychosocial Study [21]. Using structured interview data from the eating disorder examination-bariatric surgery version (EDE-BSV) the prevalence of multiple pathological eating behaviors declined following Roux-en-Y gastric bypass (RYGB) or laparoscopic adjustable band (LAGB) insertion and remained lower than presurgery throughout the 3-year follow-up period. However, post-surgery LOC eating, hunger, and problematic eating and body-related attitudes as reflected by the EDE global score were related to less favourable weight change after surgery. Post-surgery LOC eating was associated with regaining 20% of maximum weight loss. These findings are consistent with the literature that problematic eating behaviours and experiences may contribute to suboptimal weight loss and this becomes more apparent over time. These findings regarding the impact of LOC eating on suboptimal weight loss and regain in conjunction with the lack of predictive power based on pre-op BED, emphasise the clinical importance of routinely and proactively assessing pathological eating behaviour following bariatric surgery.

A grazing pattern of eating (also known as picking and nibbling or snacking) is also associated with less weight loss following surgery. Furthermore, there is some evidence that those with pre-surgery BED, are more likely to develop issues with grazing following surgery. This in turn is associated with a different weight loss trajectory and poorer weight loss outcomes [20]. It is important to make a distinction between compulsive and non-compulsive grazing. Compulsive grazing overlaps with LOC eating and is also significantly associated with anxiety disorders [25].

The problematic eating behaviours which have been outlined above focus on their negative impact on suboptimal weight loss and regain. It is important to note that a small group of individuals may experience other types of disordered eating following surgery—namely, anorexia or bulimic presentations. A study which interviewed individuals about their eating behaviours following gastric bypass, found that 12% regularly induced vomiting and this was motivated by weight and shape concerns (rather than involuntary or due to epigastric pain) [26]. Research has suggested that the changes experienced following bariatric surgery (i.e. rapid weight loss and dietary restraint) may trigger, or lead to the development of, restrictive 'anorexia nervosa-like' eating pathology. This is characterised by greater than usual weight loss after surgery, fear of weight regain, dietary restriction, and disturbances in self-perception of shape and weight [27, 28]. Due to the under-researched nature of this area, the estimated prevalence of restricted eating disordered behaviour after bariatric surgery is unknown, however these types of presentations are becoming more common [28]. It is important to identify these difficulties early as they can quickly become entrenched problems. It is possible that individuals may need onward referral to a specialist eating disorder unit for input. Furthermore, educating the wider multidisciplinary team is important so that they do not inadvertently reinforce behaviour by congratulating patients on their greater than expected weight loss. Whilst these are rare problems, they tend to be under-reported and under-recognised.

19.5 Mental Health Difficulties Following Bariatric Surgery

As mentioned previously, there are generally positive improvements and shifts in mental health but it is important to recognise that the cohort of individuals seeking bariatric surgery has a greater burden of psychological difficulties and distress. The past experiences of psychological difficulties place individuals at greater risk of experiencing future difficulties.

There are a couple of issues specifically arising from bariatric surgery that can contribute to post-operative mental health difficulties. It is worth bearing in mind that psychotropic medication should be reviewed following surgery as there can be changes in absorption, particularly following surgical procedures that affect absorption (RYGB and OAGB). This means that medication may less effective and doses may need to be adjusted accordingly. In addition, there are a number of nutritional deficiencies that can occur following surgery which may have a direct impact on mental health. For example one of the symptoms associated with low levels of iron, B12, and copper is low mood. Anecdotally, the experience of surgical complications that may require lengthy or frequent hospitalisations can also be a risk factor for mood and coping problems post-surgery. Some individuals may experience a destabilisation of their mental health when they are no longer able to regulate their emotions through food (Obviously pre-operative preparation should aim to address this although in reality, it is not always fully apparent until after surgery). It is also important to liaise closely with mental health services in order to maintain continuity of care and to provide any additional information they may require about bariatric-specific issues.

So, what does the empirical literature tell us about how individuals with premorbid mental health conditions fare after bariatric surgery? Mental health disorders obviously vary in their severity and the impact they have on the individual. Historically, there has been an assumption that individuals with severe mental health difficulties are likely to have a poor or worse outcome after surgery and as a result, may even have been excluded from surgery because of a mental health condition. A very important study [29] looked at the impact of different types of mental health difficulties on weight loss trajectories following surgery. A subgroup analysis compared individuals with (1) no mental illness (2) mild–moderate anxiety and depression (3) severe anxiety and depression and (4) individuals with bipolar/psychotic conditions. The authors found no differences in weight loss outcomes 2 years after surgery. However, the groups with more severe mental health difficulties (those with severe anxiety/depression or bipolar/psychotic conditions) tended to have more healthcare utilisation, i.e. more attendances at the Emergency Dept and more hospital days throughout the 2-year follow-up period. It is likely that this reflects the greater support requirements because of the additional challenges in terms of implementing and adjusting to new behaviours and reinforces the need to identify and offer tailored post-operative psychosocial support.

19.6 Mood Issues

A history of pre-operative mood disorder does not appear to be consistently associated with weight loss outcomes after surgery. However, a number of studies have found that consistent with much of the bariatric literature, experiencing these difficulties post-surgery was associated with suboptimal weight loss or weight regain over time. White et al. [30] reported that rates of depression improved after surgery but gradually started to increase again 6 months following surgery (Although they still remain lower than their baseline, pre-surgery levels). These post-surgery mood difficulties were associated with poorer weight loss outcomes, greater eating disorder pathology and reduced quality of life. This suggests that a subgroup of individuals will have mood issues following surgery and that the prevalence of these increases over time. Mitchell et al. [31] also reported improvement in depression in the first year after surgery but then a steady increase in depression from years 1 to 3 following surgery.

In another study, Kalarchian et al. [13] reported a decrease in the most common psychiatric conditions (anxiety, depression, and disordered eating) in the first 3 years following surgery with high rates of remission. Furthermore, the authors found that a pre-operative history of these difficulties was not associated with poorer weight loss. A recent paper which presents 7 years follow-up data from the same cohort demonstrated that rates of mental health disorders remain lower than pre-surgery levels but that for patients who had RYGB, by year 7, this difference was no longer statistically significant (34.7% vs. 29.1%) [32]. The rates of mental health disorders had started to return to their pre-surgery levels. Furthermore, the authors found that having a concurrent mood disorder post-surgery was associated with the greater weight regain and reduced quality of life, although the causality of this relationship has not been established.

There have been some efforts to identify the potential causal factors involved in the recurrence of depression in a subgroup and various ideas have been suggested including unmet weight loss expectations, recurrence of physical comorbidities, nutritional deficiencies and changes in absorption of psychotropic medication [31]. Symptoms of depression include poor self-care, lack of volition, motivational issues, withdrawal, and cognitions which revolve around failure and helplessness. It is easy to see how these symptoms may map onto the individual's ability to implement and maintain behaviour changes following bariatric surgery.

Earlier in this chapter, the high prevalence of trauma, abuse, and neglect was highlighted amongst individuals living with obesity. A number of studies have focused on whether a history of trauma has any impact on weight loss following bariatric surgery. Steinig et al. [33], in their systematic analysis of the available data, reported that there may be some initial differences in the rate of weight loss whereby those with a history of sexual abuse lose less weight initially, but these differences disappear with longer term follow-up. A recent study by King et al. found that a history of childhood trauma was not associated with the degree of weight loss or regain [34]. However, they did find that a history of childhood trauma was associated with less improvement in depression and eating disorder pathology post-surgery. This means that individuals with a history of childhood trauma may benefit from specific psychological intervention to address these issues in order to improve their psychosocial functioning and outcomes. Providing this type of intervention could potentially minimise the impact of depression and disordered eating on long-term weight outcomes. Anecdotally, those with a history of interpersonal trauma may struggle more with changes to their body image and feeling more 'visible' and noticeable to others. This can activate worries about interpersonal threat, feelings of anxiety and avoidance. It is obviously important to provide psychological intervention to address these issues and to help individuals update their perception of threat to reflect their current circumstances. Furthermore, helping individuals recognise that this is usually a transition phase, and normalising these experiences can be valuable.

19.7 Suicide

A number of studies have reported increased rates of suicide following bariatric surgery. For example Peterhansel et al. [35] reported a fourfold increase compared to the general population. Tindle et al. [36] reported that suicide rates amongst individuals post-surgery in Pennsylvania over 10 years were 6.6/10,000. These are much higher than age and sex-matched US rates. Furthermore, studies have also reported an increase in self-harm following bariatric surgery [37]. One of the issues leading to difficulties in interpreting this data is the fact that rates of self-harm and suicidality are higher amongst those seeking bariatric surgery compared to the general population [38]. For example a large study reported that 25% of individuals pre-surgery had a history of suicidality and that 4% had attempted suicide compared to rates of 3.3% suicidal ideation and 0.6% suicide attempts in the general population [38]. Past occurrence of suicidal behaviours is the best predictor of future occurrence of suicidal behaviours.

A recent paper [38] focused on suicidal behaviour and suicide in individuals who had either a gastric bypass or gastric band in their first 5 years post-surgery (this was data from the Longitudinal Assessment of Bariatric Surgery cohort). In the first 5 years after surgery, 15% reported suicidality and the vast majority of these had a pre-surgery history. In terms of the timing of suicidality post-surgery, the authors report an initial decrease in the first year after surgery but then a steady increase from this time point onwards with most suicides occurring in the fourth year after surgery. This finding was also reported by Tindle et al. [36] who found that most suicides occurred in the final year of the 3 year follow-up period.

The authors identified specific factors that were associated with increased suicidality. Individuals with a pre-surgery history of suicidality were 17× more likely to experience suicidality (self-harm/suicidal ideation) post-surgery. Other risk factors included male gender, smoking, greater pain severity, antidepressant medication use, input from mental health services, and lifetime history of psychiatric hospitalisation were independently associated with a greater risk of self-harm/suicidal ideation in years 1–5 post-surgery.

Of those that completed suicide, all occurred in individuals who had RYGB but the numbers are too small to confidently draw conclusions regarding increased risk of suicide following RYGB specifically. This would be worthy of further investigation given the potential impact of changed/inadequate absorption of psychotropic medication and increased rates of alcohol use following this procedure.

19.8 Alcohol and Other 'Addictions'

Whilst there is a lay discourse around 'habit transfer' following bariatric surgery, this is no empirical evidence to support this concept. The current empirical data indicates that alcohol is the only addictive behaviour that consistently increases following bariatric surgery. Alcohol use disorder (AUD) is a pattern of alcohol use that involves problems controlling alcohol intake, being preoccupied with alcohol, continuing to use alcohol even when it causes problems, having to drink more to get the same effect, or having withdrawal symptoms upon rapidly decreasing or stop drinking. AUD can be mild, moderate, or severe.

King et al. [39] analysed data from the LABS-2 study which is a prospective, observational longitudinal study of >2000 individuals having a primary bariatric procedure between 2006 and 2009 (note that the sleeve gastrectomy was not included). The researchers collected baseline data about a range of psychological variables, including alcohol and illicit drug use, and followed up on an annual basis. The study found that the prevalence of AUD increased substantially over time after RYGB from approximately 7% pre-surgery to 16% at year 7, while remaining stable for those who had a gastric band (from 6% to 8%). There was a slight increase in illicit drug use (primarily marijuana) following the bypass compared to the band, but there is a need for further research due to measurement/screening issues and lack of inclusion of a range of drugs (including opiates).

Azam et al. [40] conducted a systematic review of alcohol use pre- and post-bariatric surgery and found that the prevalence of AUD post-bypass increases over time. Furthermore, those individuals having a gastric bypass are at increased risk for AUD. Those who have a gastric bypass (compared to the gastric band) are at double the risk for developing AUD post-surgery [39]. This is because bariatric surgery procedures lead to different alcohol pharmokinetics. Studies show that individuals who have had a bypass reach higher peak alcohol concentration more quickly after surgery and take more time to return to a sober state. In addition, there are changes in alcohol reward sensitivity following RYGB [41]. There is currently uncertainty regarding alcohol problems following sleeve gastrectomy. A number of pre-operative factors have been found to independently increase the risk of post-operative AUD symptoms. These risk factors include male gender, younger age, smokers, low social support, those who have pre-op hx of substance use, and those who have had recent psychiatric treatment were at increased risk [39, 42].

It is important to note that AUD can be a *new* problem. King et al. (2012) reported that 60.5% of those who developed AUD did not have a history of AUD prior to surgery. Another study reported 43.8% did not have a history [41]. Contrary to the 'addiction transfer' hypothesis, binge eating and loss of control eating are not associated with the development of problematic alcohol or substance use outcomes [39].

In terms of mental health issues that may arise following surgery, it is obviously overly simplistic to relate all negative changes in mental health to bariatric surgery as some psychological conditions (e.g. bipolar, psychosis, depression) have a significant rate of relapse. Alternatively, bariatric surgery could be conceptualised as a stressor and according to the stress-diathesis model of psychological distress, individuals with a premorbid psychological vulnerability (condition) are more likely to experience a relapse or worsening of their difficulties when stress exceeds a particular threshold. The evidence and data provided in this chapter so far clearly point to the importance of proactive assessment and long-term monitoring for psychological difficulties following bariatric surgery. It is also noteworthy that some of the difficulties (e.g. AUD and LOC eating) can be new issues following surgery.

19.9 Adjustment Issues

The empirical evidence base regarding psychological difficulties that may occur following bariatric surgery does not always fully translate to the issues that arise in clinical practice. One of the reasons for this is that most research studies have focused on diagnosable mental health problems and this leads to significant limitations in accurately reflecting the psychological and emotional issues that occur after surgery. Most people are likely to experience psychological challenges following surgery as it results in changes in multiple domains of an individual's life. These include shifting relationship with food, changes in body image, changes in intimate relationships and friendships. Individuals often make a demarcation between their life before surgery and their life after surgery. Following surgery, individuals may need to develop new skills to manage situations that they have not previously faced or avoided (e.g. relationships, managing compliments, etc.). Whilst bariatric surgery is associated with multiple positive changes, it also creates tensions and challenges to negotiate [3]. Whilst these do not necessarily meet diagnostic criteria for mental health disorders, they can cause a lot of distress and impact on functioning. It is important that clinicians are aware of these issues so that they can facilitate discussions regarding these as well as normalising these adjustment experiences.

19.10 Altered Relationship with Food

Individuals often describe a different relationship with food after bariatric surgery—some may lose interest and pleasure from food and this can almost be experienced as a loss/bereavement in the early days after surgery. For some individuals, eating may become a chore rather than a pleasure. On the other hand, many individuals describe feeling 'liberated' from obsessive thoughts about food and at least in the short term after surgery, this is often a source of relief.

19.11 Body Image and Excess Skin

The multiple changes and improvements in weight and health following bariatric surgery are associated with improvements in quality of life and body image following surgery [43]. Whilst there is a positive shift in pre-to post-op body image, it still tends to remain lower than normative levels amongst the general population [44]. There are some specific challenges in terms of body image adjustment that occur following surgery. There is often a time lag on individuals updating their body image which means that they still perceive themselves to be the same weight that they were prior to surgery, despite 'knowing' that they have lost weight. In addition, individuals who have experienced abuse may feel more visible and vulnerable as they lose weight, leading to anxiety and possible sabotage attempts.

Research on whether the amount of weight lost following bariatric surgery impacts on body image is mixed. However, there is a trend towards greater weight loss being associated with improved body image [44]. Furthermore, there are a number of studies which indicate that poor body image post-operatively is associated with problematic eating behaviors, such as loss of control (binge) eating and night eating. Post-operative body image disturbance and dissatisfaction may potentially impact on long-term weight loss outcomes [45] and could be an important area for intervention.

Excess skin following massive weight loss is very common and causes multiple physical and psychosocial issues. This can be extremely psychologically distressing and disabling. Individuals often feel ashamed and self-conscious about their excess skin and may go to great lengths to camouflage it. They may also avoid situations (e.g. gyms, activity, socialising) and relationships because of concern about judgement from others. Kitzinger et al. [46] found that 75% of women and 68% of men wanted body contouring surgery. Research which compares individuals who have body contouring, versus those who have not, report improvements in various body image dimensions. However, a study found that a significant proportion of individuals were dissatisfied with the results of the procedure (27% dissatisfied with abdominoplasty) [47].

Individuals seeking bariatric surgery have high levels of body image distress before surgery. As a result of weight loss, body image improves to some extent following bariatric surgery but there are additional and new body image adjustments and challenges to negotiate.

19.12 Relationship Issues

There are often changes in peer/friendship relationships and also changes in intimate relationships following bariatric surgery and weight loss. Bruze et al. [48] analysed data from the SOS prospective study of bariatric surgery and focused on changes in relationships over a 20 year follow-up period. Bariatric surgery was associated with increased incidence of divorce (compared to the general population and controls with obesity) for those individuals who were in a relationship at the time of surgery. They also found an increased incidence of marriages and new relationships compared to controls with obesity. Changes in relationship status were more common amongst those with larger weight loss. The increased incidence of divorce and separation after bariatric surgery might be associated with increased tension in already vulnerable relationships or to improvements that empower patients to leave problematic relationships.

Important qualitative studies conducted by Romo et al. [49, 50] shed light on some of the changes in the dynamics of relationships when one partner engages in weight loss efforts. Positive changes including increased attraction, shared activities, viewing weight loss as a team effort are documented. However, it is clear that some challenges and tensions arise in some of the relationships because of factors such as partner insecurity, criticism of the other partner's lack of change/continued weight issues, partner no longer feeling needed.

Individuals who have had surgery often describe changes in their friendships and social relationships after surgery. Research has focused on exploring these changes and the factors that may arise include jealousy/envy attempts to sabotage weight loss by encouraging or putting pressure on the individual to eat inappropriate foods and a wish to maintain the status quo in the relationship [49].

19.13 Conclusions

This chapter has provided an overview of the psychological difficulties which can recur or occur after bariatric surgery. Whilst there are often significant psychological improvements in psychosocial outcomes in the short-term following surgery, the data indicates that these problems often start to re-emerge with longer term follow-up. These psychosocial difficulties are not always 'diagnosable' mental health problems and often reflect the adjustment process. Most of the data reviewed shows a similar pattern of short-term improvements in psychological problems which appear to dwindle over time with increased difficulties re-emerging as the follow-up period extends. It is clearly important to proactively assess and provide psychological interventions over an extended time period in order to identify psychosocial difficulties which may impact on an individual's weight outcome as well as their psychological health.

Key Points

- *Individuals seeking bariatric surgery have a higher incidence of psychological issues than the general population as well as those who are obese but do not seek surgery.*
- *Past experience of mental health difficulties is the strongest predictor of future mental health problems; hence, psychological evaluation, instead of serving a 'gate-keeping' function, can help make available additional support to these patients in post-operative period.*
- *The most common psychological difficulties encountered in people seeking bariatric surgery are mood disorders and binge eating disorders (BED).*
- *While a pre-operative diagnosis BED is not itself associated with poorer weight loss outcomes after bariatric surgery, pre-operative BED may be associated with post-operative loss of control (LOC) eating and LOC may be associated with less weight loss post-bariatric surgery.*
- *Suicide rates are high post-bariatric surgery, particularly in those individuals who have previously attempted suicide.*
- *Alcoholism is the only addiction that increases post-bariatric surgery.*
- *Patients may experience a number of adjustment issues post-bariatric surgery especially with respect to their body image, their social and intimate (spouse/partner) relationships and their relation to food. Adjustment issues are subtle and hard to diagnose but may lead to significant distress in daily life.*
- *Assessment of psychological difficulties and providing timely support is of the essence.*

References

1. Sarwer DB, Allison KC, Wadden TA, Ashare R, Spitzer JC, McCuen-Wurst C, et al. Psychopathology, disordered eating, and impulsivity as predictors of outcomes of bariatric surgery. Surg Obes Relat Dis. 2019;15(4):650–5.
2. De Panfilis C, Generali I, Dall'Aglio E, Marchesi F, Ossola P, Marchesi C. Temperament and one-year outcome of gastric bypass for severe obesity. Surg Obes Relat Dis. 2014;10(1):144–8.
3. Bocchieri LE, Meana M, Fisher BL. Perceived psychosocial outcomes of gastric bypass surgery: a qualitative study. Obes Surg. 2002 Dec;12(6):781–8.
4. Sogg S, Lauretti J, West-Smith L. Recommendations for the presurgical psychosocial evaluation of bariatric surgery patients. Surg Obes Relat Dis. 2016;12(4):731–49.
5. Mühlhans B, Horbach T, de Zwaan M. Psychiatric disorders in bariatric surgery candidates: a review of the literature and results of a German prebariatric surgery sample. Gen Hosp Psychiatry. 2009;31(5):414–21.
6. Kalarchian M, Marcus MD, Levine MD, Courcoulas AP, Pilkonis P, Ringham RM, et al. Psychiatric disorders among bariatric surgery candidates: relationship to obesity and functional health status. Am J Psychiatry. 2007 Feb;164(2):328–34.
7. Mitchell JE, Selzer F, Kalarchian MA, Devlin MJ, Strain GW, Elder KA, et al. Psychopathology before surgery in the Longitudinal Assessment of Bariatric Surgery-3 (LABS-3) Psychosocial Study. Surg Obes Relat Dis. 2012;8(5):533–41.
8. Dawes AJ, Maggard-Gibbons M, Maher AR, Booth MJ, Miake-Lye I, Beroes JM, et al. Mental health conditions among patients seeking and undergoing bariatric surgery: a meta-analysis. JAMA. 2016;315(2):150–63.
9. Luppino FS, de Wit LM, Bouvy PF, Stijnen T, Cuijpers P, Penninx BW, Zitman FG. Overweight, obesity, and depression. Arch Gen Psychiatry. 2013;67(3):220–9.
10. Orcutt M, King WC, Kalarchian MA, Devlin MJ, Marcus MD, Garcia L, et al. The relationship between childhood maltreatment and psychopathology in adults undergoing bariatric surgery. Surg Obes Relat Dis. 2019;15(2):295–303.
11. Danese A, Tan M. Childhood maltreatment and obesity: systematic review and meta-analysis. Mol Psychiatry. 2014;19(5):544–54.
12. Sogg S, Friedman KE. Getting off on the right foot: the many roles of the psychosocial evaluation in the bariatric surgery practice. Eur Eat Disord Rev. 2015;23(6):451–6.
13. Kalarchian MA, King WC, Devlin MJ, Marcus MD, Garcia L, Chen JY, et al. Psychiatric disorders and weight change in a prospective study of bariatric surgery patients: a 3-year follow-up. Psychosom Med. 2016;78(3):373–81.
14. Magro DO, Geloneze B, Delfini R, Pareja BC, Callejas F, Pareja JC. Long-term weight regain after gastric bypass: a 5-year prospective study. Obes Surg. 2008;18(6):648–51.
15. Courcoulas AP, Christian NJ, Belle SH, Berk PD, Flum DR, Garcia L, et al. Weight change and health outcomes at 3 years after bariatric surgery among individuals with severe obesity. Jama. 2013;310(22):2416–25.
16. Dawes AJ, Maggard-Gibbons M, Maher AR, Booth MJ, Miake-Lye I, Beroes JM, et al. Mental health conditions among patients seeking and undergoing bariatric surgery. JAMA. 2016;315(2):150.
17. Goldschmidt AB, Conceição EM, Thomas JG, Mitchell JE, Raynor HA, Bond DS. Conceptualizing and studying binge and loss of control eating in bariatric surgery patients—time for a paradigm shift? Surg Obes Relat Dis. 2016;12(8):1622–5.
18. Livhits M, Mercado C, Yermilov I, Parikh J, Dutson E, Mehran A, et al. Preoperative predictors of weight loss following bariatric surgery: systematic review. Obes Surg. 2012;22(1):70–89.
19. White MA, Kalarchian MA, Masheb RM, Marsha D, Grilo CM. Loss of control over eating predicts outcomes in bariatric surgery: a prospective 24-month follow up study. J Clin Psychiatry. 2010;71(2):175–84.

20. Conceição EM, Mitchell JE, Pinto-Bastos A, Arrojado F, Brandão I, Machado PPP. Stability of problematic eating behaviors and weight loss trajectories after bariatric surgery: a longitudinal observational study. Surg Obes Relat Dis. 2017;13(6):1063–70.
21. Devlin MJ, King WC, Kalarchian MA, White GE, Marcus MD, Garcia L, et al. Eating pathology and experience and weight loss in a prospective study of bariatric surgery patients: 3-year follow-up. Int J Eat Disord. 2016;49(12):1058–67.
22. Smith KE, Orcutt M, Steffen KJ, Crosby RD, Cao L, Garcia L, et al. Loss of control eating and binge eating in the 7 years following bariatric surgery. Obes Surg. 2019:1773–80.
23. Scholtz S, Bidlake L, Morgan J, Fiennes A, Bs MB, Ei-etar A, et al. Long-term outcomes following laparoscopic adjustable gastric banding: postoperative psychological sequelae predict outcome at 5-year. Obes Surg. 2007:1220–5.
24. White MA, Kalarchian MA, Masheb RM, Marsha D, Grilo CM. Loss of control over eating predicts outcomes in bariatric surgery: a prospective 24-month follow up study. J Clin. Psych. 2010;71(2):175–84.
25. Goodpaster K, Marek R, Ashton K, Lavery M, Merrell Rish J, Heinberg L. Grazing eating among bariatric surgery candidates: prevalence and psychosocial correlates. Surg Obes Relat Dis. 2015;11(6):S50–1.
26. de Zwaan M, Hilbert A, Swan-Kremeier L, Simonich H, Lancaster K, Howell LM, et al. Comprehensive interview assessment of eating behavior 18-35 months after gastric bypass surgery for morbid obesity. Surg Obes Relat Dis. 2010;6(1):79–85.
27. Conceição E, Vaz A, Bastos AP, Ramos A, Machado P. The development of eating disorders after bariatric surgery. Eat Disord. 2013;21(3):275–82.
28. Conceição E, Orcutt M, Mitchell J, Engel S, LaHaise K, Jorgensen M, Woodbury K, Hass N, Garcia L, Wonderlich S. Characterization of eating disorders after bariatric surgery: a case series study. Int J Eat Disord. 2013;46:274–9.
29. Fisher D, Coleman KJ, Arterburn DE, Fischer H, Yamamoto A, Young DR, et al. Mental illness in bariatric surgery: a cohort study from the PORTAL network. Obesity. 2017;25(5):850–6.
30. White MA, Kalarchian MA, Marcus MD, Grilo CM. Prognostic significance of depressive symptoms on weight loss and psychosocial outcomes following gastric bypass surgery: a prospective 24-month follow-up study. Obes Surg. 2015;25:1909–16.
31. Mitchell JE, King WC, Chen JY, Devlin MJ, Flum D, Garcia L, et al. Course of depressive symptoms and treatment in the longitudinal assessment of bariatric surgery (LABS-2) study. Obesity. 2014;22(8):1799–806.
32. Kalarchian MA, King WC, Devlin MJ, Hinerman A, Marcus MD, Yanovski SZ, et al. Mental disorders and weight change in a prospective study of bariatric surgery patients: 7 years of follow-up. Surg Obes Relat Dis. 2019;17(3):1–10.
33. Steinig J, Wagner B, Shang E, Dölemeyer R, Kersting A. Sexual abuse in bariatric surgery candidates – impact on weight loss after surgery: a systematic review. Obes Rev. 2012;13(10):892–901.
34. King W, Hinerman A, Kalarchian MA, Devlin MJ, Marcus MD, Mitchell JE. The impact of childhood trauma on change in depressive symptoms, eating pathology, and weight after Roux-en-Y gastric bypass. Surg Obes Relat Dis. 2019;1–9. (article in press).
35. Peterhänsel C, Petroff D, Klinitzke G, Kersting A, Wagner B. Risk of completed suicide after bariatric surgery: a systematic review. Obes Rev. 2013;14(5):369–82.
36. Tindle H, Omalu B, Courcoulas A, Marcus M, Hammers J, Kuller LH. Risk of suicide after long-term follow-up from bariatric surgery. Am J Med. 2010;123(11):1036–42.
37. Bhatti JA, Nathens AB, Thiruchelvam D, Grantcharov T, Goldstein BI, Redelmeier DA. Self-harm emergencies after bariatric surgery. JAMA Surg. 2015:E1–7.
38. Gordon KH, King WC, White GE, Belle SH, Courcoulas AP, Ebel FE, et al. A longitudinal examination of suicide-related thoughts and behaviors among bariatric surgery patients. Surg Obes Relat Dis. 2019;15(2):265–74.

39. King WC, Chen J, Courcoulas AP, et al. Alcohol and other substance use after bariatric surgery: prospective evidence from a U. S. multicenter cohort study. Surg Obes Relat Dis. 2017;13:1392–402.
40. Azam H, Shahrestani S, Phan K. Alcohol use disorders before and after bariatric surgery: a systematic review and meta-analysis. Ann Transl Med. 2018;6(8):148.
41. Mitchell JE, Steffen K, Engel S, King WC, Chen JY, Winters K, et al. Addictive disorders after Roux-en-Y gastric bypass. Surg Obes Relat Dis. 2015;11(4):897–905.
42. King WC, Chen J-Y, Mitchell JE, Kalarchian M, Steffen KJ, Engel SG, et al. Prevalence of alcohol use disorders before and after bariatric surgery. JAMA. 2012;307(23):2516–25.
43. Sarwer DB, Steffen KJ. Quality of life, body image and sexual functioning in bariatric surgery patients. Eur Eat Disord Rev. 2015;23(6):504–8.
44. Ivezaj V, Grilo CM. The complexity of body image following bariatric surgery: a systematic review of the literature. Obes Rev. 2018;19(8):1116–40.
45. van den Berg P, Neumark-Sztainer D, Palmeira AL, Markland DA, Silva MN, Branco TL, et al. Preventing weight regain: what's the importance of body image change after bariatric surgery? J Adolesc Heal. 2017;10(4):139–51.
46. Kitzinger HB, Abayev S, Pittermann A, Karle B, Bohdjalian A, Langer FB, et al. After massive weight loss: patients' expectations of body contouring surgery. Obes Surg. 2012;22(4):544–8.
47. de Zwaan M, Georgiadou E, Stroh CE, Teufel M, Köhler H, Tengler M, et al. Body image and quality of life in patients with and without body contouring surgery following bariatric surgery: a comparison of pre- and post-surgery groups. Front Psychol. 2014;5(Nov).
48. Bruze G, Holmin TE, Peltonen M, Ottosson J, Sjöholm K, Näslund I, et al. Associations of bariatric surgery with changes in interpersonal relationship status results from 2 swedish cohort studies. JAMA Surg. 2018;153(7):654–61.
49. Romo LK. An examination of how people who have lost weight communicatively negotiate interpersonal challenges to weight management. Health Commun [Internet]. 2017;0236:1–9.
50. Kluever Romo L, Dailey RM. Weighty dynamics: exploring couples' perceptions of post-weight-loss interaction. Health Commun. 2014;29(2):193–204.

20 Drug Related Complications After Bariatric Surgery

Chih-Kun Huang and Chia-Chia Liu

All things are poison, for there is nothing without poisonous qualities. It is only the dose which makes a thing poison.

—*Paracelsus*

20.1 Introduction

The gastrointestinal tract, the largest endocrine and exocrine system, controls the functions of food digestion, secretion, absorption, and production of barriers in our human body. It can also modulate environmental factors, food composition, and metabolic state which would be altered by bariatric surgery. Alterations in incretin secretions after bariatric surgeries are well characterized and lead to sustainable weight loss and remission of type II diabetes mellitus [1].

The anatomical and physiological alterations in the GI tract following bariatric surgery may change a wide variety of factors involved in the oral bioavailability of drugs [2, 3]. These may have some adverse effects while taking drugs after the bariatric surgery. This chapter is focused on this change and what should we do to prevent some drug-related complications after bariatric surgery.

C.-K. Huang (✉) · C.-C. Liu
Body-Science and Metabolic Disorders International (B.M.I) Medical Center, China Medical University and Hospital, Taichung, Taiwan

A. G. Bhasker et al. (eds.), *Management of Nutritional and Metabolic Complications of Bariatric Surgery*,
https://doi.org/10.1007/978-981-33-4702-1_20

20.2 Bariatric Surgery

Bariatric surgery gives excellent results for long-lasting weight loss and associated improvement in comorbidities. In 2016, laparoscopic sleeve gastrectomy (LSG) accounted for approximately 54% and laparoscopic Roux-en-Y gastric bypass (LRYGB) for another 30% of global bariatric surgeries. Other surgical procedures: biliopancreatic diversion (BPD), biliopancreatic diversion with duodenal switch (BPD-DS) were also performed to a lesser extent [4]. LRYGB is still considered the golden standard procedure. It bypasses 95% of the stomach and the proximal small intestine [5]. LSG, however, results in the removal of most of the fundus and part of the stomach body without alteration of intestinal absorption and is considered a restrictive procedure, which is relatively safe with low long-term morbidity [6–10].

Bariatric surgeries manipulate gastric luminal contents by accelerating gastric emptying time and decreasing gastric acid secretion. In LRYGB, the chyme directly passes from the small pouch of the stomach into distal intestinal part of the jejunum thus bypassing the duodenum and proximal jejunum. These changes of the gastrointestinal tract affect the absorption of orally administered drugs [3, 11–13]. Practitioners involved in taking care of weight loss procedure patients should pay more attention on oral medication use. Knowing acid dissociation constant (pKa) and the partition coefficient (log P), as well as the localization of intestinal drug transporters, is very critical to prevent drug-related complications after bariatric surgery.

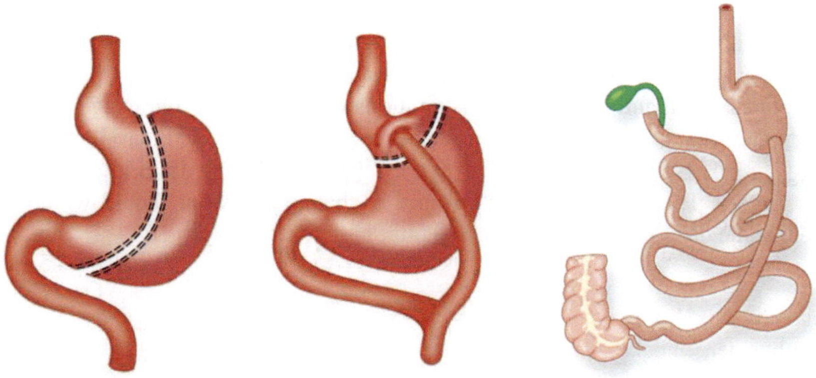

Laparoscopic sleeve gastrectomy

Laparoscopic Roux-en-Y gastric bypass

Duodenal switch

20.3 Drugs in GI Tract: The Pharmacokinetics

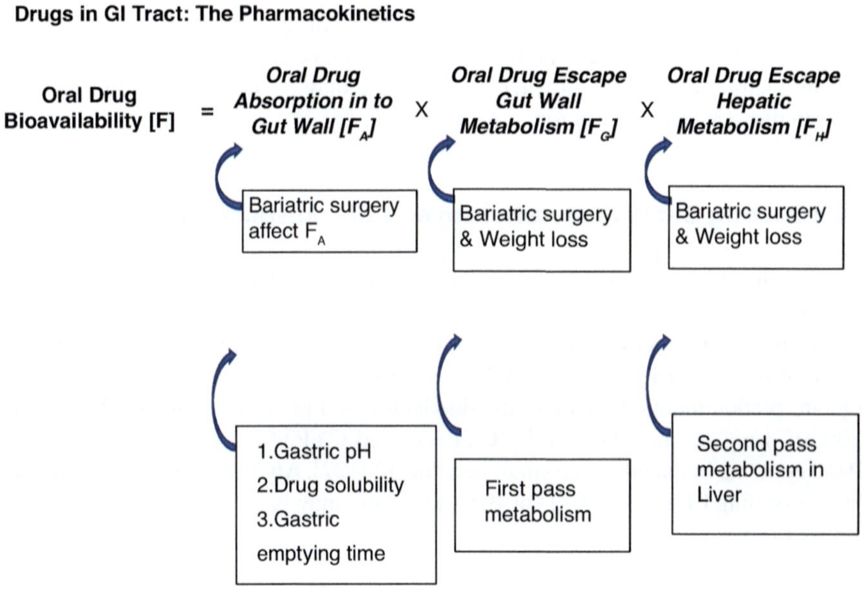

Table 20.1 Acid-base drugs physiochemical properties in normal state [17–21]

	Stomach (pH1~2)	Small intestine (pH6~8)
Weak base drugs	Fully charged and high solubility in water	Fully uncharged and absorbed rapidly from the small intestine → easily pass through GI mucosa
Weak acid drugs	Fully uncharged and absorbed rapidly from stomach → easily pass through GI mucosa	Fully charged and high solubility in water

20.3.1 Solubility, Gastric pH, Gastric Emptying Time, and Drug Absorption

Drug solubility, lipophilicity, molecular size and polarity are major components of drug physiochemical properties. The pKa, drug-specific acid dissociation constant, is a key physiochemical parameter influencing many biopharmaceutical characteristics. pKa determines a drug's ability to cross a range of pH in the GI tract. If the pKa of a drug is close to the pH of the medium, the molecule is charged and its gastrointestinal diffusion is delayed. In summary, increasing gastric pH should decrease the solubility of basic drugs and increase the solubility of acidic drugs [14].

The pH of gastrointestinal fluid has been shown to significantly affect the fraction of the dose absorbed of a drug [15, 16] (Table 20.1).

Changes in the GI tract following bariatric surgery will have different effects on different drugs [22]. After bariatric surgery, a changed gastric pH may affect drug dissolution and solubility, as well as pre-absorptive drug stability [11]. After bariatric surgery, the new stomach pouch has a reduction of gastric acid secretion. After bariatric surgeries, altered gastric emptying time may be another rate-limiting step of systemic drug absorption for some drugs [22, 23].

20.3.2 Drug Gut Wall Metabolism and GI Transporters

Duodenum and proximal part of the small intestine are rich in metabolizing enzymes which is bypassed in LRYGB, BPD, BPD-DS patients. Hence, in these patients, higher oral bioavailability is easily noted because they bypassed the "first pass metabolism." Cytochrome P450 (CYP) enzymes, especially the CYP3A4 subfamily, are predominant enzymes in the duodenum and proximal jejunum. More than 50% of drugs are metabolized by CYP3A4 and CYP3A4 accounts for 80% total P450 contents in the proximal small intestine [24–27]. After rearranging the GI tract by performing LRYGB or BPD or BPD-DS, there may be an elevated oral bioavailability (Table 20.2).

20.3.3 Oral Drug Escaping Hepatic Metabolism

Obesity is a low-grade inflammatory state which results in increased circulation of inflammatory cytokines, chemokines, and adipokines. Besides, nonalcoholic fatty liver diseases (NAFLD), nonalcoholic steatohepatitis (NASH) are both prevalent in obese populations. This will contribute to reduced activity of CYP450 activity in the liver. So, in obese individuals, second pass metabolism is weaker than in those in the normal weight range. However, weight loss by bariatric surgery and amelioration of NAFLD or NASH, will increase the CYP450 function in the liver and second pass effect in the human body [37–41].

In conclusion, weight loss and the physical adaption of the GI tract following bariatric surgeries are the main contributing factors that cause complicated and time-dependent interplay in restricting oral drug bioavailability.

Table 20.2 Intestinal transporter proteins can accelerate drug absorption [26, 28–36]

GI transporters	Corresponding medications
OATP1A2	Expressed on duodenum Thyroid, steroid hormones, fluoroquinolones, statins
PEPT1	Beta-lactamines, angiotensin converting enzymes inhibitors (ACEI), thrombin inhibitors, antineoplastics medications
P-glycoprotein	Expressed most on distal ileum and colon Digoxin, verapamil, diltiazem, sotalol

20.4 Drugs Related Complications After Bariatric Surgery

20.4.1 Analgesics

Analgesics are very important medications after bariatric surgery. It includes non-steroidal anti-inflammatory drugs (NSAIDs). According to the Clinical Practice Guidelines for the Perioperative Nutritional, Metabolic, and Nonsurgical Support of the Bariatric Surgery Patient, NSAIDs should be completely avoided after bariatric surgery. In gastric bypass patients, even a zero-tolerance policy towards the use of an NSAID is advocated [42–44]. Because pKa of NSAID is about 3–5, the elevation of gastric pH after bariatric surgery increased the absorption rate in the stomach and that is the cause of higher risks of gastric and anastomotic perforations and ulcerations. We can use paracetamol or tramadol as alternatives if possible as they are absorbed in the jejunum and the area under curve (AUC) for these drugs is not changed after bariatric surgery [45–47].

20.4.2 Anticoagulants

Anticoagulants may be affected significantly after bariatric surgery. Too low level of anticoagulants may cause massive thrombotic effects; too high level of anticoagulants may have profound bleeding risks.

20.4.2.1 Aspirin

Aspirin activity is blunted in the obese population. According to Nicholas B. Norgard et al., aspirin activity is increased after bariatric surgery. The aspirin-induced platelet inhibition may be more potent following bariatric surgery [48]. Adjustment of aspirin dose is needed after bariatric surgery in case of uncontrollable bleeding or newly formed ulcerations.

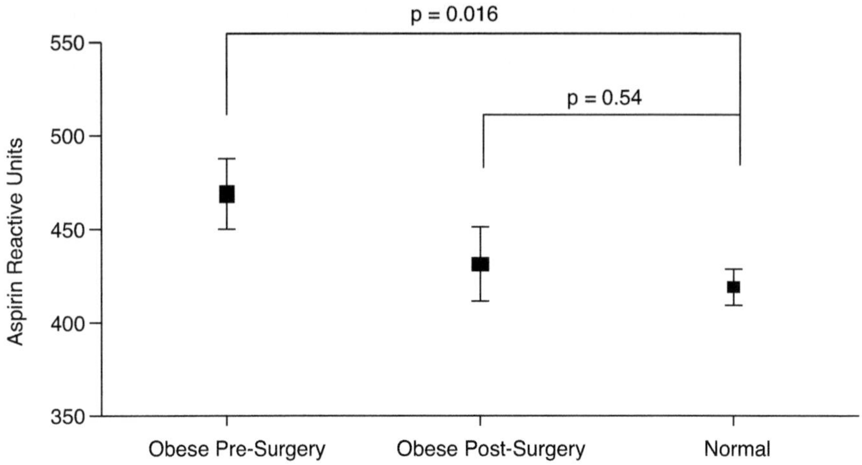

20.4.2.2 Warfarin (Vitamin K Antagonists)

Warfarin dosage requirements change transiently after bariatric surgery. During the first 1–3 months, a significant reduction in the median weekly dose was noted [ranging from 7.7 mg/week decrease at days 8–14 after surgery to a 30 mg/week decrease at days 50–56 ($p < 0.01$)]. Interestingly, the weekly dose requirement returned to and remained at pre-surgery doses 90–180 days postoperatively [49]. The possible mechanism of reduced dose requirements after surgery was due to anatomic changes or lower vitamin K intake [50]. Also a more alkaline stomach pH value resulting in more unionized warfarin available for passive absorption is another possible reason [51]. Overall, the literature suggests that warfarin dosing is reduced in the immediate postoperative period (within 3–4 weeks), with a trend towards increased dose requirements as patients are further out from surgery. Regularly monitoring of INR is necessary.

20.4.2.3 Direct Oral Anticoagulants

There is not much data regarding the use of direct oral anticoagulants in the post-bariatric surgery patients. There is only one case report showing successful use rivaroxaban on patients after bariatric surgery. Table 20.3 below is the summary of characteristics of oral antithrombotic [49]:

Table 20.3 Characteristics of oral antithrombotic

Antithrombotic agent	location of absorption	Volume of distribution[a]	Biopharmaceutics classification system[b]	Concurrent food intake impact on drug absorption
Apixaban	Primarily proximal small intestine: some gastric absorption [17, 18, 45]	21 L [46] (03 L/kg)	BCS Class III (high solubility, low permeability)	No effect Take without regard to food
Dabigatran	Lower stomach and duodenum [20]	50–70 L [47] (0.7–1 L/kg)	BCS Class II (low solubility, high permeability)	No effect Take without regard to food
Edoxaban	Proximal small intestine [14]	107 L [48] (1.5 L/kg)	BCS Class IV (low solubility, low permeability) [49]	+6–22% [50] Take without regard to food
Rivaroxaban	Primarily proximal small intestine: some gastric absorption [9, 11]	50 L (0.7 L/kg)	BCS Class II (low solubility, high permeability) [29]	+39% [10, 11] Take 15 and 20 mg dose with food to improve bioasailability
Warfarin	Proximal [25]	0.14 L/g [51] (10 L)	BCS Class II (low solubility, high permeability) [52]	No effect

[a]Reported values obtained from the prescribing information (calculated values based on 70 kg patient)
[b]BCS class is a FDA classification system that classifies drugs based on their solubility and intestinal permeability [53]

20.4.3 Psychotropic Medications

There is scanty literature about post-bariatric psychiatric medications. However, there are many patients who still need psychiatric medications for controlling diseases after surgery. Cunningham et al. found that 23% of the patients had an increase in their antidepressant use, 40% continued to require the same antidepressant, 18% had a change in antidepressant medication, and only 16% had a decrease or discontinued their antidepressant [52]. Higher level of these drugs may cause terrible toxicity. Severe episodes of the psychiatric diseases may be occurred if lower level of the medications is used. Adequate dosage and dosage form are very important in psychiatric patients.

There are some psychotropic medications that need to be changed after bariatric surgery. Many medications may cause severe side effects even lead to mortality. Tricyclic antidepressants (TCAs) and selective serotonin reuptake inhibitors (SSRIs) are highly lipophilic and may change to lower volume of distribution after bariatric surgery due to less adipose tissue [53] (Table 20.4).

20.4.4 Antimetabolic Syndrome Medications

20.4.4.1 Antidiabetic Medications

Metformin may increase bioavailability by 50% and glucose levels are thus decreased by 15% in RYGB patients, and these differences were statistically significant. AUC showed a statistically non-significant trend of 21% increase in RYGB patients compared with controls. Patients treated with metformin should be monitored after RYGB in order to prevent toxicity [54].

20.4.4.2 Statin

Statins may have side effects on liver function. There are some changes in statin levels after bariatric surgery. Atorvastatin is a typical statin medication. Careful use of statin dosage is critical (Table 20.5):

Table 20.4 Psychotropic medications and bariatric surgery

Medications	Change after LRYGB
Midazolam	CYP3A4 substrate Increased bioavailability after LRYGB
Citalopram, buspirone, diazepam,lorazepam, trazodone, zolpidem, haloperidol, oxcarbazepine	No change in vitro
Venlafaxine	No change in vitro
Amitriptyline, fluoxetine, paroxetine, sertraline, clozapine, olanzapine, quetiapine, risperidone, ziprasidone	Less dissolution in vitro after LRYGB

Table 20.5 Statin medications after bariatric surgery [55–57]

Medications	Change after bariatric surgery
Atorvastatin	Gastric bypass surgery showed a variable effect on systemic exposure to atorvastatin, ranging from a 2.9-fold decrease to a 2.3-fold increase [55]. Biliopancreatic diversion with duodenal switch, found increased twofold bioavailability of atorvastatin [56]
Simvastatin	Unknown
Pravastatin	Bariatric surgery hardly affects the pharmacokinetics of this drug. Research is needed to establish whether pravastatin from a pharmacokinetic point of view may be the most appropriate statin after bariatric surgery [57]

20.4.4.3 Antihypertensive

Wójcicki et al. investigated the pharmacokinetics of propranolol and atenolol in patients after partial gastric resection. Propranolol showed decrease in AUC by 32% and a decrease in $C_{\max}$ by 20%. There is no need to change the dose of atenolol. Propranolol is a lipophilic drug and atenolol is a hydrophilic compound. The lipophilicity of propranolol may be responsible for the observed impairment of drug absorption in patients after partial gastrectomy [58, 59]. Beta-blockers may have severe effects on the heart and asthma conditions. Close clinical monitoring of these medications is very important.

20.4.5 Antibiotics

It has been proved that using standardized dose of moxifloxacin cannot attain adequate levels in post-bariatric surgery population [60]. The same situation is for both amoxicillin and nitrofurantoin [61].

A recent study characterized the pharmacokinetics of intravenous and oral linezolid before and 3 months after RYGB surgery [62]. The bioavailability of the drug was not impaired (1.14 before and after LRYGB), however, the mean AUC with oral linezolid before RYGB was 41.6 mg·h/l compared with 98.9 mg·h/l after RYGB ($p < 0.001$). The serum exposure of the drug was more than 50% lower after bariatric surgery suggesting that dose modification may be needed.

Inadequate doses of antibiotics may cause serious complications even sepsis and mortality.

20.4.6 Antiarrhythmics

Chan et al. compared the pattern and magnitude of oral absorption of digoxin in obese patients before and after RYGB. The median time to peak concentration for digoxin decreased from 40 min at baseline to 30 and 20 min at 3 and 12 months after RYGB, respectively. The mean AUC for digoxin, heart rate, and electrocardiogram patterns were similar across the study phases [63].

20.4.7 Oral Contraceptives

Rapid weight loss in the months after bariatric surgery increases fertility, while maternal and fetal risks from rapid weight loss remain elevated [64]. Consequently, effective contraception is critical in the postoperative period. In the postoperative period of surgical weight loss there may be a reduction in the bioavailability of oral contraceptives and thus compromise contraceptive protection [65].

20.4.8 Thyroid Drugs

Significant delay of absorption of levothyroxine was noted after LRYGB patients. Hence, increased total T4 and free T4 was noted in post-bariatric patients. Obese patients scheduled for bariatric surgery should be screened for thyroid dysfunction and, if replacement therapy is necessary, strict monitoring of thyroid function and drug level is very important [66].

20.5 Conclusion

Literature assessing the change in the use of medication before and after bariatric surgery is needed. Changed in GI anatomy and post-bariatric surgical adaptation of the GI tract afterwards will cause change in the absorption of medicine, which might cause adverse drug events or result in an inadequate therapeutic effect. Theoretically, reduced drug absorption may occur after bariatric surgery. Until now, only sparse studies focus on the pharmacokinetics of frequently used drugs. Before more data emerges, close monitoring of medication formulations may still be critical to ensure adequate absorption and to prevent drug-related complications after bariatric surgery [44, 67].

Key Points

1. Bariatric surgery results in anatomical changes in the GI tract which affect the oral bioavailability of many drugs due to changes in GI lumen pH, distribution of GI transporters and enzymes in the bypassed gut, and altered first and second pass metabolism.
2. Due to altered body composition, there may be changes in drug distribution in the body.
3. These changes may lead to normal pre-surgery doses being inadequate for therapeutic effect post-surgery or excessive resulting in complications.
4. Some drugs like NSAIDs should be avoided as far as possible while others would need dose modification.

References

1. Ribeiro-Parenti L, et al. Intestinal adaptations following bariatric surgery: towards the identification of new pharmacological targets for obesity-related metabolic diseases. Curr Opin Pharmacol. 2017;37:29–34.
2. Santry HP, Gillen DL, Lauderdale DS. Trends in bariatric surgical procedures. JAMA. 2005;294:1909–17.
3. Schlatter J. Oral contraceptives after bariatric surgery. Obes Facts. 2017;10:118–26.
4. Angrisani L, Santonicola A, Iovino P, et al. IFSO Worldwide Survey 2016: primary, endoluminal, and revisional procedures. Obes Surg. 2018;28(12):3783–94.
5. Buchwald H, Oien DM. Metabolic/bariatric surgery worldwide 2011. Obes Surg. 2013;23:427–36.
6. Kansou G, Lechaux D, Delarue J, et al. Laparoscopic sleeve gastrectomy versus laparoscopic mini gastric bypass: one year outcomes. Int J Surg. 2016;22:18–22.
7. Schroeder R, Harrison TD, McGraw SL. Treatment of adult obesity with bariatric surgery. Am Fam Physician. 2016;93:31–7.
8. Li P, Fu P, Chen J, et al. Laparoscopic Roux-en-Y gastric bypass vs. laparoscopic sleeve gastrectomy for morbid obesity and diabetes mellitus: a meta-analysis of sixteen recent studies. Hepatogastroenterology. 2013;60:132–7.
9. Moloney BM, Hynes DA, Kelly ME, et al. The role of laparoscopic sleeve gastrectomy as a treatment for morbid obesity; review of outcomes. Ir J Med Sci. 2017;186:143–9.
10. Ruiz-Tovar J, Llavero C, Zubiaga L, et al. Maintenance of multivitamin supplements after sleeve gastrectomy. Obes Surg. 2016;26:2324–430.
11. Custodio JM, Wu CY, Benet LZ. Predicting drug disposition, absorption/elimination/transporter interplay and the role of food on drug absorption. Adv Drug Deliv Rev. 2008;60:717–33.
12. Mahawar KK, Sharples AJ. Contribution of malabsorption to weight loss after Roux-en-Y gastric bypass: a systematic review. Obes Surg. 2017.
13. Batterham RL, Cummings DE. Mechanisms of diabetes improvement following bariatric/metabolic surgery. Diabetes Care. 2016;39:893–901.
14. Hogben CM, Schenker LS, Tocco DJ, et al. Absorption of drugs from the stomach II: the human. J Pharmacol Exp Ther. 1957;120:540–5.
15. Russell TL, Berardi RR, Barnett JL, et al. pH-related changes in the absorption of dipyridamole in the elderly. Pharm Res. 1994;11:136–43.
16. Blum RA, D'Andrea DT, Florentino BM, et al. Increased gastric pH and the bioavailability of fluconazole and ketoconazole. Ann Intern Med. 1991;114:755–7.
17. Charman WN, Porter CJ, Mithani S, et al. Physiochemical and physiological mechanisms for the effects of food on drug absorption: the role of lipids and pH. J Pharm Sci. 1997;86:269–82.
18. Yamashita S, Kataoka M, Higashino HS, et al. Measurement of drug concentration in the stomach after intragastric administration of drug solution to healthy volunteers: analysis of intragastric fluid dynamics and drug absorption. Pharm Res. 2013;30:951–8.
19. Lahner E, Annibale B, Delle Fave G. Systematic review: impaired drug absorption related to the co-administration of antisecretory therapy. Aliment Pharmacol Ther. 2009;29:1219–29.
20. Mitra A, Kesisoglou F. Impaired drug absorption due to high stomach pH: a review of strategies for mitigation of such effect to enable pharmaceutical product development. Mol Pharm. 2013;10:3970–9.
21. Miller AD, Smith KM. Medication and nutrient administration considerations after bariatric surgery. Am J Health Syst Pharm. 2006;63:1852–7.
22. Wallden J, Thorn SE, Wattwil M. The delay of gastric emptying induced by remifentanil is not influenced by posture. Anesth Analg. 2004;99(2):429–34. Table of contents.
23. Sioka E, Tzovaras G, Perivoliotis K, et al. Impact of laparoscopic sleeve gastrectomy on gastrointestinal motility. Gastroenterol Res Pract. 2018;2018:4135813.
24. Dresser GK, Spence JD, Bailey DG. Pharmacokinetic-pharmacodynamic consequences and clinical relevance of cytochrome P450 3A4 inhibition. Clin Pharmacokinet. 2000;38(1):41–57.

25. Guengerich FP. Cytochrome P-450 3A4: regulation and role in drug metabolism. Annu Rev Pharmacol Toxicol. 1999;39:1–17.
26. Paine MF, Khalighi M, Fisher JM, et al. Characterization of interintestinal and intraintestinal variations in human CYP3A-dependent metabolism. J Pharmacol Exp Ther. 1997;283(3):1552–62.
27. Angeles PC, et al. The influence of bariatric surgery on oral drug bioavailability in patients with obesity: a systemic review. Obes Rev. 2019;20:1299–311.
28. Glaeser H, Bailey DG, Dresser GK, et al. Intestinal drug transporter expression and the impact of grapefruit juice in humans. Clin Pharmacol Ther. 2007;81:362–70.
29. Maeda T, Takahashi K, Ohtsu N, et al. Identification of influx transporter for the quinolone antibacterial agent levofloxacin. Mol Pharm. 2007;4:85–94.
30. Inui K, Tomita Y, Katsura T, et al. H+ coupled active transport of bestatin via the dipeptide transport system in rabbit intestinal brush-border membranes. J Pharmacol Exp Ther. 1992;260:482–6.
31. Walter E, Kissel T, Reers M, Dickneite G, et al. Transepithelial transport properties of peptidomimetic thrombin inhibitors in monolayers of a human intestinal cell line (Caco-2) and their correlation to in vivo data. Pharm Res. 1995;12:360–5.
32. Adibi SA. Regulation of expression of the intestinal oligopeptide to transport (Pept-1) in health and disease. Am J Physiol Gastrointest Liver Physiol. 2003;285:G779–88.
33. Adibi SA. The oligopeptide to transport (Pept-1) in human internal: biology and function. Gastroenterology. 1997;113:332–40.
34. Matheny CJ, Lamb MW, Brouwer KR, et al. Pharmacokinetic and pharmacodynamic implications of P-glyco-protein modulation. Pharmacotherapy. 2001;21:778–96.
35. Mouly S, Paine MF. P-glycoprotein increases from proximal to distal regions of human small intestine. Pharm Res. 2003;20:1595–9.
36. Darwich AS, Pade D, Ammori BJ, et al. With mechanistic pharmacokinetic model to assess modified oral drug bioavailability post bariatric surgery in morbidly obese patients: interplay between CYP3A gut wall metabolism, permeability and dissolution. J Pharm Pharmacol. 2012;64:1008–24.
37. Rao SR. Inflammatory markers and bariatric surgery: a meta-analysis. Inflamm Res. 2012;61(8):789–807.
38. Schmitt C, Kuhn B, Zhang X, Kivitz AJ, Grange S. Disease-drug-drug interaction involving tocilizumab and simvastatin in patients with rheumatoid arthritis. Clin Pharmacol Ther. 2011;89(5):735–40.
39. Tchernof A, Despres JP. Pathophysiology of human visceral obesity: an update. Physiol Rev. 2013;93(1):359–404.
40. Kolwankar D, Vuppalanchi R, Ethell B, et al. Association between non-alcoholic hepatic steatosis and hepatic cytochrome P-450 3A activity. Clin Gastroenterol Hepatol. 2007;5(3):388–93.
41. Ferslew BC, Johnston CK, Tsakalozou E, et al. Altered morphine glucuronide and bile acid disposition in patients with nonalcoholic steatohepatitis. Clin Pharmacol Ther. 2015;97(4):419–27.
42. Mechanick JI, Youdim A, Jones DB, et al. Clinical practice guidelines for the perioperative, nutritional, metabolic, and nonsurgical support of the bariatric surgery patient—2013 update: cosponsored by American Association of Clinical Endocrinologists, The Obesity Society, and American Society for Metabolic & Bariatric Surgery. Surg Obes Relat Dis. 2013;9:159–91.
43. Sasse KC, Ganser J, Kozar M, et al. Seven cases of gastric perforation in Roux-en-Y gastric bypass patients: what lessons can we learn? Obes Surg. 2008;18:530–4.
44. Yska JP, et al. NSAID use after bariatric surgery: a randomized controlled intervention study. Obes Surg. 2016.
45. Fleisher D, Li C, Zhou Y, Pao LH, et al. Drug, meal and formulation interactions influencing drug absorption after oral administration. Clinical implications. Clin Pharmacokinet. 1999;36:233–54.
46. Tesserommatis C, Saranteas T, Chatzijanni E, et al. Modifications off clonidine binding to rabbit liver protein under the influence off not-steroid-anti-inflammatory drugs in vitro. Eur J Drug Metab Pharmacokinet. 2003;28:245–7.

47. Terry SI, Gould JC, McManus JP, et al. Absorption of penicillin and paracetamol after small intestinal bypass surgery. Eur J Clin Pharmacol. 1982;23:245–8.
48. Norgard NB, et al. Aspirin responsiveness changes in obese patients following bariatric surgery. Cardiovasc Ther. 2017 Aug;35(4).
49. Martin KA, et al. Oral anticoagulant use after bariatric surgery: a literature review and clinical guidance. Am J Med. 2017 May;130(5):517–24.
50. Slater GH, Ren CJ, Siegel N, et al. Serum fat-soluble vitamin deficiency and abnormal calcium metabolism after malabsorptive bariatric surgery. J Gastrointest Surg. 2004;8:48–55. discussion 54-45. [PubMed: 14746835].
51. Smith A, Henriksen B, Cohen A. Pharmacokinetic considerations in Roux-en-Y gastric bypass patients. Am J Health-Syst Pharm. 2011;68:2241–7.
52. Cunningham JL, Merrell CC, Sarr M, et al. Investigation of anti-depressant medication usage after bariatric surgery. Obes Surg. 2012;22:530–5.
53. Voelker M, Foster TG. Nursing challenges in the administration of oral antidepressant medications in gastric bypass patients. J Perianesth Nurs. 2007;22:108–24.
54. Padwal RS, Gabr RQ, Sharma AM, et al. Effect of gastric bypass surgery on the absorption and bioavailability of metformin. Diabetes Care. 2011;34:1295–300.
55. Skottheim IB, Stormark K, Christensen H, et al. Significantly altered systemic exposure to atorvastatin acid following gastric bypass surgery in morbidly obese patients. Clin Pharmacol Ther. 2009;86:311–8.
56. Skottheim IB, Jakobsen GS, Stormark K, et al. Significant increase in systemic exposure of atorvastatin after biliopancreatic diversion with duodenal switch. Clin Pharmacol Ther. 2010;87:699–705.
57. Schachter M. Chemical, pharmacokinetic and pharmacodynamic properties of statins: an update. Fundam Clin Pharmacol. 2005;19:117–25.
58. Wójcicki J, Wojciechowski G, Wójcicki M, et al. Pharmacokinetics of propranolol and atenolol in patients after partial gastric resection: a comparative study. Eur J Clin Pharmacol. 2000;56:75–9.
59. Valdivieso A, Calvo R, Gonzalez JP, et al. Influence of several surgical techniques in peptic ulcer disease on the oral kinetic of a basic drug. Acta Chir Belg. 1993;93:88–91.
60. Colin P, Eleveld DJ, Struys MM, et al. Moxifloxacin dosing in post-bariatric surgery patients. Br J Clin Pharmacol. 2014;78:84–93.
61. Magee SR, Shih G, Hume A. Malabsorption off oral antibiotics in pregnancy after gastric bypass surgery. J Am Board Fam Med. 2007;20:310–3.
62. Hamilton R, Thai XC, Ameri D, et al. Oral bioavailability of linezolid before and after Roux-en-Y gastric bypass surgery: is dose modification necessary in obese subjects? J Antimicrob Chemother. 2013;68:666–73.
63. Chan LN, Lin YS, Tay-Sontheimer JC, et al. Proximal Roux-en-Y gastric bypass alters drug absorption pattern but not systemic exposure of CYP3A4 and P-glycoprotein substrates. Pharmacotherapy. 2015;35:361–9.
64. Merhi ZO. Challenging oral contraception after weight loss by bariatric surgery. Gynecol Obstet Invest. 2007;64:100–2.
65. Paulen ME, Zapata LB, Cansino C, et al. Contraceptive use among women with a history of bariatric surgery: a systematic review. Contraception. 2010;82:86–94.
66. Rubio IGS, Galrão AL, Santo MA, et al. Levothyroxine absorption in morbidly obese patients before and after Roux-en-Y gastric bypass (RYGB) surgery. Obes Surg. 2012;22:253–8.
67. Lizer MH, Papageorgeon H, Glembot TM. Nutritional and pharmacologic challenges in the bariatric surgery patient. Obes Surg. 2010;20:1654–9.

21 Weight Regain After Bariatric Metabolic Surgery

Mohit Bhandari, Manoj Khurana, and M. A. L. Fobi

Weight regain is a bigger issue than just calorie in and calorie out.

21.1 Introduction

Obesity is a worldwide health problem of epidemic proportions [1, 2]. Causes of obesity are multifactorial [3]. Persons inherit silenced genes. Epigenetic modulation occurs dynamically and continuously throughout the life of an individual and is influenced by the environment, exercise habit, food, medications, sleep, and stress. Obesity is understood to be a pathologic process resulting in excess body fat. It is the result of the interaction of inherited genetics and with the environment mediated by epigenetic changes in those genes or their expressed proteins. Sixty-seven percent of the variability in body mass index (BMI) is attributable to inheritance. Of the total variability, 40% is due to genes that control food intake, 12% is due to metabolic rate, 5% to fat oxidation, and 10% to spontaneous physical activity. There is definitely a genetic predisposition that is enhanced by environmental, cultural, and psychosocial factors [4, 5].

Obesity is also a multisystem disease that spares no body organ [6]. Conditions associated with obesity include CAD, T2D, cancers (endometrial, breast, and colon), HTN, dyslipidemia (high total cholesterol, high triglycerides), stroke, liver, and gallbladder disease, sleep apnea and respiratory disorders, osteoarthritis, gynecologic problems (infertility, abnormal menses, and polycystic ovary) and pseudotumor cerebri.

M. Bhandari (✉) · M. Khurana · M. A. L. Fobi
Mohak Bariatrics and Robotics Surgery Center, Indore, India

A. G. Bhasker et al. (eds.), *Management of Nutritional and Metabolic Complications of Bariatric Surgery*,
https://doi.org/10.1007/978-981-33-4702-1_21

Intentional weight loss, even to a modest degree (5–10%), has a significant impact on the morbidity and mortality associated with obesity. There are many strategies for nonsurgical weight reduction, including diet, exercise, hospital supervised, commercially available, and psychiatric-behavior modification programs and medications. Unfortunately, although many people can lose weight successfully through dietary manipulation, only 5–10% of patients with extreme obesity are able to sustain significant weight reduction. The National Institutes of Health (NIH) Technology Assessment Conference in 1992 concluded that dietary management of severe obesity, with or without behavioral modification, failed to provide acceptable evidence of long-term efficacy [7].

Bariatric surgery has been shown to provide the most effective long-term treatment option for patients with obesity, particularly severe obesity, resulting in improved obesity-related comorbidities and increased overall life expectancy [8]. Weight regain, is part of the natural history of any intentional weight loss effort [9].

21.2 Definition

Weight regain occurs after almost all strategies for nonsurgical weight reduction but only in a subset of patients who lose weight surgically. Weight regain after surgery has been defined variably. There is some weight regain after the nadir weight in all patients due to the adaptation of the patient to the operation. This is usually a regain of 1–10 kg after which the patient's weight stabilizes. Significant weight regain is defined as either weight gain of >10 kg, weight gain of 25% of weight loss, recurrence of weight loss status to <50% EBWL, BMI status >35 kg/m^2 for class III obesity, or BMI > 40 kg/m^2 for patients with super obesity and super-super obesity [10–15].

21.3 Causes of Weight Regain

Significant weight regain that occurs in a subset of patients after surgical treatment appears to be multifactorial. Overlapping aetiologies are categorized as patient-specific (presence of psychiatric disorders, physical inactivity, use of medications that cause weight gain, endocrinopathies, and dietary non-compliance and eating disorders) and operation-specific (the choice of bariatric surgical procedure performed and the duration of follow-up after the operation—physiologic adaptation) [16, 17].

21.4 Patient-Specific Causes of Weight Regain

Patient-specific causes of weight regain are well documented in many studies. Loss of dietary control with grazing behaviors (defined as consumption of smaller amounts of foods over extended periods of time) are factors identified in studies [17,

18]. Colles et al. [18] reported that over a 1-year follow-up of 129 AGB patients, uncontrolled eating with grazing was associated with decreased weight loss. Uncontrolled eaters lost 21.6 kg compared to 26.7 kg in controlled eaters, and "grazers" lost 17.3% of their initial weight versus 22.9% in patients with controlled eating habits. Kofman et al. [19] found a significant relationship between loss of control when eating and weight regain. Approximately half of all respondents reported they deviated from their dietary plan, and the frequency of grazing was positively correlated with weight recidivism post-RYGB. Food indiscretion was a major contributing factor to weight regain in a survey of 100 morbidly obese patients who were followed up for 85 months in a study by Freire et al. [20]. These authors demonstrated that poor diet quality, characterized by an excessive intake of calories, snacks, and sweets, as well as oils and fatty foods, was statistically higher in patients experiencing weight regain. Finally, both Magro et al. and Freire et al. demonstrated the importance of appropriate nutritional counseling on long-term weight maintenance wherein the lack of appropriate nutritional follow-up was significantly associated with weight regain post-surgery [10, 20].

Another patient-specific cause of weight regain is the mental status of the patient. Kalarchian et al. followed 96 RYGB patients for 2–7 years post-surgery and reported that those classified as binge eaters increased their BMI by 5.3 kg/m^2 compared to a 2.4-kg/m^2 increase in non-binge eaters [21].

Depression, alcohol, and drug use, food urges, and fewer follow-up visits were reported to be predictors of weight gain in RYGB patients at a mean follow-up of 28.1 months by Odom et al. [22]. Colles et al. [18] suggested that the presence of an eating disorder increased in over 1 year in patients following AGB from 26.3% to 38.0% and correlated with poorer weight loss. Bond et al. [23] suggested that impulsive behavioral traits were a risk factor for weight regain following bariatric surgery at 2-years follow-up. Finally, a study of 60 adult veterans who were followed with a multidisciplinary evaluation for 24 months post-surgery found 18 participants experienced weight regain between the 12- and 24-months measurement points and weight regain increased in a dose-response pattern in relation to increasing number of psychiatric diagnoses [24]. Further, patients with two or more psychiatric conditions were approximately six times more likely to either lose no further weight or regain the weight.

Hormonal imbalances have been causes of weight regain in some patients. Studies commented on potential hormonal or metabolic imbalances that could explain weight regain post-bariatric surgery. The study of Engstrom et al. of 40 RYGB patients with a mean follow-up of 42.5 months reported that post-prandial suppression of plasma ghrelin level was correlated with weight loss and maintenance of weight loss [25]. Ghrelin was also implicated as a factor influencing weight maintenance and ultimately failure of weight loss in a 5-year trial conducted by Bohdjalian et al. [26]. Herein, weight regain was observed in 19.2% of patients post-LSG, and measurements of plasma ghrelin demonstrated that the levels were higher in weight regain patients compared to those who experienced appropriate weight loss or maintenance post-surgery.

Orexigenic medications have also been reported as causes of weight regain after surgical treatment. These include steroids, antihistamines. Anti-depressants and antidiabetic agents.

Inadequate physical activity has been identified as a contributing factor for weight regain in the survey study of 100 patients post-RYGB by Freire et al. Patients who performed physical exercises had the lowest weight regain incidence compared to those who were relatively inactive [20].

A patient with significant weight regain needs to be evaluated looking at the dietary history, physical activity levels, and orexigenic medications use. Anatomical causes of weight regain should also be investigated with radiological tests and endoscopic evaluation as determined by the prior surgical procedure and medical history.

Based on these findings, the initial alteration of the patient's medications with psychological and nutritional counseling may be tried. In some cases, trial of anorexic drugs with psychological and nutritional counseling may be indicated.

Occasionally, patients respond to this nonsurgical management with good weight loss and maintenance. However, in most cases, the outcome of nonsurgical management is short lived.

21.5 Operation Specific Causes of Weight Regain

Significant weight regain has been documented in subset of patients within all of the most commonly performed bariatric surgeries. The incidence is least after vertical gastrectomy with a duodenal switch (BPD-DS), banded gastric bypass (BGBP), and one anastomosis gastric bypass (OAGB). The incidence increases after Roux-en-Y gastric bypass (RYGB), vertical sleeve gastrectomy (VSG), and laparoscopic adjustable gastric banding (LAGB), respectively.

In cases where obvious anatomic findings are determined to be the cause of the weight regain, correction of the anatomic derangement should be considered. This may entail endoscopic intervention or surgical intervention. Endoscopic intervention may involve pouch and/or stoma reduction or in the case of a fistula, endoscopic closure of the fistula. If surgical intervention is indicated because of anatomic derangement, revising the anatomy to that of the original operation or conversion to another operation may be the options.

In cases with an intact anatomic configuration of the initial operation, surgical revision to another operation by enhancing one or more of the various mechanisms responsible for weight loss and/or maintenance are the options. The outcome of surgical reintervention, weight loss, weight loss maintenance, and resolution of comorbid conditions depend on the initial operation and the choice of the revision operation. Generally speaking, surgical reintervention with the revision to a particular operation results in the suboptimal outcome than the primary operation and also has a higher complication rate. Surgical reversal in all cases results in almost all weight regain and even more.

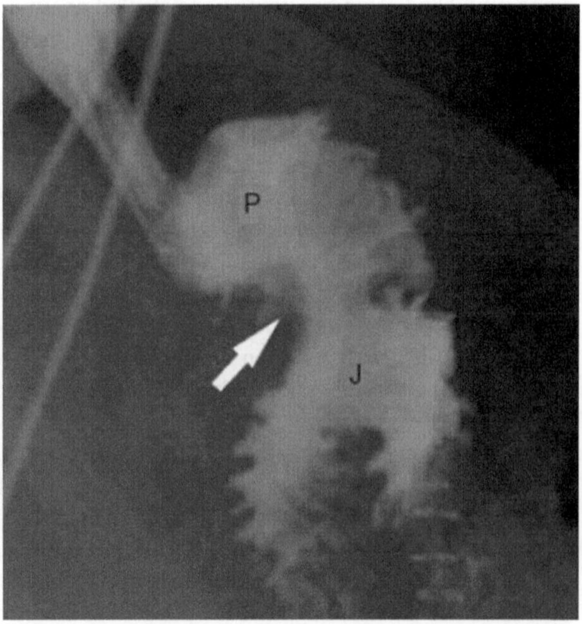

Fig. 21.1 Dilated gastric pouch and stoma

Gastric Bypass There are many possible causes of weight regain after a gastric bypass operation. Pouch dilatation, increase in stoma size, and gastro-gastric fistula are recognized causes of weight regain after RYGB. Pouch dilatation is considered, if the pouch is >6 cm long or >5 cm wide [27] (Fig. 21.1). However, these measurements are empirical, and little scientific evidence exists to support them. Henegan et al. have evaluated a selected cohort of patients who underwent gastroscopy after RYGB for functional symptoms or weight loss problems. The patients were divided into two groups, those who had an optimal weight loss (n = 175) and those who regained weight (n = 205). There was no significant difference in average pouch width and average pouch volume between the groups. Only the average length of pouch reached significant difference and was 5.0 and 5.8 cm, respectively. Of note, the average pouch in the weight regain group was 26 cm^2 as compared to 21.8 cm^2 in the optimal weight loss group [28].

Topart et al. have estimated pouch size after barium swallow in 107 patients on average 3 years after operation and found no correlation between the pouch size and %EWL. Patients who had large pouches (>50 mL) had similar weight loss to those who had normal-sized pouches, 68 vs. 66%EWL, respectively. Even in patients with pouches >100 mL in size weight loss was comparable to that with smaller pouches [29].

A wide gastrojejunostomy is considered one which exceeds 2 cm [28]. Different techniques are used to create gastrojejunostomy in RYGB and result in different stoma size. Hand-sewn anastomosis is usually 12–14 mm wide, circular stapled anastomosis maybe 21 or 25 mm in diameter depending on instrument size and linear stapled anastomosis maybe up to 45 mm. Recent meta-analysis of studies comparing hand-sewn anastomosis to stapled anastomosis did not find any difference on weight loss after 12 months. However, more long-term follow-up data is needed to estimate the impact of initial stoma size on weight regain [30].

Different endoscopic procedures have been used for gastroenterostomy reduction including sclerotherapy or transoral outlet reduction (Tore) by placing sutures around dilated stoma. Other techniques, such as Restorative Obesity Surgery Endoscopic (ROSE) and endoscopic gastric plication, aim at creating tissue folds that reduce pouch and stoma size. Endoscopic plication achieves the intended pouch and stoma size at 3 months. However, after 12 months it returns to pre-interventional size and patients fail to achieve sustainable weight loss [31]. The other option is laparoscopic refashioning of the gastric pouch. Different techniques were suggested including longitudinal gastric pouch resection on 34 Fr boogie [32], resection of the gastric pouch with complementary resection of blind end of the alimentary (AL) limb at gastroenterostomy [33] or proximal jejunum [34], or resection of the gastric pouch with a new gastroenterostomy anastomosis [35]. The highest 69 %EWL after a mean follow-up of 20 months was reported by Iannelli et al. [32]. Twenty patients had gastric pouch resection on 34 Fr boogie. Of note is that all patients in this study had a dilated stomach, but normal 12–14 mm gastroenterostomies. Furthermore, a 30% complication rate was observed in this study including three patients with intra-abdominal abscesses. The other two studies, in which the pouch was resected together with a part of the small bowel, found much lower 11.4–29.1 %EWL after 1 year [33, 34].

Hamdi et al. resected gastric pouch and created a new gastroenterostomy in 25 patients. The % excess body mass index loss (%EBMIL) was 43.3 at 1 year, but decreased to 14% at 3 years [35]. Recently, León et al. [36] suggested laparoscopic double-layer gastro jejunal plication for patients with weight regain after RYGB. In a series of four patients, average %EWL after the procedure was 46.2% at 6 months. The results of the presented studies suggest that surgical refashioning of the gastric pouch may achieve acceptable short-term results. However, more studies with longer follow-up are needed in order to evaluate the efficiency of pouch and stoma reduction, as there are data about substantial weight regain 3 years after these procedures.

Recent systematic literature review of salvage banding with the adjustable or non-adjustable band as a treatment method for weight regain after RYGB included 94 patients from seven studies with 12–42 months follow-up. Further weight loss after salvage banding varied from 28 to 65 %EBMIL. Long-term complications requiring revision were observed in 17% of patients. All studies, except one, included in the review used an adjustable gastric band [37]. Long-term follow-up studies are needed to find out, if weight loss is sustainable after this procedure and what will be the rate of band removal.

Systematic review of four randomized studies and several retrospective series have concluded that surgeons should focus on the length of the common channel rather than on the length of the Roux Limb or biliopancreatic (BP) limb in order to reduce failure rates in RYGB [38]. Distal gastric bypass with a common channel of 50–150 cm was proposed for the treatment of obesity. However, despite superior long-term weight loss it caused frequent severe metabolic derangements requiring revisions and should not be used as a primary operation for obesity [39]. Distalization of the RYGB has also been used for the treatment of weight regain. Basically, there are two modifications of distalization of the RYGB. The first modification is when the Roux limb is divided close to entero-enterostomy anastomosis and moved it distally to create a long BP limb. Different authors suggest different place for AL limb anastomosis. Rawlins et al. [40] re-anastomosed the AL limb 100 cm and Sugarman et al. [41] 150 cm proximal to the ileocecal valve. Fobi et al. [42] selected the place for anastomosis by estimating that the length of the AL limb and common channel together would consist of 50% of all small bowel length.

In the second modification, BP limb is divided close to the entero-enterostomy anastomosis and moved distally and re-anastomosed 75 cm proximal to the ileocecal valve, creating a very long AL limb [43]. The %EBMIL was similar between two modifications after 1 year (55% vs. 52%). However, the protein-calorie malnutrition (PCM) tended to be lower after the second modification, 7% vs. 8–31%. Caruana et al. [44] have analyzed weight loss results according to the percentage of intestine bypassed in the first modification. %EWL after 2 years was significantly higher in patients with ≥70% of intestine bypassed, 47% vs. 26%, respectively. However, no PCM was observed in the group with <70% of bypassed intestine while PCM reached 44% in the other group. More studies are needed to determine an optimal length of different limbs while performing distalization of the RYGB for weight regain. As PCM is a frequent complication after distalization of the RYGB, the longer common channel might be considered to reduce the risk of PCM.

Another important anatomic change that has been shown to reduce the effectiveness of the RYGB is the presence of a gastro-gastric fistula (GGF) (Fig. 21.2). A GGF is an abnormal communication between the gastric pouch and the excluded stomach. GGF is an uncommon, but potentially significant complication after divided laparoscopic Roux-en-Y gastric bypass, with an incidence ranging between 1.5% and 6% [45]. Gastro-gastric fistulas may reduce both the restrictive and malabsorptive components of RYGB by allowing food to travel through alternative routes and thus not passing through the surgically created gastric pouch, gastrojejunostomy and bypassed intestine. Ergo, most commonly, patients with a GGF present with weight regain in the long term [46].

21.6 Sleeve Gastrectomy

Weight regain after the sleeve is due to either an inappropriately performed operation leaving behind a large sleeve, retained antrum, retained fundus, a dilated sleeve, increased ghrelin levels, or inadequate follow-up support and maladaptive eating behavior. Obeidant et al. [47] performed a retrospective review of prospectively collected data of 125 consecutive patients who underwent SG. Of the 110 patients with available data, 54 had the antrum divided 6 cm from the pylorus and 56 patients at 2 cm. At 2 years following surgery, 12 patients (22%) with a 6-cm remnant antrum had regained weight (again defined as at least 10 kg from nadir weight) compared with only two patients (4%) with a 2-cm antral remnant ($p = 0.003$).

Long-term follow-up is important in preventing weight regain and Sarala et al. [48] proposed that the lifelong follow-up provided by the National Health Service in the UK is responsible for less weight regain in the long term (Fig. 21.3).

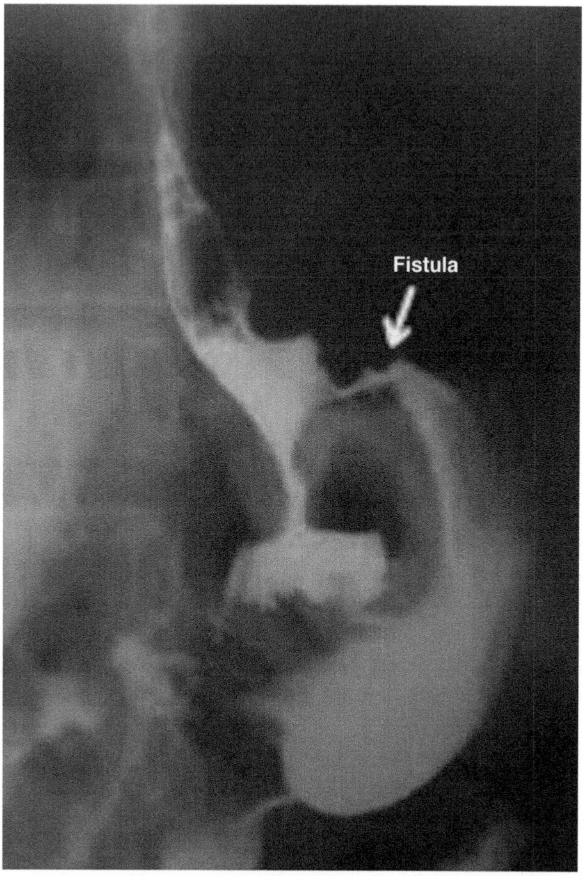

Fig. 21.2 Gastro-gastric fistula

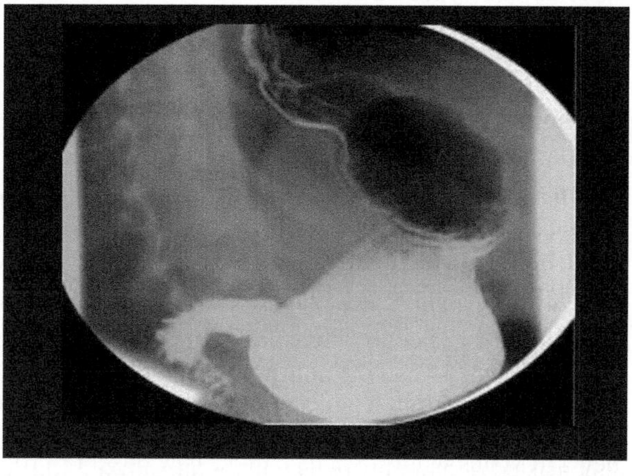

Fig. 21.3 Dilated sleeve gastrectomy

Lombardo et al. [49] performed the only study that specifically aimed to investigate whether or not more frequent follow-up visits prevent weight regain. In their series of 71 patients that included 43 patients who had undergone SG with a baseline BMI of 49.8 kg/m^2, they compared a group of patients who had follow-up visits at 9, 12, 15, 18, 24, 30, and 36 months with a group that had follow-up at only 12, 18, 24, and 36 months. They concluded that more follow-up visits may help reduce weight regain based on significant differences between the groups for change in body weight, change in BMI, and change in %EWL. However, no definition or rate was reported pertaining to weight regain in this retrospective non-randomized study.

Liu et al. [50] have been the only group to report weight regain rates yearly alongside other outcome data. When they employed their definition of weight regain (an increase in %EWL of 25), they had regained rates of 0, 1.0, 11.6, 19.2, and 29.5% at 1, 2, 3, 4, and 5 years postoperatively, respectively. This clearly demonstrates the increasing susceptibility to weight regain experienced by patients as time from surgery increases.

Sleeve anatomy is commonly proposed as a mechanism for weight regain following SG [51–54]. It is difficult to understand how an initially "large" sleeve, or primary dilation is a cause of weight regain rather than insufficient weight loss, but the answer may lie in the fact that this often results from an incompletely excised fundus, the most distensible part of the stomach, which may then increasingly distend and release larger amounts of ghrelin. It does seem logical, however, that progressive sleeve dilatation or secondary dilatation would contribute to weight regain [53, 55, 56].

Deguines et al. [57] have demonstrated a correlation between residual gastric volume and SG success as defined by %EWL > 50%, BAROS > 3, BMI < 35 kg/m^2, and/or the Biron criteria. Yet, to date, the association between sleeve dilation and weight regain has not been convincing [58]. Although long-term weight loss data after SG is rare, some studies have noted that weight regain may be a significant issue.

A systematic review reported that the percentage of people who regained weight ranged from 5.7% at 2 years to 75.6% at 6 years after SG [59]. Beyond 7 years, the weight regain rate was estimated to be 27.8% with a range of 14–37% [60].

Ellatif et al. [61] analyzed data from 1395 individuals who underwent SG and reported that weight regain occurred in 29 people (3.5%) in the group using a larger bougie size (_44F) and 8 people (1.4%) in the group using a smaller bougie size (_36F). The difference between the bougie sizes was statistically significant, suggesting that a thinner bougie may be a protective factor against post-SG weight regain. One major flaw of this study is that it did not provide definition of weight regain; instead, the authors confused the concept of insufficient weight loss and weight regain, which could influence the outcome interpretation.

Obeidant et al. [47] compared the surgical outcomes between two groups; group A consisted of 54 individuals with 6-cm antral remnant and group B was composed of 56 individuals with 2-cm antral remnant. After 2 years, the rate of weight regain was 12% and 2% for groups A and B, respectively ($p = 0.003$), which indicated that a more radical antral resection may be more useful in preventing weight regain. These findings were replicated in another study conducted by Abdallah et al. [61]. Similarly, 105 individuals were divided into two groups and followed for 2 years; significant weight regain after SG occurred in 9.4% of the group, with the higher residual gastric volume compared with 1.9% of the group with a smaller gastric remnant.

21.7 BPD-DS

There are very few reports of weight regain after the BPD-DS operation. Report of resleeving the pouch to enhance the restrictive mechanism has been used by some. Shortening the common limb has also been rarely used. The duodenal switch in most cases is a safe operation for patients who have failed other bariatric operation.

21.8 LAGB

The gastric band has been shown to slip proximally in 8% of patients, releasing the intended compressive and restrictive effects [62]. Thus, it is important for patients who are experiencing weight recidivism after band placement to be assessed for potential pouch distension or slippage of the band as factors contributing to failure. Pouch distension can oftentimes be managed by complete band deflation, a low-calorie diet, reinforcement of portion size, and follow-up contrast study in 4–6 weeks [63]. This conservative management strategy is successful in over 70% of patients. Band slippage can be managed similarly, but oftentimes, surgical intervention is required with band re-positioning or band replacement [63].

21.9 OAGB

There have been very few reports on managing weight regain after OAGB. At our center, we have revised the OAGB to a banded gastric bypass with good outcome. Some surgeons have reported lengthening the biliopancreatic limb at the expense of the common channel. This results in severe PCM and thus not recommended.

21.10 Adjuvant Pharmaceutical Therapy Use in Bariatric Surgery

Phentermine is one of the treatments with a consistent presence in the market on FDA-approved weight loss treatments, as it has been in prescription use in the USA for over 50 years as a short-term adjunct in a weight reduction regimen. Orlistat is an approved weight loss treatment as it was designed to block the absorption of dietary fat, rather than suppress the appetite or increase the feeling of fullness as with other weight loss medications. Qsymia was approved on July 17, 2012, as an adjunct to a reduced-calorie diet and increased physical activity for chronic weight management in adults with an initial body mass index (BMI) of 30 kg/m^2 or greater (obese) or 27 kg/m^2 or greater (overweight) when accompanied by weight-related comorbidities such as hypertension, type 2 diabetes mellitus, or dyslipidemia. Qsymia is a combination of phentermine and topiramate, a drug approved as a single-agent for the treatment of migraines and epilepsy. Also in 2012, FDA-approved Belviq (lorcaserin) and, in 2014, Contrave, a fixed-dose combination of bupropion and naltrexone, both as an adjunct to a reduced-calorie diet and increased physical activity for chronic weight management. As of this writing, there has been a request by the FDA on Feb 13, 2020, to remove Lorcaserin from the market because of its carcinogenic potential. Liraglutide/Saxenda®, a GLP agonist, was also approved for weight loss in 2015 and has the distinction of being the only anti-obesity medication to have data beyond 1 year [65–67]. Bariatric surgery effectiveness may be enhanced by the use of perioperative, adjuvant pharmaceutical therapy.

21.11 Consequences of Weight Regain

Weight regain, also referred to as secondary weight gain or recidivism, is a complication of bariatric surgery evidenced by a gradual decline in the percentage of weight change observed in longitudinal studies. It is associated with the recurrence of obesity-related comorbidities including type 2 diabetes and is likely to have a significant economic burden.

In addition to a return of comorbid illnesses, weight regain is also associated with worsening QOL. Specifically, the studies show that bariatric patients who regain at least 15% of the maximal weight lost seem to have similar QOL as patients with morbid obesity who have not undergone bariatric surgery despite an overall weight loss and a lower BMI. Additionally, studies also show that the amount of weight regain is negatively and linearly correlated with post-bariatric QOL [67].

While surgical revision has traditionally been used to treat weight regain, the procedure is associated with limited efficacy data and higher complication rates than that of the index surgery [68]. Thus, it is critical that health practitioners understand that there is weight recidivism post-bariatric surgery and develop a strategy to manage these patients and to guide future planning of diminishing health resources.

21.12 Conclusion

Weight regain is part of natural history after bariatric metabolic surgery. However, significant weight regain after surgical treatment occurs only in a subset of patients. There are many possible causes of weight regain after metabolic surgery. The incidence and magnitude of weight regain vary with the choice of operation and the time from the original operation. Weight regain, depending on the magnitude can occasionally be managed nonsurgically however, in many cases surgical intervention is a good option.

Key Points *Weight regain is part of natural history after bariatric metabolic surgery.*

- *Significant weight regain after surgical treatment occurs in a subset of patients.*
- *Significant weight regain is defined as either weight gain of >10 kg, weight gain of 25% of weight loss, recurrence of weight loss status to <50% EBWL, BMI status >35 kg/m² for class III obesity, or BMI > 40 kg/m² for patients with super obesity and super-super obesity.*
- *Weight regain may have overlapping aetiologies which are categorized as patient-specific (presence of psychiatric disorders, physical inactivity, use of medications that cause weight gain, endocrinopathies, and dietary non-compliance and eating disorders) and operation-specific.*
- *Bariatric surgery effectiveness may be enhanced by the use of perioperative, adjuvant pharmaceutical therapy.*
- *In addition to a return of comorbid illnesses, weight regain is also associated with worsening QOL.*
- *it is critical that health practitioners understand that there is weight recidivism post-bariatric surgery and develop a strategy to manage these patients and to guide future planning of diminishing health resources.*

References

1. Obesity: preventing and managing the global epidemic. Report of a WHO consultation. World Health Organ Tech Rep Ser. 2000;894:i–xii, 1–253.
2. Popkin BM, Doak CM. The obesity epidemic is a worldwide phenomenon. Nutr Rev. 1998 Apr;56(4 Pt 1):106–14.
3. Flegal KM, Carroll MD, Kuczmarski RJ, Johnson CL. Overweight and obesity in the United States: prevalence and trends, 1960-1994. Int J Obes Relat Metab Disord J Int Assoc Study Obes. 1998 Jan;22(1):39–47.
4. Ozanne SE. Epigenetic signatures of obesity. N Engl J Med. 2015 Mar 5;372(10):973–4.
5. Ravussin E, Bogardus C. Energy balance and weight regulation: genetics versus environment. Br J Nutr. 2000 Mar;83(Suppl 1):S17–20.
6. Health implications of obesity. National Institutes of Health Consensus Development Conference Statement. Ann Intern Med. 1985 Dec;103(Pt 2):1073–7.
7. Methods for voluntary weight loss and control. NIH Technology Assessment Conference Panel. Ann Intern Med. 1992 Jun 1;116(11):942–9.
8. Gastrointestinal surgery for severe obesity. National Institutes of Health Consensus Development Conference Statement. Am J Clin Nutr. 1992;55(2 Suppl):615S–9S.
9. Christou NV, Look D, MacLean LD. Weight gain after short- and long-limb gastric bypass in patients followed for longer than 10 years. Ann Surg. 2006 Nov;244(5):734–40.
10. Magro DO, Geloneze B, Delfini R, Pareja BC, Callejas F, Pareja JC. Long-term weight regain after gastric bypass: a 5-year prospective study. Obes Surg. 2008 Jun 1;18(6):648–51.
11. Baig SJ, Priya P, Mahawar KK, Shah S. Indian Bariatric Surgery Outcome Reporting (IBSOR) Group. Weight regain after bariatric surgery-a multicentre study of 9617 patients from Indian bariatric surgery outcome reporting group. Obes Surg. 2019 May;29(5):1583–92.

12. Carmeli I, Golomb I, Sadot E, Kashtan H, Keidar A. Laparoscopic conversion of sleeve gastrectomy to a biliopancreatic diversion with duodenal switch or a Roux-en-Y gastric bypass due to weight loss failure: our algorithm. Surg Obes Relat Dis Off J Am Soc Bariatr Surg. 2015 Feb;11(1):79–85.
13. Homan J, Betzel B, Aarts EO, van Laarhoven KJHM, Janssen IMC, Berends FJ. Secondary surgery after sleeve gastrectomy: Roux-en-Y gastric bypass or biliopancreatic diversion with duodenal switch. Surg Obes Relat Dis Off J Am Soc Bariatr Surg. 2015 Aug;11(4):771–777.
14. Jiménez A, Casamitjana R, Flores L, Viaplana J, Corcelles R, Lacy A, et al. Long-term effects of sleeve gastrectomy and Roux-en-Y gastric bypass surgery on type 2 diabetes mellitus in morbidly obese subjects. Ann Surg. 2012 Dec;256(6):1023–9.
15. Brethauer SA, Aminian A, Romero-Talamás H, Batayyah E, Mackey J, Kennedy L, et al. Can diabetes be surgically cured? Long-term metabolic effects of bariatric surgery in obese patients with type 2 diabetes mellitus. Ann Surg. 2013 Oct;258(4):628–36; discussion 636–637.
16. Karmali S, Brar B, Shi X, Sharma AM, de Gara C, Birch DW. Weight recidivism post-bariatric surgery: a systematic review. Obes Surg. 2013 Nov;23(11):1922–33.
17. Sjöström L, Lindroos A-K, Peltonen M, Torgerson J, Bouchard C, Carlsson B, et al. Lifestyle, diabetes, and cardiovascular risk factors 10 years after bariatric surgery. N Engl J Med. 2004 Dec 23;351(26):2683–93.
18. Colles SL, Dixon JB, O'Brien PE. Grazing and loss of control related to eating: two high-risk factors following bariatric surgery. Obes Silver Spring Md. 2008 Mar;16(3):615–22.
19. Kofman MD, Lent MR, Swencionis C. Maladaptive eating patterns, quality of life, and weight outcomes following gastric bypass: results of an Internet survey. Obes Silver Spring Md. 2010 Oct;18(10):1938–43.
20. Freire RH, Borges MC, Alvarez-Leite JI, Toulson Davisson Correia MI. Food quality, physical activity, and nutritional follow-up as determinant of weight regain after Roux-en-Y gastric bypass. Nutr Burbank Los Angel Cty Calif. 2012 Jan;28(1):53–8.
21. Kalarchian MA, Marcus MD, Wilson GT, Labouvie EW, Brolin RE, LaMarca LB. Binge eating among gastric bypass patients at long-term follow-up. Obes Surg. 2002 Apr;12(2):270–5.
22. Odom J, Zalesin KC, Washington TL, Miller WW, Hakmeh B, Zaremba DL, et al. Behavioral predictors of weight regain after bariatric surgery. Obes Surg. 2010 Mar;20(3):349–56.
23. Bond DS, Phelan S, Leahey TM, Hill JO, Wing RR. Weight-loss maintenance in successful weight losers: surgical vs non-surgical methods. Int J Obes. 2009 Jan;33(1):173–80.
24. Rutledge T, Groesz LM, Savu M. Psychiatric factors and weight loss patterns following gastric bypass surgery in a veteran population. Obes Surg. 2011 Jan;21(1):29–35.
25. Engström BE, Öhrvall M, Sundbom M, Lind L, Karlsson FA. Meal suppression of circulating ghrelin is normalized in obese individuals following gastric bypass surgery. Int J Obes. 2007 Mar;31(3):476–80.
26. Bohdjalian A, Langer FB, Shakeri-Leidenmühler S, Gfrerer L, Ludvik B, Zacherl J, et al. Sleeve gastrectomy as sole and definitive bariatric procedure: 5-year results for weight loss and ghrelin. Obes Surg. 2010 May;20(5):535–40.
27. Brethauer SA, Nfonsam V, Sherman V, Udomsawaengsup S, Schauer PR, Chand B. Endoscopy and upper gastrointestinal contrast studies are complementary in evaluation of weight regain after bariatric surgery. Surg Obes Relat Dis Off J Am Soc Bariatr Surg. 2006;2(6):643–8; discussion 649–650.
28. Heneghan HM, Yimcharoen P, Brethauer SA, Kroh M, Chand B. Influence of pouch and stoma size on weight loss after gastric bypass. Surg Obes Relat Dis Off J Am Soc Bariatr Surg. 2012 Aug;8(4):408–15.
29. Topart P, Becouarn G, Ritz P. Pouch size after gastric bypass does not correlate with weight loss outcome. Obes Surg. 2011 Sep;21(9):1350–4.
30. Jiang H-P, Lin L-L, Jiang X, Qiao H-Q. Meta-analysis of hand-sewn versus mechanical gastrojejunal anastomosis during laparoscopic Roux-en-Y gastric bypass for morbid obesity. Int J Surg Lond Engl. 2016 Aug;32:150–7.
31. Gallo AS, DuCoin CG, Berducci MA, Nino DF, Almadani M, Sandler BJ, et al. Endoscopic revision of gastric bypass: Holy Grail or Epic fail? Surg Endosc. 2016;30(9):3922–7.

32. Iannelli A, Schneck A-S, Hébuterne X, Gugenheim J. Gastric pouch resizing for Roux-en-Y gastric bypass failure in patients with a dilated pouch. Surg Obes Relat Dis Off J Am Soc Bariatr Surg. 2013 Apr;9(2):260–7.
33. Al-Bader I, Khoursheed M, Al Sharaf K, Mouzannar DA, Ashraf A, Fingerhut A. Revisional laparoscopic gastric pouch resizing for inadequate weight loss after Roux-en-Y gastric bypass. Obes Surg. 2015;25(7):1103–8.
34. Parikh M, Heacock L, Gagner M. Laparoscopic "gastrojejunal sleeve reduction" as a revision procedure for weight loss failure after Roux-en-Y gastric bypass. Obes Surg. 2011 May;21(5):650–4.
35. Hamdi A, Julien C, Brown P, Woods I, Hamdi A, Ortega G, et al. Midterm outcomes of revisional surgery for gastric pouch and gastrojejunal anastomotic enlargement in patients with weight regain after gastric bypass for morbid obesity. Obes Surg. 2014 Aug;24(8):1386–90.
36. León F, Maiz C, Daroch D, Quezada N, Gabrielli M, Muñoz C, et al. Laparoscopic hand-sewn revisional gastrojejunal plication for weight loss failure after Roux-en-Y gastric bypass. Obes Surg. 2015 Apr;25(4):744–9.
37. Vijgen GHEJ, Schouten R, Bouvy ND, Greve JWM. Salvage banding for failed Roux-en-Y gastric bypass. Surg Obes Relat Dis Off J Am Soc Bariatr Surg. 2012 Dec;8(6):803–8.
38. Stefanidis D, Kuwada TS, Gersin KS. The importance of the length of the limbs for gastric bypass patients–an evidence-based review. Obes Surg. 2011 Jan;21(1):119–24.
39. Kellum JM, Chikunguwo SM, Maher JW, Wolfe LG, Sugerman HJ. Long-term results of malabsorptive distal Roux-en-Y gastric bypass in superobese patients. Surg Obes Relat Dis Off J Am Soc Bariatr Surg. 2011 Apr;7(2):189–93.
40. Rawlins ML, Teel D, Hedgcorth K, Maguire JP. Revision of Roux-en-Y gastric bypass to distal bypass for failed weight loss. Surg Obes Relat Dis Off J Am Soc Bariatr Surg. 2011 Feb;7(1):45–9.
41. Sugerman HJ, Kellum JM, DeMaria EJ. Conversion of proximal to distal gastric bypass for failed gastric bypass for superobesity. J Gastrointest Surg Off J Soc Surg Aliment Tract. 1997;1(6):517–24; discussion 524–526.
42. Fobi MA, Lee H, Igwe D, Felahy B, James E, Stanczyk M, et al. Revision of failed gastric bypass to distal Roux-en-Y gastric bypass: a review of 65 cases. Obes Surg. 2001 Apr;11(2):190–5.
43. Brolin RE, Cody RP. Weight loss outcome of revisional bariatric operations varies according to the primary procedure. Ann Surg. 2008 Aug;248(2):227–32.
44. Caruana JA, Monte SV, Jacobs DM, Voytovich C, Ghanim H, Dandona P. Distal small bowel bypass for weight regain after gastric bypass: safety and efficacy threshold occurs at <70% bypass. Surg Obes Relat Dis Off J Am Soc Bariatr Surg. 2015 Dec;11(6):1248–55.
45. Cucchi SG, Pories WJ, MacDonald KG, Morgan EJ. Gastrogastric fistulas. A complication of divided gastric bypass surgery. Ann Surg. 1995 Apr;221(4):387–91.
46. Filho AJB, Kondo W, Nassif LS, Garcia MJ, Tirapelle RA, Dotti CM. Gastrogastric fistula: a possible complication of Roux-en-Y gastric bypass. JSLS. 2006 Sep;10(3):326–31.
47. Obeidat F, Shanti H, Mismar A, Albsoul N, Al-Qudah M. The magnitude of antral resection in laparoscopic sleeve gastrectomy and its relationship to excess weight loss. Obes Surg. 2015 Oct;25(10):1928–32.
48. Sarela AI, Dexter SPL, O'Kane M, Menon A, McMahon MJ. Long-term follow-up after laparoscopic sleeve gastrectomy: 8-9-year results. Surg Obes Relat Dis Off J Am Soc Bariatr Surg. 2012 Dec;8(6):679–84.
49. Lombardo M, Bellia A, Mattiuzzo F, Franchi A, Ferri C, Elvira P, et al. Frequent follow-up visits reduce weight regain in long-term management after bariatric surgery. Bariatr Surg Pract Patient Care. 2015 Aug 3;10(3):119–25.
50. Liu SY-W, Wong SK-H, Lam CC-H, Yung MY, Kong AP-S, Ng EK-W. Long-term results on weight loss and diabetes remission after laparoscopic sleeve gastrectomy for a morbidly obese Chinese population. Obes Surg. 2015 Oct;25(10):1901–8.
51. Braghetto I, Cortes C, Herquiñigo D, Csendes P, Rojas A, Mushle M, et al. Evaluation of the radiological gastric capacity and evolution of the BMI 2-3 years after sleeve gastrectomy. Obes Surg. 2009 Sep;19(9):1262–9.

52. Braghetto I, Csendes A, Lanzarini E, Papapietro K, Cárcamo C, Molina JC. Is laparoscopic sleeve gastrectomy an acceptable primary bariatric procedure in obese patients? Early and 5-year postoperative results. Surg Laparosc Endosc Percutan Tech. 2012 Dec;22(6):479–86.
53. Noel P, Nedelcu M, Nocca D, Schneck A-S, Gugenheim J, Iannelli A, et al. Revised sleeve gastrectomy: another option for weight loss failure after sleeve gastrectomy. Surg Endosc. 2014 Apr;28(4):1096–102.
54. Baltasar A, Serra C, Pérez N, Bou R, Bengochea M. Re-sleeve gastrectomy. Obes Surg. 2006 Nov;16(11):1535–8.
55. Nedelcu M, Noel P, Iannelli A, Gagner M. Revised sleeve gastrectomy (re-sleeve). Surg Obes Relat Dis Off J Am Soc Bariatr Surg. 2015 Dec;11(6):1282–8.
56. Yehoshua RT, Eidelman LA, Stein M, Fichman S, Mazor A, Chen J, et al. Laparoscopic sleeve gastrectomy–volume and pressure assessment. Obes Surg. 2008 Sep;18(9):1083–8.
57. Deguines J-B, Verhaeghe P, Yzet T, Robert B, Cosse C, Regimbeau J-M. Is the residual gastric volume after laparoscopic sleeve gastrectomy an objective criterion for adapting the treatment strategy after failure? Surg Obes Relat Dis Off J Am Soc Bariatr Surg. 2013 Oct;9(5):660–6.
58. Langer FB, Bohdjalian A, Felberbauer FX, Fleischmann E, Reza Hoda MA, Ludvik B, et al. Does gastric dilatation limit the success of sleeve gastrectomy as a sole operation for morbid obesity? Obes Surg. 2006 Feb;16(2):166–71.
59. Lauti M, Kularatna M, Hill AG, MacCormick AD. Weight regain following sleeve gastrectomy—a systematic review. Obes Surg. 2016 Jun 1;26(6):1326–34.
60. Clapp B, Wynn M, Martyn C, Foster C, O'Dell M, Tyroch A. Long term (7 or more years) outcomes of the sleeve gastrectomy: a meta-analysis. Surg Obes Relat Dis. 2018 Jun 1;14(6):741–7.
61. Abd Ellatif ME, Abdallah E, Askar W, Thabet W, Aboushady M, Abbas AE, et al. Long term predictors of success after laparoscopic sleeve gastrectomy. Int J Surg. 2014 May 1;12(5):504–8.
62. DeMaria EJ, Sugerman HJ, Meador JG, Doty JM, Kellum JM, Wolfe L, et al. High failure rate after laparoscopic adjustable silicone gastric banding for treatment of morbid obesity. Ann Surg. 2001 Jun;233(6):809–18.
63. Eid I, Birch DW, Sharma AM, Sherman V, Karmali S. Complications associated with adjustable gastric banding for morbid obesity: a surgeon's guides. Can J Surg J Can Chir. 2011 Feb;54(1):61–6.
64. Jirapinyo P, Dayyeh BKA, Thompson CC. Weight regain after Roux-en-Y gastric bypass has a large negative impact on the Bariatric Quality of Life Index. BMJ Open Gastroenterol. 2017 Sep 1;4(1):e000153.
65. Jester L, et al. Obesity Medications. Obes Surg. 1996;6:412–542.
66. Schwartz J, et al. Obesity medications. Obes Surg. 2016;26:452–8.
67. Hanipah ZN, et al. Obesity medications. SOARD. 2018;14:93–8.
68. Brethauer SA, Kothari S, Sudan R, Williams B, English WJ, Brengman M, et al. Systematic review on reoperative bariatric surgery: American Society for Metabolic and Bariatric Surgery Revision Task Force. Surg Obes Relat Dis. 2014 Sep 1;10(5):952–72.

Re-emergence of Comorbidities After Bariatric Surgery

22

Tejal Bipin Lathia and Vishakha Jain

There is nothing permanent except change.

—Heraclitus

22.1 Introduction

The advent of bariatric surgery (BS) has changed the way obesity is managed. Rapid advances in the field of bariatric surgery have opened up newer avenues with better surgical modalities, lesser complications, and better outcomes in people with obesity. Judicious selection of patient and procedure are of paramount importance. This determines both short-term as well as long-term outcomes post-surgery. There is no doubt that bariatric surgery results in significant weight loss. However, we cannot equate the trajectory of weight loss with that of the accompanying comorbidities. The remission as well as re-emergence of comorbidities are impacted by factors other than weight loss alone.

Recent meta-analyses on outcomes in patients who undergo sleeve gastrectomy (SG) and Roux-en-Y-gastric bypass (RYGB) surgeries, the commonest surgeries performed now, demonstrate primarily a loss of excess body weight and amelioration or remission of diabetes mellitus. Other comorbidities like dyslipidemia, metabolic syndrome (MetS), cardiovascular disease (CVD), polycystic ovarian syndrome (PCOS), obstructive sleep apnea (OSA) syndrome, non-alcoholic steatohepatitis (NASH) all show improvement to a great extent. But many pre-existing

T. B. Lathia (✉)
Department of Endocrinology, Apollo and Fortis Hospitals, Navi Mumbai, India

V. Jain
All India Institute of Medical Sciences, Bibinagar, Hyderabad, India

A. G. Bhasker et al. (eds.), *Management of Nutritional and Metabolic Complications of Bariatric Surgery*,
https://doi.org/10.1007/978-981-33-4702-1_22

comorbidities like hypertension, chronic kidney disease, non-alcoholic fatty liver disease (NAFLD), and osteoarthritis do not resolve but may show some improvement.

Discussing the re-emergence of comorbidities after bariatric surgery is a daunting task as there are limited studies with inadequate long-term follow-up of patients. Most of the evidence looks at either uncontrolled case series or cohorts with variable follow-ups. Furthermore, follow-up rates decline from year 1 to year 5 post-surgery and only 4% of studies report more than 80% follow-up rates. Hence comorbidities re-emerging after surgery may be missed or inadequately reported.

With the limited data available to us, the earliest co-morbidity probably to re-emerge is mental health issues while the major late comorbidity to re-emerge is diabetes mellitus. Post-bariatric surgery follow-ups are vital—support group meetings, behavioral intervention, and ongoing psychological support are key to prevent re-emergence of comorbidities. Further research is needed to document the late re-emergence of comorbidities.

In this chapter, we will discuss the resolution and re-emergence of comorbidities for which data is available namely mental health disorders and diabetes mellitus. We briefly describe comorbidities that remit to varying degrees after surgery but in whom data on re-emergence is lacking and is needed. We further discuss the factors that impact the re-emergence of comorbidities and medical interventions that may prevent weight regain which is the chief factor modifying their evolution. We also recommend strategies that may help to prevent the re-emergence of comorbidities.

22.2 Mental Health Disorders

Mental health evaluation and diagnosis of pre-existing psychological and psychiatric comorbidities are mandatory prior to performing any bariatric surgery, many of which are ameliorated by the surgery. Depression improves after surgery [1] and may lead to lasting improvements in cognition [2].

Anecdotal evidence exists that alcohol and substance abuse disorders increase after bariatric surgery. King et al. [3] conducted the first prospective multicentre cohort study on the prevalence of these disorders before and after bariatric surgery. In this cohort, the prevalence of alcohol use disorder (AUD) was greater in the second postoperative year (9.6%) than the year prior to surgery (7.6%) or in the first postoperative year (7.3%). It was associated with male sex, younger age, smoking, regular alcohol consumption, recreational drug use, and lower interpersonal support, and undergoing RYGB versus laparoscopic adjustable gastric banding (LAGB) (AOR, 2.07). The authors hypothesized that this increase in AUD was due to an increase in alcohol sensitivity following RYGB combined with the resumption of higher levels of alcohol consumption in the second postoperative year. However, they did not find a significant association between preoperative mental health, depressive symptoms, binge eating, or past-year treatment for psychiatric or emotional problems, poor weight loss or weight regain, and postoperative AUD.

The Longitudinal Assessment of Bariatric Surgery-2 (LABS) was an observational cohort study [4] which conducted assessments pre-surgery, 6 months post-surgery, and annually post-surgery for up to 7 years. Prevalence of opioid use decreased after surgery from 14.7% (95% CI: 13.3–16.2) at baseline to 12.9% (95% CI: 11.5–14.4) at month 6 but then increased to 20.3%, above baseline levels, as time progressed (95% CI: 18.2–22.5) at year 7.

After bariatric surgery, the prevalence of prescribed opioid analgesic use initially decreased but then increased to surpass baseline prevalence. Studies have shown that drugs, alcohol, and food trigger similar reward responses in the brain, and binge eating can be construed as an "addiction." Alcohol and drugs could substitute for overeating following bariatric surgery.

Several studies have demonstrated that a subgroup of patients after weight loss surgery will develop or redevelop subjective binge or "loss of control" eating, and rarely even self-induced vomiting for weight and shape reasons. deZwaan et al. [5] interviewed a sample of 59 patients in-person who had undergone RYGB about a range of eating behaviors, including binge eating, chewing, and spitting out food, picking at and nibbling food, and nocturnal eating and compensatory behaviors such as vomiting and laxative and diuretic misuse. Subjective bulimic episodes were reported by 25% and vomiting for weight and shape reasons by 12% of the participants, on average, 2 years after surgery. Subjective bulimic episodes were significantly associated with a preoperative binge eating disorder, with more eating-related and general psychopathology after surgery, and with less weight loss. The authors concluded that a substantial subgroup of patients with a preoperative eating disorder will develop binge eating after surgery that might be associated with less weight loss. A subsample will start vomiting for weight and shape reasons after bariatric surgery. This is the classic example of re-emergence of a comorbidity after surgery mainly due to weight loss less than anticipated.

A study [6] examined the clinical significance of the loss of control over eating (LOC) in bariatric surgery over 24 months of prospective multi-wave follow-ups. 361 gastric bypass surgery patients completed a battery of assessments before surgery and at 6, 12, and 24 months following surgery. Prior to surgery, 61% of patients reported LOC; post-surgery, 31% reported LOC at 6-month follow-up, 36% reported LOC at 12-month follow-up, and 39% reported LOC at 24-month follow-up. Postoperative LOC is a prospective predictor of significantly poorer post-surgical weight and psychosocial outcomes at 12- and 24-month following surgery. Thus, after an initial reduction in LOC at 6 months, the behavior worsened by end of 2 year follow-up.

Another study [7] indicated that over 60% of patients who met criteria for binge eating disorder before surgery developed graze eating (i.e., eating small/modest amounts of food continuously throughout the day) after surgery. Graze eating is particularly problematic because the postoperative stomach does not preclude it, and it can contribute to weight regain. Graze eating seems to be an emergent comorbidity to substitute for previous binge eating which is not possible post-surgery.

A systematic review and meta-analysis by Adams et al. [8] suggested that mortality by suicide was significant after bariatric surgery while analyzing all-cause and cause-specific mortality in post-bariatric surgery patients. Backman et al. [9] examined the prevalence of diagnosis and treatment for alcohol and substance use disorders, depression, and suicide attempts before and after RYGB in a nationwide cohort study in Sweden, compared with that in a large unselected population cohort (who had not undergone bariatric surgery) using several national databases.

Patients who underwent RYGB also had an increased risk of attempted suicide after surgery compared with before. There was no such increase in the reference cohort. The increase in suicides was previously studied by Tindle et al. [10]. Medical data following bariatric operations performed on Pennsylvania residents between 1995 and 2004. About 30% of suicides occurred within the first 2 years following surgery, with almost 70% occurring within 3 years. For every age category except the youngest, suicide rates were higher among men versus women.

Increase in alcohol and substance use, LOC eating, graze eating as well as increase in suicides are early remerging comorbidities within the first 1–2 years post-surgery. Addiction transfer, change in the pharmacokinetics of alcohol post-RYGB, failure to achieve expected weight gain, failure of comorbidities, or quality of life to improve are some of the reasons for these mental health problems.

22.3 Type 2 Diabetes Mellitus

A systematic review and meta-analysis published in 2013 by Gloy et al. [11] that included 11 randomized controlled trials (RCTs) ($n = 796$) in patients with Body Mass Index (BMI) between 30 and 52 kg/m^2 found that surgeries including RYGB, LAGB, SG, and Biliopancreatic diversion (BPD) result in greater remission of type 2 diabetes mellitus (T2DM) [Relative Risk (RR) of T2DM remission: 22.1; 95% CI: 3.2–154.3] compared to a variety of non-surgical treatment options.

22.4 Diabetes Relapse

Observational studies show that the sustainability of the metabolic effects of BS on type 2 diabetes is highly variable.

Using retrospective electronic chart analyses of 4434 patients, Arterburn et al. [12] showed that type 2 diabetes remission occurred in 68% of subjects within 5 years of the surgery. Of these, 35% relapsed within 5 years of initial remission, with a median time to relapse after surgery of 8.3 years. Factors associated with relapse included preoperative HbA1c levels above 6.5%, prior insulin use, and longer duration of type 2 diabetes. Preoperative BMIs did not predict type 2 diabetes remission or relapse and, interestingly, weight regain after RYGB was not a predictor of relapse.

Mingrone et al. [13] studied the durability of the effects of BPD, RYGB, and conventional medical therapy (MT) in 60 patients randomized to one of the three interventions. At 5 years, type 2 diabetes remitted in 37% of patients after RYGB, in 63% after BPD, and in none of the medically treated patients. About 44% of the surgical patients who remitted after 2 years relapsed by year 5. However, despite the relapse, 80% of the surgical patients were able to maintain HbA1c levels below

7.0% through diet or metformin alone, suggesting good type 2 diabetes control with minimal therapy. In this study, weight changes did not predict type 2 diabetes remission or relapse after surgery.

In the STAMPEDE trial [14], 90% completed the 5-year follow-up. At baseline, HbA1c was 9.2 ± 1.5%, and the mean BMI was 37 ± 3.5. Patients who underwent surgical procedures had a greater mean percentage reduction from baseline in HbA1c level than did patients who received MT alone (2.1% vs. 0.3%, $P = 0.003$). At 5 years, changes from baseline observed in the RYGB and SG groups were superior to the changes seen in the MT group with respect to body weight (−23%, −19%, and −5% in the RYGB, SG, and MT groups, respectively), triglyceride level (−40%, −29%, and −8%), high-density lipoprotein cholesterol level (+32%, 30%, and 7%), use of insulin (−35%, −34%, and −13%) ($P < 0.05$ for all comparisons).

In the 7 year outcome of the LABS (Longitudinal study of Bariatric Surgery) study [15], of 2348 participants, 1738 underwent RYGB (74%) and 610 underwent LAGB (26%). Among those with diabetes at baseline (RYGB [28%]; LAGB [29%]), the proportion in remission at 1, 3, 5, and 7 years were 70%, 70%, 65% and 60%, respectively, for RYGB and 31%, 30%, 30%, and 20% for LAGB. The incidence of diabetes at all follow-up assessments was less than 1.5% for RYGB. After both procedures, greater post-surgical weight loss was associated with remission. However, even after controlling for differences in the amount of weight lost, relative diabetes remission rates remained nearly twofold higher after RYGB than LAGB.

Overall, these studies show a high rate of type 2 diabetes remission after BPD and RYGB as compared with SG. Relapse usually occurs in 5 years or later. The risk factors for relapse of type 2 diabetes after BS are indicators of low beta-cell function: longer duration of type 2 diabetes, insulin use, poor diabetes control, and higher preoperative A1C levels. In addition, less weight loss after surgery and/or greater weight regain have been associated with diabetes relapse in some but not all studies.

Given the progressive nature of type 2 diabetes and its increased rate with aging, it is not entirely surprising that diabetes relapse occurs after BS. By inducing sustained weight loss, these procedures significantly improve diabetes control and appear to alter the trajectory of the disease without resulting in a permanent cure. Type 2 diabetes after BS seems to return in a less severe form, and patients require less insulin and fewer oral medications to achieve control.

22.5 Comorbidities That Remit After Bariatric Surgery

Obesity is an established risk factor for various cardiovascular disease and bariatric surgery not only leads to substantial weight loss but also the remission of cardiovascular disease (CVD) risk factors like diabetes mellitus, dyslipidaemia, and hypertension. It seems almost intuitive that bariatric surgery not only reduces overall CV mortality by almost 50% but reduces the incidence of myocardial infarction and stroke by 30% [16].

It does not mean there will be no cardiovascular events or deaths after bariatric surgery. There is a persistent residual risk of heart disease and death in spite of weight loss. This is probably because cardiovascular disease is a multifactorial in nature and some of these factors are non-modifiable like gender and heredity while some factors like smoking may have residual effect in spite of discontinuation. It is thus not possible to classify CV disease as re-emergent or persistent.

In the recent GATEWAY trial [17], 100 patients with obesity and hypertension (the majority of whom did not have diabetes mellitus) were randomized to gastric bypass or medical therapy alone. Patients randomized to gastric bypass were six times more likely to reduce ≥30% of the total number of antihypertensive medications while maintaining controlled blood pressure levels. In addition, 51% of the patients submitted to gastric bypass showed remission of hypertension in post-hoc analysis. However, there is no data available on the re-emergence of hypertension once it has remitted post-surgery.

The type of surgery was the strongest independent predictor for all lipid level improvements or remissions in a study by Spivak et al. [18] Normal total cholesterol (TC) levels of below 200 mg/dL and low density lipoproteins (LDL) were achieved by 76% post-RYGB patients compared with 43.5% post-SG patients (odds ratio [OR] = 6.24, 95% confidence interval [CI]: 3.69–10.53) and 25.6% post-LABG patients (OR = 9.66, 95% CI: 4.11–22.67; $P < 0.01$).The levels of high-density-lipoprotein cholesterol (HDL) were most improved post-SG, reaching normal levels in 58.1% of SG male patients versus 39.5% of RYGB male patients (OR = 1.56, $P = 0.02$). The lowering of triglyceride levels by approximately 75% was comparable after SG and RYGB procedures. There is no data on the re-emergence of dyslipidaemia and the need for restarting statin therapy after bariatric surgery in those who have remitted post-surgery.

In a study [19] reporting the resolution of metabolic syndrome (MetS) post-RYGB in 3795 patients, MetS was diagnosed in 60% of the predominantly (80%) female patients. At baseline, 28% of patients had impaired glucose metabolism, 40% hypertension, and 30% dyslipidaemia.

Postoperative follow-up rate after 5 years was 70%. The authors found that 86% had resolution of MetS. After 5–9 years, complete remission of type 2 diabetes was achieved in 78%, hypertension in 51%, and dyslipidaemia in 89%. Elevated uric acid levels also reduce by 50% after surgery [20]. There is no data that addresses the re-emergence of metabolic syndrome per se after remission.

Obstructive sleep apnea (OSA) is a highly prevalent disorder in obese patients and has strong association with increase in cardiovascular mortality and other metabolic abnormalities. In a prospective multicentre study [21], the prevalence of OSA decreased from 71% at baseline to 44% at 12 months after surgery ($P < 0.001$). OSA was cured in 45% and cured or improved in 78% of the patients. But moderate or severe OSA still persisted in 20% of the patients after the operation, probably as factors other than weight alone play a role in the development of OSA.

However, de novo OSA occurred in 8% of the patients at the end of 12 months which may actually signal an early re-emergence of this comorbidity.

In severely obese patients submitted to bariatric surgery, obesity-associated gonadal dysfunction was very prevalent: polycystic ovarian disease (PCOS) was present in 36% of women and male-obesity secondary hypogonadism (MOSH) was present in 64% of men. After bariatric surgery, there was resolution of PCOS in 96% of affected women and the resolution of MOSH occurred in 87% of affected men [22]. No long-term data about re-emergence of PCOS or MOSH in the long term after surgery is available.

Until recently, most of the literature [23] suggested a protective effect of bariatric surgery on cancer incidence and mortality, till the study by Derogar et al. [24]which suggested increase incidence of colorectal cancer after bariatric surgery (RYGB). If this finding is validated in other studies, this would signal an emerging co-morbidity as a result of bariatric surgery. However, in a review of literature of all studies till date, Maestro et al. [25] conceded that the overall cancer risk was reduced after bariatric surgery especially in women, but more appropriately designed studies would be necessary since the existing studies do not reach the highest levels of evidence.

To summarize, there is meaningful reduction, resolution, or prevention of several comorbidities associated with obesity after bariatric surgery but very scarce data on re-emergence of these comorbidities.

22.6 Factors That Affect the Re-emergence of Comorbidities

1. Type of surgery
2. Weight regain
3. Delayed surgery
4. Mental health
5. Patient factors
6. Support post-surgery

22.6.1 Type of Initial Surgery

The greater the malabsorption in the initial surgery, the greater the remission of metabolic abnormalities and less the chances of relapse or re-emergence of comorbidities. Thus, if degree of malabsorption BPD > RYGB > SG > LAGB follows this sequence, the re-emergence of comorbidities would follow the reverse order—LAGB > SG > RYGB > BPD. Patients undergoing less malabsorptive surgery will require more frequent follow-up in order to detect early re-emergence of comorbidities like diabetes.

A review by Tice et al. [26] comparing RYGB with LAGB finds diabetes resolution in 78% after RYGB and 50% after LAGB. A meta-analysis by Buchwald et al. [27] also echoed the same finding and suggested an average of 78% achieved complete resolution without any anti-diabetic medications. Furthermore, 87% had either diabetes improved or resolved and required fewer anti-diabetic medications following bariatric surgery and diabetes resolution were greatest for patients undergoing BPD/DS, followed by RYGB, and least for LAGB.

Another meta-analysis by Buchwald and Oien [28] involving 1846 diabetic patients finds diabetes resolution in 99%, 84%, 72%, and 48% patients after BPD/BPD-DS, RYGB, gastroplasty, and gastric banding respectively. A recent meta-analysis by Chang et al. [29] reported an overall diabetes remission of around 90% after bypass surgeries (pooled data of RYGB and BPD) and 70% after gastric banding.

The "perfect" bariatric procedure remains the topic of debate. A study by Wharton et al. [30] evaluated the impact of self-selection of bariatric procedure on weight loss and diabetes remission. After the multidisciplinary team's assessment, the patients could make their own choice of procedures (self-selected, SS), unless medical/surgical conditions limited this (medically restricted, MR). A total of 303 patients were included and 271 of them made their own choice (SS 90%). Self-selected bariatric procedures yield excellent weight loss and metabolic outcome. Providing an information-dense environment augments the choice of the right operation and could improve patients' compliance with weight loss surgery programs.

22.6.2 Weight Regain

Weight regain has been seen as a factor in relapse for diabetes mellitus in some but not all studies. Poorer beta-cell function at the time of surgery equally predicts relapse. However, weight regain will also predict the worsening of OSA, osteoarthritis, and PCOS symptomatology. There is little or no data to support these observations frequently seen in clinical practice.

22.6.3 Delayed Surgery

Often bariatric surgery is chosen for weight loss after most comorbidities have been present for many years. Thus, advanced knee osteoarthritis, long-standing hypertension, and diabetes (requiring insulin), renal failure (either because of diabetes or hypertension or both) do not resolve.

Long-standing hypertension can cause permanent and irreversible changes in vasculature. Even patients with pheochromocytoma, primary hyperaldosteronism, and acromegaly fail to be cured of hypertension post-surgery when there is a delay in diagnosis and treatment. Similarly, beta-cell exhaustion cannot be overcome by weight loss alone. Renal failure is irreversible and will mandate renal replacement therapy.

22.6.4 Patient Selection

This is probably the most important predictor of re-emergence of comorbidities. Patients with unresolved mental health issues, dependence on alcohol or smoking, depression would be less likely to comply with Health care practitioner (HCP) recommendations for follow-up visits, lifestyle modifications, and nutritional supplementation. This would in turn result in poorer weight loss, greater weight regain, and re-emergence of comorbidities.

22.6.5 Mental Health

A paper by Meany et al. [31] reviewed the data on the development of binge eating (BE), binge eating disorder (BED), and loss of control (LOC) eating after bariatric surgery and the impact of these problems on long-term weight outcome. Fourteen of the available 15 studies suggest that the development of problems with BE, BED, or LOC eating post-bariatric surgery is associated with less weight loss and/or more weight regain post-bariatric surgery. These data suggests that it is important to identify individuals at high risk for these problems, to follow them post-operatively, and if appropriate interventions can be developed if such behaviors occur in order to maximize weight loss outcomes.

A systematic review on psychosocial predictors of success following bariatric surgery [32] found greater success in patients who are young and female, and have a high self-esteem, good mental health, a satisfactory marriage, and high socioeconomic status, who are self-critical and cope in a direct and active way, are not too obese, were obese before the age of 18, suffer from and are concerned about their obesity, have realistic expectations and undisturbed eating behaviors.

Conceição et al. [33] reported three cases where eating disorder developed anew after bariatric surgery. These case reports suggest that gastric restriction and requirements after surgery may create conditions that trigger eating disordered-like symptoms The following factors may contribute to this effect: the rapid weight loss; food restriction and even vomiting that are considered to be normal in the post-surgery period; the ritualized eating and rigorous eating schedule required at post-surgery; patients will get frequent reminders of the importance of controlling food ingestion to prevent the weight regain. All these conditions may make patients susceptible to a pattern of extreme control and rigid dietary rules. Ultimately, malnutrition and inadequate intake may help maintain the problem. The number of eating disorders that develop after bariatric surgery, particularly partial cases, is probably underreported.

22.6.6 Patient Continued Healthcare/Support Group Contact

Patients undergoing bariatric surgery need ongoing support in numerous ways even after surgery for nutrition, exercise, etc. Other unresolved comorbidities also require ongoing care like knee osteoarthritis, obstructive sleep apnea, chronic kidney disease.

A significant linear relationship was found between support group meeting attendance and the percentage of excess weight loss with simple regression analysis (adjusted R^2 0.061, P 0.007), with age (adjusted R^2 0.100, P 0.002) and the baseline body mass index added to the model (adjusted R^2 0.072, P 0.011) in a group of 102 patients [34], predominantly women with mean BMI of 46 kg/m^2.

The challenge is getting patients to maintain contact. A nationwide cohort study in France [35] aimed to assess 5 year follow-up post-bariatric surgery. Some 16,620 patients were included in the study. The percentage of patients with one or more visits to a surgeon decreased between the first and fifth years, from 87 to 29% ($P < 0.001$); similar decreases were observed for visits to a nutritionist/endocrinologist (from 23 to 12%; $P < 0.001$) or general practitioner (from 93 to 83%; $P < 0.001$). The mean number of visits to a general practitioner was 7 and 6 in the first and fifth years, respectively.

In multivariable analyses, male sex, younger age, absence of type 2 diabetes, and poor 1-year follow-up were predictors of poor 5-year follow-up. This suggests that re-emergence of many comorbidities may be underreported as a result of this poor follow-up.

22.7 Prevention of Re-emergence of Comorbidities

Three key factors impact the risk of re-emergence of comorbidities—mental health and weight regain.

1. *Continued Contact with Mental Health Professional*: As alcohol use disorders and depression re-emerge as early as 3 years post-bariatric surgery, identifying and treating these conditions is imperative. This will necessitate visits with qualified mental health professionals not only in the immediate post-bariatric surgery setting but for the foreseeable future. It will also ensure that patients comply with post-bariatric surgery treatment recommendations like regular healthcare contact and nutritional recommendations to avoid complications ensuing from the surgery.
2. *Avoiding Weight Regain*: Reappearance of metabolic syndrome and diabetes mellitus is influenced by weight regain. Continuance of adherence to lifestyle modification with regular exercise, consistent healthy diet will greatly mitigate weight regain. This in turn necessitates long-term follow-up and consistent contact with health care personnel to ensure this.
3. *Continuing Care in MDT Setting*: Most guidelines strongly recommend performing surgery in MDT setting. In response to the growing popularity of bariatric surgery in France, the HAS issued guidelines in January 2009 with a view to monitoring this activity and preventing unnecessary surgery. These guidelines recommended the establishment of MDT meetings attended by obesity specialists, in order to (1) validate or refuse bariatric surgery, (2) define preoperative management, if required, and (3) simply check that the patients satisfied the criteria for surgical treatment of obesity.

   There exist other best practice guidelines which define very clearly what constitutes an MDT and describes in detail what needs to be done both preoperatively and postoperatively. However, very little is said about long-term follow-up, documentation of comorbidity resolution and relapse and mental health evaluations postoperatively.

In a national survey in the USA [36], although 95% of respondents reported using a multidisciplinary team, only 53% had a general physician, nutritionist, and mental health specialist (NIH-recommended team). Just 47% mandated primary care, nutrition, and mental health evaluations (NIH-recommended evaluations). The authors concluded that inconsistent and unpredictable patterns of multidisciplinary methods were found. Further research should explore the impact of different methods on outcomes.

Compliance with a multidisciplinary team meeting's decision prior to bariatric surgery protects against major postoperative complications. Rebibo et al. [37] found that following the introduction of MDT meetings, although the overall complication rate remained similar, the major complication rate and the reoperation rate decreased (5.8% vs. 3.2%; $P \leq 0.05$) with no deaths following the implementation of MDT meetings. However, again the paper failed to discuss what should be done by MDT for long-term monitoring and follow-up and whether the MDT has any role in the reduction of weight regain, what is the impact on mental health outcomes and impact on resolution and relapse of comorbidities.

A bariatric surgery performed without inputs from nutritionist, endocrinologist, psychologist, and psychiatrist carries a risk of poor resolution and early re-emergence of comorbidities as the patient selection may be faulty, and unresolved eating disorders, depression, and more severe psychiatric comorbidities may be missed.

Our recommendation is that bariatric surgery should not be performed outside of the multidisciplinary team approach setting. This would ensure consistency of care. However, this may not always be done in practice.

22.8 Weight Regain and Liraglutide

In the context of preventing or treating weight regain, we discuss in brief the use of Liraglutide for the same. Phentermine-Topiramate is not available in many countries such as ours (India), and Lorcaserin was recently withdrawn from the market in view of the suspected increase in cancer risk and Orlistat is minimally effective.

There is limited data which is mostly retrospective. Recent prospective studies available were designed with the primary objective being the treatment of Type 2 diabetes mellitus not treatment of weight regain per se but give us some insight on weight loss that can be achieved with the use of Liraglutide.

A retrospective study from UAE by Alameri et al. reviewed 59 patients who were given Liraglutide. Seven patients discontinued the medication (five due to nausea and vomiting and two due to pregnancy). Mean weight at Liraglutide initiation (0.6–3.0 mg/day) was 95.1 ± 13.3 kg and mean BMI of 36.9 ± 4.4 kg/m^2. After 3 months, mean weight and BMI reduction were 5.4 ± 9.8 kg and 1.3 ± 1.1 kg/m^2 respectively ($P < 0.01$).

Rye et al. [38] performed a retrospective chart review of 33 consecutive patients, aged 18–65, who received Liraglutide for weight loss in the setting of any previous bariatric surgery. Indications were weight recidivism (>10% weight regain from the lowest post-surgical weight), inadequate weight loss (<20% weight loss from initial clinic assessment, or pre-surgical weight if unavailable), and plateau (patient desires further weight loss but does not fit into either other category). At 16 weeks median percentage weight loss was 7.1%, and at 28 weeks 9.7%. Median BMI change was 3.5 kg/m^2 (16 weeks) and 4.7 kg/m^2 (28 weeks). There were no major adverse events.

GRAVITAS [39] was a randomized double-blind, placebo-controlled trial that enrolled adults who had undergone Roux-en-Y gastric bypass or vertical sleeve gastrectomy and had persistent or recurrent type 2 diabetes with HbA1c levels higher than 6.5% at least 1 year after surgery. Participants were randomly assigned to either subcutaneous liraglutide 1.8 mg once daily or placebo, both given together with a reduced-calorie diet, aiming for a 500 kcal/day deficit from baseline energy intake, and increased physical activity.

Significant improvements in body weight from baseline in the liraglutide group were already apparent at week 6 (–2 · 38 kg) and this weight reduction trend continued through weeks 10 (–3 · 71 kg, weeks 18 (–4 · 46 kg), and 26 (–5 · 26 kg), with no apparent plateauing of effect. Overall, 46% in the liraglutide group lost 5% or more of their baseline body weight, 15% lost 10% or more of their baseline body weight, and 4% lost 15% or more. The proportion of patients in the liraglutide group with weight loss of 5% or greater steadily increased: 17% at week 6, 33% at week 10, 38% at week 18, and 46% at week 26.

One hundred seventeen post-bariatric surgery patients from the Wharton Medical Clinic [40] were analyzed for changes in weight while taking Liraglutide 3.0 mg were examined post-bariatric surgery (Roux-en-Y gastric bypass—45%, gastric banding—43%, and gastric sleeve—22%). Over 7.6 ± 7.1 months taking liraglutide 3.0 mg, patients lost a statistically significant amount of weight (−6.3 ± 7.7 kg, $P < 0.05$) regardless of the type of surgery they had ($P > 0.05$). This decrease in weight remained significant after 1-year of taking liraglutide 3.0 mg ($P < 0.05$). Nausea was the most prevalent side effect, reported by 29.1% patients. While options for excess weight management in post-bariatric surgery patients are limited, the results of this study suggest that post-bariatric surgery patients can lose a significant amount of weight while taking liraglutide 3.0 mg regardless of the type of surgery they had. Further, similar to non-surgical populations, post-bariatric surgery patients taking liraglutide 3.0 mg may experience gastrointestinal side effects such as nausea and can continue to lose weight for up to 1 year.

Key Points

1. *Psychological issues are amongst the earliest comorbidities to re-emerge after BS.*
2. *The major late comorbidity to re-emerge is diabetes mellitus, often in a less severe form than the original disease.*
3. *Certain diseases like Hypertension, dyslipidemia, OSA, PCOS & MOSH improve post-bariatric surgery but may not resolve completely and there is limited research available regarding their re-emergence post BS.*

4. *In case of cardiovascular and renal disease, there may be irreversible damage to vasculature that precludes remission.*
5. *The relationship between weight regain and re-emergence of comorbidities is complex and not as yet fully elucidated.*

References

1. de Zwaan M, Enderle J, Wagner S, et al. Anxiety and depression in bariatric surgery patients: a prospective, follow-up study using structured clinical interviews. J Affect Disord. 2011;133(1–2):61–8. https://doi.org/10.1016/j.jad.2011.03.025.
2. Alosco ML, Galioto R, Spitznagel MB, et al. Cognitive function after bariatric surgery: evidence for improvement 3 years after surgery. Am J Surg. 2014;207(6):870–6. https://doi.org/10.1016/j.amjsurg.2013.05.018.
3. King WC, Chen J-Y, Mitchell JE, et al. Prevalence of alcohol use disorders before and after bariatric surgery. JAMA. 2012;307(23) https://doi.org/10.1001/jama.2012.6147.
4. King WC, Chen J-Y, Belle SH, et al. Use of prescribed opioids before and after bariatric surgery: prospective evidence from a U.S. multicenter cohort study. Surg Obes Relat Dis. 2017;13(8):1337–46. https://doi.org/10.1016/j.soard.2017.04.003.
5. de Zwaan M, Hilbert A, Swan-Kremeier L, et al. Comprehensive interview assessment of eating behavior 18–35 months after gastric bypass surgery for morbid obesity. Surg Obes Relat Dis. 2010;6(1):79–85. https://doi.org/10.1016/j.soard.2009.08.011.
6. White MA, Kalarchian MA, Masheb RM, Marcus MD, Grilo CM. Loss of control over eating predicts outcomes in bariatric surgery patients: a prospective, 24-month follow-up study. J Clin Psychiatry. 2010;71(02):175–84. https://doi.org/10.4088/JCP.08m04328blu.
7. Pizato N, Botelho P, Gonçalves V, Dutra E, de Carvalho K. Effect of grazing behavior on weight regain post-bariatric surgery: a systematic review. Nutrients. 2017;9(12):1322. https://doi.org/10.3390/nu9121322.
8. Adams TD, Mehta TS, Davidson LE, Hunt SC. All-cause and cause-specific mortality associated with bariatric surgery: a review. Curr Atheroscler Rep. 2015;17(12):74. https://doi.org/10.1007/s11883-015-0551-4.
9. Backman O, Stockeld D, Rasmussen F, Näslund E, Marsk R. Alcohol and substance abuse, depression and suicide attempts after Roux-en-Y gastric bypass surgery. Br J Surg. 2016;103(10):1336–42. https://doi.org/10.1002/bjs.10258.
10. Tindle HA, Omalu B, Courcoulas A, Marcus M, Hammers J, Kuller LH. Risk of suicide after long-term follow-up from bariatric surgery. Am J Med. 2010;123(11):1036–42. https://doi.org/10.1016/j.amjmed.2010.06.016.
11. Gloy VL, Briel M, Bhatt DL, et al. Bariatric surgery versus non-surgical treatment for obesity: a systematic review and meta-analysis of randomised controlled trials. BMJ. 2013;347:f5934. https://doi.org/10.1136/bmj.f5934.
12. Arterburn DE, Bogart A, Sherwood NE, et al. A multisite study of long-term remission and relapse of type 2 diabetes mellitus following gastric bypass. Obes Surg. 2013;23(1):93–102. https://doi.org/10.1007/s11695-012-0802-1.
13. Mingrone G, Panunzi S, De Gaetano A, et al. Bariatric surgery versus conventional medical therapy for type 2 diabetes. N Engl J Med. 2012;366(17):1577–85. https://doi.org/10.1056/NEJMoa1200111.
14. Schauer PR, Bhatt DL, Kirwan JP, et al. Bariatric surgery versus intensive medical therapy for diabetes — 5-year outcomes. N Engl J Med. 2017;376(7):641–51. https://doi.org/10.1056/NEJMoa1600869.
15. Courcoulas AP, King WC, Belle SH, et al. Seven-year weight trajectories and health outcomes in the longitudinal assessment of bariatric surgery (LABS) study. JAMA Surg. 2018;153(5):427–34. https://doi.org/10.1001/jamasurg.2017.5025.
16. Sjöström L, Peltonen M, Jacobson P, et al. Bariatric surgery and long-term cardiovascular events. JAMA. 2012;307(1):56. https://doi.org/10.1001/jama.2011.1914.

17. Schiavon CA, Bersch-Ferreira AC, Santucci EV, et al. Effects of bariatric surgery in obese patients with hypertension: the GATEWAY randomized trial (gastric bypass to treat obese patients with steady hypertension). Circulation. 2018;137(11):1132–42. https://doi.org/10.1161/CIRCULATIONAHA.117.032130.
18. Spivak H, Sakran N, Dicker D, et al. Different effects of bariatric surgical procedures on dyslipidemia: a registry-based analysis. Surg Obes Relat Dis. 2017;13(7):1189–94. https://doi.org/10.1016/j.soard.2017.03.013.
19. Shah K, Johnny Nergard B, Stray Frazier K, Geir Leifsson B, Aghajani E, Gislason H. Long-term effects of laparoscopic Roux-en-Y gastric bypass on metabolic syndrome in patients with morbid obesity. Surg Obes Relat Dis Off J Am Soc Bariatr Surg. 2016;12(8):1449–56. https://doi.org/10.1016/j.soard.2016.03.017.
20. Maglio C, Peltonen M, Neovius M, et al. Effects of bariatric surgery on gout incidence in the Swedish Obese Subjects study: a non-randomised, prospective, controlled intervention trial. Ann Rheum Dis. 2017;76(4):688. https://doi.org/10.1136/annrheumdis-2016-209958.
21. Peromaa-Haavisto P, Tuomilehto H, Kössi J, et al. Obstructive sleep apnea: the effect of bariatric surgery after 12 months. A prospective multicenter trial. Sleep Med. 2017;35:85–90. https://doi.org/10.1016/j.sleep.2016.12.017.
22. Escobar-Morreale HF, Santacruz E, Luque-Ramírez M, Botella Carretero JI. Prevalence of 'obesity-associated gonadal dysfunction' in severely obese men and women and its resolution after bariatric surgery: a systematic review and meta-analysis. Hum Reprod Update. 2017;23(4):390–408. https://doi.org/10.1093/humupd/dmx012.
23. Adams TD, Stroup AM, Gress RE, et al. Cancer incidence and mortality after gastric bypass surgery. Obes Silver Spring Md. 2009;17(4):796–802. https://doi.org/10.1038/oby.2008.610.
24. Derogar M, Hull MA, Kant P, Östlund M, Lu Y, Lagergren J. Increased risk of colorectal cancer after obesity surgery. Ann Surg. 2013;258(6):983–8. https://doi.org/10.1097/SLA.0b013e318288463a.
25. Maestro A, Rigla M, Caixàs A. Does bariatric surgery reduce cancer risk? A review of the literature. Endocrinol Nutr Engl Ed. 2015;62(3):138–43. https://doi.org/10.1016/j.endoen.2014.12.005.
26. Tice JA, Karliner L, Walsh J, Petersen AJ, Feldman MD. Gastric banding or bypass? A systematic review comparing the two most popular bariatric procedures. Am J Med. 2008;121(10):885–93. https://doi.org/10.1016/j.amjmed.2008.05.036.
27. Buchwald H, Estok R, Fahrbach K, et al. Weight and type 2 diabetes after bariatric surgery: systematic review and meta-analysis. Am J Med. 2009;122(3):248–256.e5. https://doi.org/10.1016/j.amjmed.2008.09.041.
28. Buchwald H, Oien DM. Metabolic/bariatric surgery worldwide 2011. Obes Surg. 2013;23(4):427–36. https://doi.org/10.1007/s11695-012-0864-0.
29. Chang S-H, Stoll CRT, Song J, Varela JE, Eagon CJ, Colditz GA. The effectiveness and risks of bariatric surgery: an updated systematic review and meta-analysis, 2003-2012. JAMA Surg. 2014;149(3):275–87. https://doi.org/10.1001/jamasurg.2013.3654.
30. Wharton S, Serodio K, VanderLelie S. Morbidly obese patients self select bariatric surgery regardless of EOSS stage. Can J Diabetes. 2015;39:S73. https://doi.org/10.1016/j.jcjd.2015.01.274.
31. Meany G, Conceição E, Mitchell JE. Binge eating, binge eating disorder and loss of control eating: effects on weight outcomes after bariatric surgery. Eur Eat Disord Rev. 2014;22(2):87–91. https://doi.org/10.1002/erv.2273.
32. van Hout GCM, Verschure SKM, Van Heck GL. Psychosocial predictors of success following bariatric surgery. Obes Surg. 2005;15(4):552–60. https://doi.org/10.1381/0960892053723484.
33. Conceição E, Vaz A, Bastos AP, Ramos A, Machado P. The development of eating disorders after bariatric surgery. Eat Disord. 2013;21(3):275–82. https://doi.org/10.1080/10640266.2013.779193.
34. Kaiser KA, Franks SF, Smith AB. Positive relationship between support group attendance and one-year postoperative weight loss in gastric banding patients. Surg Obes Relat Dis. 2011;7(1):89–93. https://doi.org/10.1016/j.soard.2010.07.013.

35. Thereaux J, Lesuffleur T, Païta M, et al. Long-term follow-up after bariatric surgery in a national cohort. BJS. 2017;104(10):1362–71. https://doi.org/10.1002/bjs.10557.
36. Santry HP, Chin MH, Cagney KA, Alverdy JC, Lauderdale DS. The use of multidisciplinary teams to evaluate bariatric surgery patients: results from a national survey in the U.S.A. Obes Surg. 2006;16(1):59–66. https://doi.org/10.1381/096089206775222096.
37. Rebibo L, Maréchal V, De Lameth I, et al. Compliance with a multidisciplinary team meeting's decision prior to bariatric surgery protects against major postoperative complications. Surg Obes Relat Dis. 2017;13(9):1537–43. https://doi.org/10.1016/j.soard.2017.05.026.
38. Rye P, Modi R, Cawsey S, Sharma AM. Efficacy of high-dose liraglutide as an adjunct for weight loss in patients with prior bariatric surgery. Obes Surg. 2018;28(11):3553–8. https://doi.org/10.1007/s11695-018-3393-7.
39. Miras AD, Pérez-Pevida B, Aldhwayan M, et al. Adjunctive liraglutide treatment in patients with persistent or recurrent type 2 diabetes after metabolic surgery (GRAVITAS): a randomised, double-blind, placebo-controlled trial. Lancet Diabetes Endocrinol. 2019;7(7):549–59. https://doi.org/10.1016/S2213-8587(19)30157-3.
40. Wharton S, Kuk JL, Luszczynski M, Kamran E, Christensen RAG. Liraglutide 3.0 mg for the management of insufficient weight loss or excessive weight regain post-bariatric surgery. Clin Obes. 2019;9(4) https://doi.org/10.1111/cob.12323.

Micro-nutritional, Endocrine, and Metabolic Complications in Bariatric Surgery-Case Capsules

23

Shivanshu Mishra and P. Praveen Raj

Knowing is better than wondering, waking is better than sleeping, and even the biggest failure, even the worst, beats the hell out of never trying.

—*Grey's Anatomy*

23.1 Post-RYGB Cardiomyopathy

A 56-year-old male had undergone bariatric surgery 11 months back. He was readmitted to the hospital with exertional dyspnea and bilateral lower extremity pitting edema. His preoperative BMI reduced from 43 kg/m^2 to a current BMI of 33.7 kg/m^2 (weight 112 kg to 87 kg). He had no cardiovascular risk factors. Physical examination revealed normal blood pressure and pulse rate, normal heart sounds, no jugular venous distension, no hepatojugular reflux, and no lower limb venous disease. Complete blood count, C reactive protein, renal function test, liver function tests were normal, and no proteinuria was detected. CXR and ECG were normal. N-Terminal pro-brain Natriuretic Peptide (NT pro-BNP) value was elevated at 1417 ng/l (normal value <300 ng/ml).

CT of thorax and abdomen scan revealed no features suggestive of complications post-surgery. There was no abdominal or pelvic mass, venous thrombosis, pulmonary embolism, or evidence of Budd-Chiari syndrome. A bilateral venous doppler was done to rule out any peripheral signs of deep vein thrombosis. Transthoracic echocardiography (2-D Echo) showed a reduced left ventricular ejection fraction to 50% from preoperative value of 62%. 2-D Echo also showed normal size and volume of the cardiac chambers and no pericardial disease. There was an impairment

S. Mishra (✉) · P. P. Raj
Bariatric Division, GEM Hospital and Research Center, Coimbatore, India

A. G. Bhasker et al. (eds.), *Management of Nutritional and Metabolic Complications of Bariatric Surgery*,
https://doi.org/10.1007/978-981-33-4702-1_23

of percentage left ventricular (LV) global longitudinal strain (GLS) (−12.4%). We found a "pseudo-normal" trans-mitral flow pattern in the echocardiography. Diastolic dysfunction was also noted. The right ventricular function and pulmonary artery pressure were normal. Computed tomography (CT) coronary angiogram was normal. Impaired left ventricular (LV) global longitudinal strain with evidence of increased LV-filling pressures, the diagnosis of cardiomyopathy was made. The various reasons for cardiomyopathy were evaluated. It was noted that the serum selenium concentration was low at 61 g/l (normal values range from 89 to 150 g/l). The blood levels were normal for the other micro-nutrients: vitamins A, B1, B9, B12, C, D, E, and K, iron, calcium, zinc, copper. The possible association of selenium-deficient cardiomyopathy was made. Oral supplementation with a dosage of 2 g/kg/day was initiated and was continued for three months. Congestive heart failure treatment with ACE inhibitor and furosemide was started along with the supplementation of selenium. Dyspnea and the pedal edema were reduced with 2 weeks of treatment, and the patient symptomatically improved. On follow-up of the patient after 6 months, the patient remained asymptomatic. Serum selenium and NT pro-BNP (121 ng/l) had returned to normal levels. Echocardiography findings were normal on the follow-up of the patient.

Selenium is an essential trace element and a vital constituent of antioxidant enzymes that participate in various physiological activities, protecting the cells against the harmful effects of free radicals by modulating the cell response [1]. The role of selenium has been explored in normal thyroid functioning, immune system enhancement, carcinogenesis, cardiovascular diseases, in the prevention of pre-eclampsia, diabetes mellitus, and also male reproduction. It has been documented that a significant percentage of obese individuals have pre-existing lower serum selenium levels [2, 3]. A recent study by Papamargaritis et al. showed, a reduction in selenium concentration was observed in the early postoperative period following bariatric surgery, even after adequate multivitamin and mineral supplementation [4]. The deficiency appears within 3 months post-surgery [5]. Interestingly, no specific recommendation exists for selenium replacement in the post-bariatric setting.

23.2 Causes of Selenium Deficiency After RYGB

Several mechanisms relating to selenium deficiency may occur concurrently after RYGB, which arc as follows:

Pre-existing deficiency is one of the most common reasons for clinical manifestation post-surgery (2–58%). Reduced dietary intake of selenium that may further be reduced following surgery due to the predominant restrictive nature of the operation. RYGB results in bypass of the proximal intestines (duodenum and upper jejunum), with failure to absorb the micro-nutrients, precipitating deficiencies. There is no absorption from the stomach or the remaining parts of the intestine. Therefore, malabsorption of selenium following RYGB is a possible cause of deficiencies. Discontinuation of postoperative selenium supplementation could lead to decreased levels of serum selenium. Some types of multivitamin/mineral supplements may not contain sufficient amounts of minerals, which need to look for appropriately.

Selenium deficiency is rare, but if present, it may cause myopathy, cardiomyopathy, decreased immunity, low thyroid function, skin loss, pigmentation of hair, and progressive encephalopathy [6, 7]. Selenium deficiency has also been shown to contribute to the progression of viral infections. Cardiomyopathy results from the depletion of selenium-associated enzymes, which aid in the protection of cell membranes from damage by free radicals hence exposing it to myocardial necrosis and sudden death. The time duration for the development of congestive heart failure varies from several days or weeks in patients who develop a deficiency of selenium following malabsorptive bariatric procedures. The prompt correction of the gap by selenium treatment becomes necessary to reverse the harmful effects on the myocardium.

Selenium is more effectively absorbed from plant food than animal products. Other dietary components like vitamin C and E, zinc, copper, magnesium, vitamin B, and some amino acids such as methionine, cysteine, and glutamine may play a role that affects the serum selenium levels. Selenium deficiency can be assessed by measuring plasma erythrocyte ad whole blood selenium, plasma selenoproteins P, and overall blood glutathione activity. Selenoenzyme methionine sulfoxide reductase B1 (MsrB1) assessment is considered to be the most sensitive protein marker of selenium status [8]. Plant origin food products are the primary source of selenium, and the concentration varies tremendously according to its levels in the soil. A high concentration of selenium is found in food products like walnuts, brazil nuts, peanuts, almonds, cashew nuts, hazelnuts, pistachios, grains, saltwater and freshwater fish, poultry, eggs, and mushroom. A prospective study by Freeth et al. has shown that RYGB increased the risk of selenium deficiency, leading to deranged GTP homeostasis. The study recommended supplementation of selenium at a higher dosage than the current RDA (i.e., 55 μg) during the first 3 months post-surgery [5].

A multidisciplinary team managing the increasing number of bariatric patients needs to be aware of possible micro-nutrient deficiencies, their symptoms, diagnosis, and prevention [9]. Stress should be placed on the need for lifelong supplementation and annual monitoring of nutritional laboratory values. Selenium can be supplemented as a part of a vitamin-mineral supplement regime following metabolic surgery.

23.3 Postprandial Fainting

A morbidly obese diabetic female (BMI –45.6 kg/m^2; HbA1c-8.7%) who underwent laparoscopic sleeve followed by Roux-en-Y gastric bypass for inadequate weight loss was referred with frequent episodes of lightheadedness, flushing, abdominal pain, loose stools, and frequent fainting episodes 20–30 min after meals. The symptoms began 2 months following surgery. Her BMI dropped from 45.6 kg/m^2 to 31 kg/m^2, with aa %EWL of 78%, 16 months post revisional RYGB. A multidisciplinary bariatric team comprising of a surgeon, medical gastroenterologist, endocrinologist, psychiatrist, and dietician analyzed the patient. The possible differential diagnoses were dumping syndrome, nesidioblastosis, and neuroendocrine tumors. The patient was evaluated for insulin, C-peptide, chromogranin, which were normal. Computerized tomography (CT scan), upper GI endoscopy was also normal. With a provisional diagnosis of dumping syndrome, pharmacotherapy in the form of acarbose and octreotide was initiated with dietary modifications, but there was no alleviation of the symptoms. The provocative test in the way of oral glucose tolerance test (OGTT) was done to confirm the diagnosis. The Sigstad's score was 21.

Dumping syndrome post-RYGB was made as a diagnosis. With dietary and medical options exhausted, a decision for the reversal of RYGB to sleeve gastrectomy was made. The proximal and the distal pouches were mobilized after clearing all the dense adhesions to the liver. The gastrojejunostomy complex was mobilized and divided. The biliopancreatic limb proximal to the jejunostomy was divided and anastomosed to the divided end of the roux limb. Gastro-gastrostomy was done between the proximal and the distal pouches using a linear stapler technique. The patient improved drastically with complete resolution of symptoms and Sigstad's score of 1. The patient had a minimal weight regain of 3 kg, with the static status of diabetes.

Dumping syndrome (DS) is a frequent complication observed after Roux-en-Y gastric bypass (RYGB) found in around 40–50% cases [10]. The mechanisms which lead to dumping syndrome after RYGB are numerous and remain to be fully elucidated. Early DS is observed 10–30 min after a rapid passage of hyperosmolar food into the proximal bowel, which facilitates the fast movement of fluids into the bowel lumen, causing an increased sympathetic response [11]. Hyperosmolar nutrients in the proximal gut cause a shift of fluid from the plasma to the intestinal lumen. This results in a reduction in plasma volume, tachycardia, and rarely syncope. These events are manifested by hypotension, tachycardia, dizziness, fatigue, nausea, pallor, flushing, headache, diaphoresis, crampy abdominal pain, bloating, diarrhea, and syncope. Late DS occurs 1–3 h after the passage of a highly loaded carbohydrate meal into the jejunum, causing an incretin-driven hyper-insulinemic response. A couple of GI hormones are believed to play an essential role in the incretin effect: glucose-dependent insulinotropic polypeptide or gastric inhibitory polypeptide (GIP) and GLP-1. An elevated GLP-1 response has been reported in patients following RYGB, and a positive correlation has been observed between increasing GLP-1 levels and insulin release. Therefore, an exaggerated GLP-1 response appears to be pivotal in mediating the hyper-insulinemic and hypoglycemic effect that is characteristic of late dumping syndrome [12]. Late DS is characterized by diaphoresis, weakness, tremors, dizziness, fatigue, and altered consciousness [11].

Scores such as Sigstad's score and the Arts' dumping questionnaire can be used to identify patients with clinically significant dumping symptoms. The Sigstad's scoring system allocates points to each dumping symptom, and the cumulative points are used to calculate a diagnostic index, which helps in diagnostic confirmation of DS. A score value of >7 confirms DS, while patients with score <4, another differential diagnosis should be considered [13]. Art's questionnaire is used to differentiate early, and late DS [14]. Provocative tests such as the oral glucose tolerance test (OGTT) or mixed-meal tolerance test can be used to confirm clinically suspicious DS [15]. The OGTT is considered confirmatory for early dumping syndrome based on the presence of an early (30 min) increase in hematocrit greater than 3% or an increment in pulse rate more than 10 beats/min after 30 min, the latter being regarded as the most sensitive indicator of early dumping syndrome. Test results are conclusive for late dumping based on the development of late (60–180 min post-ingestion) hypoglycemia [11].

Most (around 95%) of the DS can be treated by adequate counseling and dietary therapy [16]. Fluid intake should be delayed until at least 30 min after meals. Rapidly absorbable carbohydrates should be excluded from the diet to prevent late dumping symptoms. High fiber, protein-rich foods, consumption of fruit and vegetable should be encouraged, whereas alcoholic beverages are better avoided. Meals should be eaten slowly and chewed well. Dietary supplements which increase the viscosity of food (e.g., pectin, guar gum, and glucomannan) delays the rate of gastric emptying and inhibits glucose absorption. The above dietary modifications result in slowing gastric emptying, reducing the release of GI hormones, improving hyperglycemia, and thereby controlling dumping symptoms. [17]. Few (3–5%) need medical therapy in the form of acarbose, octreotide for the treatment [16]. Acarbose is an α-glycosidase hydrolase inhibitor. It delays carbohydrate digestion in the proximal bowel, thus blunting postprandial hyperglycemia and subsequent hypoglycemia. Acarbose usage is best suited for patients with late dumping syndrome and is associated with abdominal bloating, excessive flatulence, and loose stools [18]. Somatostatin analogs (octreotide, pasireotide) are an effective treatment option for patients with dumping syndrome who fail to respond to or do not tolerate dietary modification and acarbose management. Somatostatin analogs inhibit gastric emptying time. They also inhibit the release of GI hormones and insulin and also inhibit postprandial vasodilatation. Both short-acting and long-acting formulations of somatostatin analogs are efficient in reducing early and late dumping symptoms [18]. Other pharmacologic interventions, such as diazoxide, nifedipine, and exendin 9–39, have also been investigated for the management of dumping syndrome. However, the data supporting the efficacy of the above is limited. Intractable cases (<1%) may require endoscopic or surgical revisions for its treatment [19, 20]. Multiple surgical options have been proposed ranging from reduction of gastrojejunal anastomosis, jejunal interposition, partial pancreatectomy to the reversal of RYGB [20–24]. Weight regain, and relapse of comorbidities remain the prime cause of concern in patients undergoing reversal to normal anatomy. Reversal of RYGB to LSG, however, provides a dynamic equilibrium concerning the resolution of symptoms of DS as well as decreasing the possibility of weight regain and recurrence of obesity-associated comorbidities. However, in the case described, a reversal to sleeve was the only option available.

23.4 Liver Decompensation

A 42-year-old hypertensive female with weight and height of 141 kg and 151 cm, suffering from super-super-obese and metabolic syndrome with a BMI of 61.8 kg/m^2, had been admitted to the hospital with complaints of gradual increase in weight past 15 years. She had limited physical activity. Her lipid parameters were deranged (cholesterol-230 mg/dl, triglyceride-264 mg/dl, VLDL-180 mg/dl, LDL-180 mg/dl). She was a known case of diabetes and hypertensive past 20 years on treatment. Her glycosylated hemoglobin preoperatively was 9.3%. The liver function tests during the preoperative period were normal. Ultrasonogram (USG) of the abdomen showed grade 2 fatty liver. Upper GI endoscopy showed reflux esophagitis (Los-Angeles grade-A). The patient had a history of open hernioplasty with abdominoplasty in the year 2012. The patient had tried weight reduction measures but was not able to achieve the same. After a thorough evaluation, the patient underwent laparoscopic Roux-en-Y gastric bypass (RYGB). The patient was put on calcium (1000 g/day), multivitamin, proton pump inhibitors, Vit B-12, and ursodeoxycholic acid (UDCA) supplements for 6 months and was on regular follow-up.

Following 6 months, the patient lost 36 kg of weight and BMI change of 15 (62 kg/m^2 to 47.1 kg/m^2). Seven months post-surgery, the patient was readmitted to our hospital with decreased appetite, jaundice, and persistent vomiting. On evaluation, her total bilirubin was 10.2 mg/dl, with the direct component being 8.2 mg/dl. AST levels were abnormally high at 213 U/l? (N-up-to 40 U/l). She had a low albumin level of 1.9 g/dl. USG showed severe hepatomegaly with fatty liver. Magnetic resonance cholangiography (MRCP) abdomen showed severe fatty infiltration of the liver with hepatomegaly.

There was no evidence of gall stone disease or common bile duct stones, ruling out the possibility of cholangitis. INR was raised to 2.64. The same was corrected using fresh frozen plasma. The patient developed features of hepatic encephalopathy. Serum ammonia levels were elevated to 171.9 μg/dl (N-18.7-86.9 μg/dl). Liver biopsy to rule out any autoimmune etiology was done, which showed features suggestive of non-alcoholic steatohepatitis (NAFLD activity score-6) with periportal and perisinusoidal fibrosis (stage 2). Over time, the patient's conscious level decreased with increased stupor and drowsiness. Her serum creatinine increased to 4.2 mg/dl, with a subsequent decrease in the urine output. Hemodialysis was started because of the failing renal parameters as well as anuria. The patient developed features of sepsis and multi-organ dysfunction syndrome over the next 4 days and expired after that. The cause of the death was acute liver failure, hepatorenal syndrome post-RYGB.

Non-alcoholic fatty liver disease (NAFLD) is among the most common causes of chronic liver disease in India and worldwide and is strongly associated with obesity and metabolic syndrome [25]. NAFLD comprises a wide spectrum of conditions, characterized by macro-vesicular hepatic steatosis, prevalent in patients who are non-alcoholic [26]. The histopathological NAFLD findings varied. It ranged from steatosis, non-alcoholic steatohepatitis (NASH) to advanced fibrosis, and cirrhosis. NAFLD represents the hepatic component of the metabolic syndrome [27]. Steatohepatitis is now considered as an important cause of end-stage liver disease. It is also a predisposing cause of an unknown number of cases of cryptogenic cirrhosis. Cryptogenic liver cirrhosis has been found in around 1.4% of patients with morbid obesity [28]. In the majority of patients, metabolic surgery improves liver steatosis, inflammation, and fibrosis in NAFLD patients with obesity, the exact mechanism of the worsening is unclear. Although rare, the progression of NAFLD to liver cirrhosis and further liver damage has been reported, based upon the severity of steatosis [29]. A possible explanation of liver function worsening could be due to rapid weight loss resulting in increased free fatty acid levels due to extensive fat mobilization, thus causing liver injury.

Varying degrees of fibrosis and also cases of de novo fibrosis are seen in a few cases, which is mild, without the development of cirrhosis or liver function alteration, seen in around 16% cases. Deterioration of liver function was attributed to the type of the metabolic procedure and the extent of malnutrition and malabsorption [30]. Progressive fibrosis during the long term (>5 years follow-up) was seen in spite of the improvement of hepatic steatosis and ballooning, which occurred during the first year post-RYGB. Worsening of liver function was seen as patients with higher BMI and higher insulin resistance [30]. Only a few reports of severe liver deterioration following RYGB have been seen [31]. A recent RCT by Kalinowski et al. reported that patients with NASH undergoing RYGB were more likely to develop early transient deterioration of liver function compared to Sleeve gastrectomy (LSG) [32]. Preoperatively diagnosed liver cirrhosis, alcohol abuse, and the presence of intraoperative complications contributed to negative events after RYGB [33]. Extended excluded limbs or distal versions of RYGB also contribute to the negative impact on liver function after RYGB [34]. A systemic review by Jan et al. also highlighted the increased incidence of morbidity and mortality, post-bariatric surgery, leading to decompensatory liver disease and also fulminating acute liver failure, in Child A group of patients [33]. A "second hit," post rapid weight loss after malabsorptive procedures, that is caused due to exposure of toxins from bacterial overgrowth from intestinal mobilization, nutritional, and protein deficiencies, maybe the cause for liver injury [35]. According to a study by Sasaki et al., around 5% of the patients with morbid obesity had a component of undiagnosed cirrhosis at the time of bariatric surgery [36]. Such patients have non-specific symptoms during the preoperative period, and even intraoperative macroscopic liver disease may be easily overlooked [37]. Hence it is of utmost importance to exclude advanced liver disease before bariatric surgery. Meticulous postoperative follow-up with close monitoring of liver function tests, especially in patients with super obesity, impaired insulin resistance, and preoperative liver pathologies, have been established. Improvement or even cessation of symptoms could be achieved by elongation of the common limb or biliopancreatic limb reversal in patients who underwent RYGB.

23.5 Neuropathy

A 48-year-old woman underwent laparoscopic RYGB for morbid obesity (body mass index [BMI] of 43.7 kg/m^2) in 2017. Medical history consisted of type 2 diabetes mellitus (T2DM) and hypothyroidism and was on regular medications with HB1Ac being 6.4% and TSH being 3.9 μIU/l. Previous surgical history comprised of a classical cesarean section. She had no history of intestinal problems, coeliac disease, malabsorption, or neurological symptoms. The patient was a non-alcoholic and a non-smoker. Her nutritional intake was incongruity with the international guidelines and recommendations following bariatric surgery (BS). The patient was on over-the-counter multivitamin and mineral supplement with a calcium dosage of 1000 mg calcium-carbonate consumption every day. The patient was on a regular follow-up as per the institutional protocol. Two years after surgery, she presented for a standard follow-up review, including the required blood investigations. Her weight was stable (BMI of 26.2 kg/m^2).

She returned to our center, around 5 months later, as she started to develop multiple complaints. Her complaints included blurred vision, concentration problems, confusion, irritability, tinnitus, palpitations, tingling in the fingers and toes, behavioral changes, mood swings, decreased muscle strength, muscle weakness, ataxia, aphasia, and glossitis. A clinical diagnosis of anemia based on deficiencies of iron, folate, and vitamin B12 and also deficiency of vitamin B1, B 6, B11, B12, E, or copper a vitamin D deficiency was kept in mind owing to the peculiar clinical features of the patient. The patient was admitted and evaluated. Her blood parameters were normal except for the following deranged parameters hemoglobin (7.9 mmol/l) (N-8.5–11.0 mmol/l); borderline low hematocrit (0.35) (N-0.35–0.45); Vit D (34 nmol/l) (N > 75 nmol/l); iron (4.0 μmol/l) (N-10–25 μmol/l); ferritin (6.0 μg/l) (N-13–200 μg/l); Vit B12 (170 pmol/l) (N > 200 pmol/l); methylmalonic acid (MMA) (155 nmol/l) (N < 430 nmol/l). MCV was normal. Other vitamins like B1, B6, B11, E, and trace minerals like selenium, copper, and zinc were normal. Serum folic acid level was 11.8 nmol/l (N > 10 nmol/l).

A differential diagnosis of polyneuropathy associated with neuropsychiatric symptoms was made. Management was streamlined, taking deficiency of vitamin B12 deficiency and folic acid into the aspect. As the cause of these problems could be identified, no electromyogram was performed. The patient received an intramuscular injection directly (1000 μg hydroxocobalamin per dose). The same was repeated weekly for the next 6 weeks. Improvements were seen within 1 week of commencing the therapy. Glossitis, tingling in fingers and toes, and neuropsychiatric symptoms (irritability, mood swings, and behavioral changes) symptoms started to get alleviated with treatment. Concentration issues, confusion, blurred vision, palpitations, reduced muscle strength, weakness, aphasia, ataxia, and tinnitus improved; however, they were still present in a milder form. After 2–3 weeks of treatment, weakness, confusion, aphasia, and ataxia were entirely resolved. However, within 4–5 days of the follow-up injection, she reported improvement in the above symptoms. After that, the intramuscular injection therapy of Vit B12 was adjusted to two doses per week. Tinnitus, palpitations, and concentration problems were cured, and overall weakness had disappeared after 4 weeks of treatment. Only the blurred vision was persistent in a subtle form. All laboratory blood results mentioned in this scenario came to normalcy, while all the complaints had resolved the following 6 weeks of therapy entirely.

Laparoscopic RYGB has been the most commonly reported procedure that is associated with anemia and other nutritional deficiencies. Following RYGB, anemia can be microcytic (which is because of iron deficiency), or macrocytic (due to Vit B12 or folic acid deficiency). A recent meta-analysis by Kwon et al. have shown the high prevalence of Vit B12 deficiency following RYGB [38]. Vitamin B12 plays a pivotal role in erythropoiesis and is a key vitamin essential for proper brain development. Deficiency of Vit B12 causes leads to megaloblastic anemia and developmental disorders of the nervous system with dementia and mood disorders [39]. Vitamin B12 is essential for the initial myelination and development of the central nervous system and also for the maintenance of its normal function. Demyelination of the cervical, thoracic dorsal, and lateral columns of the spinal cord are seen in patients with cobalamin deficiency. Occasionally it is also associated with demyelination of cranial, peripheral nerves and white matter in the brain. Histopathological analysis reveals a "spongy degeneration" owing to the loss of and swelling of the myelin sheath [40].

The most frequently associated neurological symptoms encountered are symmetric paraesthesia with altered sensation over the skin and gait problems [41]. Physical examination may reveal pallor, jaundice, pigmentary changes in the skin, edema, or neurological defects such as altered proprio-reception, ataxia, and weakness. Personality changes, amnesia, psychosis, and, rarely, delirium neuropsychiatric manifestations are encountered [40]. Less prevalent conditions associated with Vit B12 deficiency include glossitis, malabsorption, and rarely thrombosis. Hematological abnormalities usually precede the onset of neurological disease [42].

Various factors have been implicated in the occurrence of anemia post metabolic surgery.

1. Existing preoperative deficiency of Vit B12 (around 13%), which is considered to be a major predictive factor for postoperative deficiency, leading to secondary anemia [43]
2. Inadequate food intake during the postoperative period, as the patients tend to avoid consumption of red meat, which acts as a good source of heme iron [44]
3. Deranged absorption following RYGB
4. Altered bioavailability of drugs
5. Increased hepcidin levels due to obesity-related inflammation [45]
6. Altered metabolism and absorption of other micro-nutrients [46]

Most (99%) of the active absorption of cobalamin is dependent on the cobalamin-binding protein intrinsic factor (IF), while only 1% of the absorption is carried out through non-specific passive absorption [40, 41]. Following RYGB, there is a loss of acid secretion and IF in the stomach. There is an exclusion of the remnant stomach, while the proximal small bowel is bypassed [47]. Altered anatomy has an influence on the absorption of cobalamin.

Serum Vit. B12 serves as a poor predictor of functional Vit B12 deficiency, as the intracellular level deficiencies are not taken into account. Increased methylmalonic acid (MMA) and total homocysteine levels are considered to be sensitive markers for Vit B12 deficiencies [48, 49]. More intense follow-up and management of Vit B12 deficiency become necessary as these deficiencies have been reported in spite of regular supplementations according to the existing guidelines. Studies have proven that oral supplementation of postoperative Vit B-12 deficiencies was successful in greater than 80% of the patients. Intramuscular injection of Vit B12 remains the gold standard in symptomatic Vit B12 deficient patients [43]. A high dose of oral cyanocobalamin can be considered in selected asymptomatic patients [50]. Dosage of 1000 μg oral Vit B12 daily or a 500 μg weekly administration of Vit B12 through the intranasal route can also be considered. Intramuscular or subcutaneous of B12 supplementation, with a dose of 1000–3000 μg every 6–12 months to 1000 μg/month is indicated if cobalamin sufficiency cannot be maintained through oral or intranasal routes [51].

23.6 Adrenal Insufficiency

A 54-year post-menopausal female, with class 3 morbid obesity (BMI 45.6 kg/m^2) was consulted and counseled for abdominoplasty along with weight loss surgery. Comorbidities included T2DM, hypertension, and was on medications. She was also a known case of bronchial asthma on treatment. Previous surgical history included an open hysterectomy for dysfunctional uterine bleeding. She had a wound infection during the hospital stay and was subsequently hospitalized for a month and a half. She had a history of osteoarthritis and used to take intra-articular steroid injection for joint pain occasionally. On examination, she had exertional dyspnea, pendulous hanging abdomen wall, which hindered her day to day activity along with severely restricted mobility. She had multiple bruises with thinned out atrophic skin with striae at numerous points all over the abdominal wall. She was assessed, evaluated, and underwent laparoscopic RYGB with concomitant abdominoplasty. Postoperatively she had wound infection, which was managed with culture-specific antibiotics. The patient was discharged on postoperative day 07. The patient was not on proper follow-up and came just once, 2 weeks following the surgery. Three months following discharge, the patient came to the hospital with dyspnea at rest, pain at the wound line with recurrent episodes of vomiting with reduced intake. She had fainting episodes on and off, past 2 weeks, and was clinically dehydrated. The patient had frequent bouts of hypotension, weakness, and inability to carry day to day activities. On examination, she was dyspneic, hypotensive along with tachycardia and tachypnea. There was an acute exacerbation of asthma. Bilateral wheeze was present, and she had wound site induration with cellulitis with wound gaping at few points of the suture line.

Transthoracic echocardiography and serum electrolytes were in normal range except for hyponatremia. Other blood parameters were in the normal range, except for mildly increased total counts and serum sodium levels being 130 mEq/l

(N-135–145 mEq/l). Serum renin and aldosterone were normal. The patient's clinical picture raised the suspicion for adrenal insufficiency. She had orthostatic hypotension, inappropriately low cortisol of 1.9 μg/dl (N-3–18 μg/dl). On performing dynamic testing with 1 μg cosyntropin (low dose ACTH stimulation test), which aided in the stimulation of the hypothalamic-pituitary-adrenal (HPA) axis, 30 min after stimulation, the values of serum cortisol increased to 10.8 μg/dl, hence confirming the AI diagnosis. Serum ACTH measured 22.8 pg/ml, confirming the diagnosis of adrenal insufficiency. MRI brain showed no abnormality of pituitary glands. Anti-adrenal antibodies were negative. Computed tomography of the abdomen revealed no mass lesions in the pancreas or the adrenals. Injectable hydrocortisone therapy (100 mg/day thrice daily) was initiated and given for a week. The patient was discharged on tablet prednisolone 40 mg continued for 10 months and was gradually weaned off later to 20 mg/day prednisolone. A 250 μg cosyntropin stimulation test was done during the follow-up. The analysis revealed an adequate serum cortisol response following which hydrocortisone therapy was discontinued. The patient has remained clinically stable to date.

BS, like many major abdominal surgeries, is surgical stress to the body [52, 53]. Adrenal insufficiency has been noted after major surgery as a consequence of surgical stress or blood loss affecting the pituitary gland [53]. Adequate absorption of oral corticosteroids plays a key role in survival in patients who have primary or secondary adrenal insufficiency. RYGB creates altered anatomy, reduced gastrointestinal transit time, which is further associated with changes in the absorption surface hence compromising the medication bioavailability [54]. Enhanced absorption following rapid gastric emptying results in excess plasma peak cortisol levels and could cause intermittent overexposure to corticosteroids, with possibly harmful long-term effects [55]. There is malabsorption of bile following RYGB, which affects cholesterol absorption. Altered absorption leads to a decreased precursor for steroid synthesis, causing adrenal insufficiency [56]. Malabsorption of trace elements and vitamins (especially selenium and vitamin B5), which are considered to be steroid biosynthesis cofactors, also leads to the reduction of the same. There is weight loss following RYGB, which causes the re-setting of the hypothalamic-pituitary-adrenal axis (HPA). Similar conditions causing adrenal insufficiency are seen in anorexia nervosa and perioperative complications such as blood loss causing pituitary/adrenal infarct or apoplexy [57–59].

The HPA axis is a major factor that determines the patient's responses to surgical trauma, and cortisol plays an important role in regulating humoral mediators during those conditions [60]. Postoperative complications are thought to be caused due to an uncontrolled inflammatory response. The increased stress leads to the overproduction of proinflammatory cytokines like TNF and IL-6 [61]. Literature suggests that severe sepsis and severe surgical stress may be associated with relative adrenal insufficiency, which may contribute to a fatal outcome [62]. Literature has also shown, that there is a direct correlation between the increase in serum cortisol levels postoperatively with the degree of surgical stress. There is a hypersecretion of IL-6 and CRP in scenarios of severe surgical stress, such as in our case. Furthermore, these variables could be directly linked to the serious postoperative complications and hence the prolonged hospitalization. Several studies have concluded that corticosteroid replacement therapy is useful in patients with relative adrenal insufficiency [63]. It has been shown that the preoperative administration of corticosteroids has been found beneficial in attenuating surgery-induced inflammatory responses and in preventing postoperative complications. A short ACTH stimulation test performed in the preoperative period helps to determine a patient's maximal cortisol response to surgical trauma.

Daily cortisol requirements are more in patients who are morbidly obese because of a higher volume distribution and accelerated clearance [64]. Literature shows that the cortisol clearance is inversely related to insulin sensitivity and that fatty liver disease is associated with enhanced cortisol clearance, possibly through alterations in the activity of the 5α-, 5β-reductase, and also 11β-hydroxysteroid dehydrogenase type 1 in the liver [65]. Since the majority of the patients who are morbidly obese have fatty liver disease as well as decreased insulin sensitivity, there are at least two factors that lead to cortisol clearance. Hence dose adjustments of serum cortisol, individualized according to the daily profiles, before as well as after surgery, in morbidly obese patients is recommended.

References

1. Hassan Zadeh M, Mohammadi Farsani G, Zamaninour N. Selenium status after Roux-en-Y gastric bypass: interventions and recommendations. Obes Surg. 2019 Nov;29(11):3743–8.
2. Mechanick JI, Apovian C, Brethauer S, Garvey WT, Joffe AM, Kim J, et al. Clinical practice guidelines for the perioperative nutrition, metabolic, and nonsurgical support of patients undergoing bariatric procedures – 2019 update: cosponsored by American Association of Clinical Endocrinologists/American College of Endocrinology. Endocr Pract. 2019.
3. Alasfar F, Ben-Nakhi M, Khoursheed M, Kehinde EO, Alsaleh M. Selenium is significantly depleted among morbidly obese female patients seeking bariatric surgery. Obes Surg. 2011 Nov;21(11):1710–3.
4. Papamargaritis D, Aasheim ET, Sampson B, le Roux CW. Copper, selenium and zinc levels after bariatric surgery in patients recommended to take multivitamin-mineral supplementation. J Trace Elem Med Biol. 2015;31:167–72.
5. Freeth A, Prajuabpansri P, Victory JM, Jenkins P. Assessment of selenium in Roux-en-Y gastric bypass and gastric banding surgery. Obes Surg. 2012 Nov;22(11):1660–5.
6. Kushner RF. Managing micronutrient deficiencies in the bariatric surgical patient. In: Treatment of the obese patient: Springer; 2014. p. 255–70.
7. Singh NK. Morbid obesity, cardiac disease, and bariatric surgery. Clin Cardiol. 2009;32:289.
8. Papp LV, Holmgren A, Khanna KK. Selenium and selenoproteins in health and disease. Antioxidants Redox Signal. 2010;12:793–5.
9. Shankar P, Boylan M, Sriram K. Micronutrient deficiencies after bariatric surgery. Nutrition. 2010;26(11–12):1031–7.
10. Lim RB, Blackburn GL, Jones DB. Benchmarking best practices in weight loss surgery. Curr Probl Surg. 2010 Feb;47(2):79–174.
11. Tack J, Arts J, Caenepeel P, De Wulf D, Bisschops R. Pathophysiology, diagnosis and management of postoperative dumping syndrome. Nat Rev Gastroenterol Hepatol. 2009 Oct;6(10):583–90.
12. Salehi M, Gastaldelli A, D'Alessio DA. Blockade of glucagon-like peptide 1 receptor corrects postprandial hypoglycemia after gastric bypass. Gastroenterology. 2014;146(3):669–80.e2.

13. Sigstad H. A clinical diagnostic index in the diagnosis of the dumping syndrome. Changes in plasma volume and blood sugar after a test meal. Acta Med Scand. 1970;188(6):479–86.
14. Arts J, Caenepeel P, Bisschops R, Dewulf D, Holvoet L, Piessevaux H, et al. Efficacy of the long-acting repeatable formulation of the somatostatin analogue octreotide in postoperative dumping. Clin Gastroenterol Hepatol. 2009 Apr;7(4):432–7.
15. van der Kleij FG, Vecht J, Lamers CB, Masclee AA. Diagnostic value of dumping provocation in patients after gastric surgery. Scand J Gastroenterol. 1996 Dec;31(12):1162–6.
16. Ukleja A. Dumping syndrome: pathophysiology and treatment. Nutr Clin Pract. 2005 Oct;20(5):517–25.
17. Kneepkens CM, Fernandes J, Vonk RJ. Dumping syndrome in children. Diagnosis and effect of glucomannan on glucose tolerance and absorption. Acta Paediatr Scand. 1988 Mar;77(2):279–86.
18. Vilarrasa N, Goday A, Rubio MA, Caixas A, Pellitero S, Ciudin A, et al. Hyperinsulinemic hypoglycemia after bariatric surgery: diagnosis and management experience from a Spanish Multicenter Registry. Obes Facts. 2016;9(1):41–51.
19. Fernandez-Esparrach G, Lautz DB, Thompson CC. Peroral endoscopic anastomotic reduction improves intractable dumping syndrome in Roux-en-Y gastric bypass patients. Surg Obes Relat Dis. 2010;6(1):36–40.
20. Dapri G, Cadiere GB, Himpens J. Laparoscopic reconversion of Roux-en-Y gastric bypass to original anatomy: technique and preliminary outcomes. Obes Surg. 2011 Aug;21(8):1289–95.
21. Himpens J, Dapri G, Cadiere GB. Laparoscopic conversion of the gastric bypass into a normal anatomy. Obes Surg. 2006 Jul;16(7):908–12.
22. Carter CO, Fernandez AZ, McNatt SS, Powell MS. Conversion from gastric bypass to sleeve gastrectomy for complications of gastric bypass. Surg Obes Relat Dis. 2016;12(3):572–6.
23. Meier JJ, Nauck MA, Butler PC. Comment to: Patti ME, McMahon G, Mun EC et al. (2005) Severe hypoglycaemia post-gastric bypass requiring partial pancreatectomy: evidence for inappropriate insulin secretion and pancreatic islet hyperplasia. Diabetologia 48:2236–2240. Diabetologia. 2006;49:607–610.
24. Thondam SK, Nair S, Wile D, Gill GV. Diazoxide for the treatment of hypoglycaemic dumping syndrome. QJM. 2013 Sep;106(9):855–8.
25. Maheshwari A, Thuluvath PJ. Cryptogenic cirrhosis and NAFLD: are they related? Am J Gastroenterol. 2006 Mar;101(3):664–8.
26. Mulhall BP, Ong JP, Younossi ZM. Non-alcoholic fatty liver disease: an overview. J Gastroenterol Hepatol. 2002 Nov;17(11):1136–43.
27. Mottin CC, Moretto M, Padoin AV, Kupski C, Swarowsky AM, Glock L, et al. Histological behavior of hepatic steatosis in morbidly obese patients after weight loss induced by bariatric surgery. Obes Surg. 2005;15(6):788–93.
28. Dallal RM, Mattar SG, Lord JL, Watson AR, Cottam DR, Eid GM, et al. Results of laparoscopic gastric bypass in patients with cirrhosis. Obes Surg. 2004 Jan;14(1):47–53.
29. Harrison SA, Torgerson S, Hayashi PH. The natural history of nonalcoholic fatty liver disease: a clinical histopathological study. Am J Gastroenterol. 2003 Sep;98(9):2042–7.
30. Mathurin P, Hollebecque A, Arnalsteen L, Buob D, Leteurtre E, Caiazzo R, et al. Prospective study of the long-term effects of bariatric surgery on liver injury in patients without advanced disease. Gastroenterology. 2009 Aug;137(2):532–40.
31. Mahawar KK, Parmar C, Graham Y, De Alwis N, Carr WRJ, Jennings N, et al. Monitoring of liver function tests after Roux-en-Y gastric bypass: an examination of evidence base. Obes Surg. 2016 Oct;26(10):2516–22.
32. Kalinowski P, Paluszkiewicz R, Ziarkiewicz-Wroblewska B, Wroblewski T, Remiszewski P, Grodzicki M, et al. Liver function in patients with nonalcoholic fatty liver disease randomized to Roux-en-Y gastric bypass versus sleeve gastrectomy: a secondary analysis of a randomized clinical trial. Ann Surg. 2017 Nov;266(5):738–45.
33. Jan A, Narwaria M, Mahawar KK. A systematic review of bariatric surgery in patients with liver cirrhosis. Obes Surg. 2015 Aug;25(8):1518–26.

34. Sugerman HJ, Kellum JM, DeMaria EJ. Conversion of proximal to distal gastric bypass for failed gastric bypass for superobesity. J Gastrointest Surg. 1997;1(6):516–7.
35. Day CP, James OF. Steatohepatitis: a tale of two "hits"? Gastroenterology. 1998;114:842–5.
36. Sasaki A, Nitta H, Otsuka K, Umemura A, Baba S, Obuchi T, et al. Bariatric surgery and non-alcoholic fatty liver disease: current and potential future treatments. Front Endocrinol (Lausanne). 2014;5:164.
37. Teixeira ARF, Bellodi-Privato M, Carvalheira JB, Pilla VF, Pareja JC, D'Albuquerque LAC. The incapacity of the surgeon to identify NASH in bariatric surgery makes biopsy mandatory. Obes Surg. 2009 Dec;19(12):1678–84.
38. Kwon Y, Kim HJ, Lo Menzo E, Park S, Szomstein S, Rosenthal RJ. Anemia, iron and vitamin B12 deficiencies after sleeve gastrectomy compared to Roux-en-Y gastric bypass: a meta-analysis. Surg Obes Relat Dis. 2014;10(4):589–97.
39. Reynolds E. Vitamin B12, folic acid, and the nervous system. Lancet Neurol. 2006 Nov;5(11):949–60.
40. Kumar N. Nutritional neuropathies. Neurol Clin. 2007 Feb;25(1):209–55.
41. Stabler SP. Clinical practice. Vitamin B12 deficiency. N Engl J Med. 2013 Jan;368(2):149–60.
42. Lindenbaum J, Healton EB, Savage DG, Brust JC, Garrett TJ, Podell ER, et al. Neuropsychiatric disorders caused by cobalamin deficiency in the absence of anemia or macrocytosis. 1988. Nutrition. 1995;11(2):181; discussion 180, 182.
43. van der Beek ESJ, Monpellier VM, Eland I, Tromp E, van Ramshorst B. Nutritional deficiencies in gastric bypass patients; incidence, time of occurrence and implications for post-operative surveillance. Obes Surg. 2015 May;25(5):818–23.
44. Salgado WJ, Modotti C, Nonino CB, Ceneviva R. Anemia and iron deficiency before and after bariatric surgery. Surg Obes Relat Dis. 2014;10(1):49–54.
45. Wisse BE. The inflammatory syndrome: the role of adipose tissue cytokines in metabolic disorders linked to obesity. J Am Soc Nephrol. 2004 Nov;15(11):2792–800.
46. Kotkiewicz A, Donaldson K, Dye C, Rogers AM, Mauger D, Kong L, et al. Anemia and the need for intravenous iron infusion after Roux-en-Y gastric bypass. Clin Med Insights Blood Disord. 2015;8:9–17.
47. Schilling RF, Gohdes PN, Hardie GH. Vitamin B12 deficiency after gastric bypass surgery for obesity. Ann Intern Med. 1984 Oct;101(4):501–2.
48. Kushner RF, Shanta RV. Emergence of pica (ingestion of non-food substances) accompanying iron deficiency anemia after gastric bypass surgery. Obes Surg. 2005;15(10):1491–5.
49. Stabler SP, Allen RH, Dolce ET, Johnson MA. Elevated serum S-adenosylhomocysteine in cobalamin-deficient elderly and response to treatment. Am J Clin Nutr. 2006 Dec;84(6):1422–9.
50. Majumder S, Soriano J, Louie Cruz A, Dasanu CA. Vitamin B12 deficiency in patients undergoing bariatric surgery: preventive strategies and key recommendations. Surg Obes Relat Dis. 2013;9(6):1013–9.
51. Mechanick JI, Youdim A, Jones DB, Garvey WT, Hurley DL, McMahon MM, et al. Clinical practice guidelines for the perioperative nutritional, metabolic, and nonsurgical support of the bariatric surgery patient–2013 update: cosponsored by American Association of Clinical Endocrinologists, The Obesity Society, and American Society for Metabolic & Bariatric Surgery. Obesity (Silver Spring). 2013 Mar;21(Suppl 1):S1–27.
52. Colquitt JL, Pickett K, Loveman E, Frampton GK. Surgery for weight loss in adults. Cochrane Database Syst Rev. 2014 Aug;8:CD003641.
53. Kashiwabara M, Miyashita M, Nomura T, Makino H, Matsutani T, Kim C, et al. Surgical trauma-induced adrenal insufficiency is associated with postoperative inflammatory responses. J Nippon Med Sch. 2007 Aug;74(4):274–83.
54. Padwal R, Brocks D, Sharma AM. A systematic review of drug absorption following bariatric surgery and its theoretical implications. Obes Rev. 2010 Jan;11(1):41–50.
55. de Heide LJM, de Boer HHR, van Borren M, Emous M, Aarts E, de Boer H. Pharmacokinetics of glucocorticoid replacement before and after bariatric surgery in patients with adrenal insufficiency. J Endocr Soc. 2018 Dec;2(12):1338–44.

56. Stephens JW, Boregowda K, Barry J, Price DE, Eyre N, Baxter JN. Adrenal insufficiency following bariatric surgery. Obes Rev. 2012 Jun;13(6):560–2.
57. Chrousos GP. The hypothalamic-pituitary-adrenal axis and immune-mediated inflammation. N Engl J Med. 1995 May;332(20):1351–62.
58. Himel AR, Cabral SA, Shaffery JP, Grayson BE. Anxiety behavior and hypothalamic-pituitary-adrenal axis altered in a female rat model of vertical sleeve gastrectomy. PLoS One. 2018;13(7):e0200026.
59. Pasquali R. The hypothalamic-pituitary-adrenal axis and sex hormones in chronic stress and obesity: pathophysiological and clinical aspects. Ann N Y Acad Sci. 2012 Aug;1264:20–35.
60. Naito Y, Fukata J, Tamai S, Seo N, Nakai Y, Mori K, et al. Biphasic changes in hypothalamo-pituitary-adrenal function during the early recovery period after major abdominal surgery. J Clin Endocrinol Metab. 1991 Jul;73(1):111–7.
61. Sakamoto K, Arakawa H, Mita S, Ishiko T, Ikei S, Egami H, et al. Elevation of circulating interleukin 6 after surgery: factors influencing the serum level. Cytokine. 1994 Mar;6(2):181–6.
62. Manglik S, Flores E, Lubarsky L, Fernandez F, Chhibber VL, Tayek JA. Glucocorticoid insufficiency in patients who present to the hospital with severe sepsis: a prospective clinical trial. Crit Care Med. 2003 Jun;31(6):1668–75.
63. Annane D, Sebille V, Charpentier C, Bollaert P-E, Francois B, Korach J-M, et al. Effect of treatment with low doses of hydrocortisone and fludrocortisone on mortality in patients with septic shock. JAMA. 2002 Aug;288(7):862–71.
64. Andrew R, Phillips DI, Walker BR. Obesity and gender influence cortisol secretion and metabolism in man. J Clin Endocrinol Metab. 1998 May;83(5):1806–9.
65. Holt HB, Wild SH, Postle AD, Zhang J, Koster G, Umpleby M, et al. Cortisol clearance and associations with insulin sensitivity, body fat and fatty liver in middle-aged men. Diabetologia. 2007 May;50(5):1024–32.

GPSR Compliance

The European Union's (EU) General Product Safety Regulation (GPSR) is a set of rules that requires consumer products to be safe and our obligations to ensure this.

If you have any concerns about our products, you can contact us on ProductSafety@springernature.com

In case Publisher is established outside the EU, the EU authorized representative is:

Springer Nature Customer Service Center GmbH
Europaplatz 3
69115 Heidelberg, Germany

Batch number: 10726133

Printed by Printforce, the Netherlands